# Atlas of Pelvic Surgery

THIRD EDITION

THIRD EDITION

# Atlas
# of
# Pelvic Surgery

Clifford R. Wheeless, Jr., M.D.
*Director, Institute for Special Pelvic Surgery*
*Sinai Hospital of Baltimore*
*Baltimore, Maryland*

*Associate Professor of Gynecology and Obstetrics*
*The Johns Hopkins University School of Medicine*
*Gynecologist-Obstetrician*
*The Johns Hopkins Hospital*
*Baltimore, Maryland*

*Consultant, Gynecologic Oncology*
*Peninsula General Hospital*
*Salisbury, Maryland*

John Parker, *Medical Illustrator*

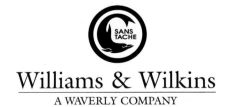

**Williams & Wilkins**
A WAVERLY COMPANY

BALTIMORE • PHILADELPHIA • LONDON • PARIS • BANGKOK
BUENOS AIRES • HONG KONG • MUNICH • SYDNEY • TOKYO • WROCLAW

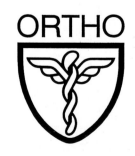

*Editor:* Charles W. Mitchell
*Managing Editor:* Marjorie Kidd Keating
*Production Coordinator:* Marette Magargle-Smith
*Copy Editor:* Bill Cady
*Designer/Illustration Planner/Composition:* Mario Fernández
*Manufacturing:* Transcontinental Printing, Inc.

Copyright © 1997

Williams & Wilkins
351 W. Camden Street
Baltimore, Maryland 21201-2436 USA

Rose Tree Corporate Center
1400 North Providence Road
Building II, Suite 5025
Media, Pennsylvania 19063-2043 USA

Accurate indications, adverse reactions, and dosage schedules for drugs are provided in this
book, but it is possible that they may change. The reader is urged to review the package information data of the manufacturers of the medications mentioned.

*Printed in Canada*

First Edition, 1981
Second Edition, 1988

**Library of Congress Cataloging-in-Publication Data**

Wheeless, Clifford R., 1938–
 Atlas of pelvic surgery / Clifford R. Wheeless, Jr., John Parker, medical illustrator
  p.   cm.
 Includes index.
 ISBN 0-683-08956-0
 1. Generative organs, Female—Surgery—Atlases. 2. Abdomen—Surgery—Atlases. I. Title
 [DNLM: 1. Genitalia, Female—surgery—atlases. WP 17 W564a 1997]
 RG104.W48 1997
 617.5'5'0222—dc20
 DNLM/DLC
 for Library of Congress                                      96-16526
                                                               CIP

To purchase additional copies of this book, call our customer service department at
**(800) 638-0672** or fax orders to **(800) 447-8438**. For other book services, including chap-
ter reprints and large quantity sales, ask for the Special Sales department.

Canadian customers should call **(800) 268-4178**, or fax **(905) 470-6780**. For all other calls originating outside of the United States, please call **(410) 528-4223** or fax us at **(410) 528-8550**.

*Visit Williams & Wilkins on the Internet:* http://www.wwilkins.com or contact our customer service department at **custserv@wwilkins.com**. Williams & Wilkins customer service
representatives are available from 8:30 am to 6:00 pm, EST, Monday through Friday, for tele-
phone access.

                                                          97 98 99
                                       1  2  3  4  5  6  7  8  9  10

My family—my wife, Missy; my son, Clifford Roberts Wheeless III, M.D.; and my daughter,
Elise Porchia Wheeless Kiely, J.D.—for their patience, understanding, and support.
My patients—for their interest, their loyalty, and their confidence.
My mentors—James H. Dorsey, M.D., Houston Everett, M.D.,
John B. Graham, M.D., Howard W. Jones, Jr., M.D., Kazumasa Masubuchi, M.D.,
Mark Ravitch, M.D., Richard W. TeLinde, M.D., Donald Woodruff, M.D.,
Nils Kock, M.D., and Donald G. Skinner, M.D.—
for their guidance and encouragement.

# Preface

In preparing the third edition of the *Atlas of Pelvic Surgery*, I have recorded procedures that I have found to be of continual use in the practice of pelvic surgery. Some of these operations cross different surgical specialties because of the interrelatedness of pelvic organs to pelvic disease.

There may be legitimate differences of opinion about some of the procedures presented and the steps used to perform them. Moreover, surgery does not always allow the surgeon the luxury of precisely performing each operation as illustrated here. Surgeons must constantly improvise, adapting their technique to the individual patient and the problem that is being treated. This atlas is intended as a general guide, a framework on which to build one's own technique.

This third edition contains operations not included in the first or second editions of the *Atlas*. I have been deeply gratified to learn that the first and second editions have encouraged many young surgeons to study and learn procedures with which they had not been familiar and which later proved beneficial to their patients.

Once again I would like to acknowledge the contributions of countless pelvic surgeons whose expertise, intelligence, and technical skill allowed the development of the operations illustrated and described here. I am personally indebted to Richard W. TeLinde, Howard W. Jones, Jr., the late John B. Graham, the late Houston Everett, Donald Woodruff, Kazumasa Masubuchi of Tokyo, Mark Ravitch, James Henderson Dorsey, Richard Shackelford, Philippe Poitout of Paris, France, Nils Kock, and Donald G. Skinner. Their patient teaching and counsel during countless hours at the operating table made it possible for me to perform these operations and thus produce this atlas.

The contribution of the medical illustrator, John Parker, cannot be adequately described in this brief preface. A master artist out of the school of Max Brödel at The Johns Hopkins University School of Medicine, John Parker has developed his artistic technique through many years of observing and drawing at the operating table.

I deeply appreciate the careful preparation of the manuscript by Peggy LeBrun and the editorial assistance of Betty Ann Howard.

Finally, I would like to thank the editors and staff of Williams & Wilkins for their interest, encouragement, resources, and advice, without which this atlas would not be available.

*Clifford R. Wheeless, Jr., M.D.*
*Baltimore, Maryland*

# Contents

# 1

## Vulva and Introitus

# Biopsy of the Vulva

Gross lesions of the vulva often seem to be benign. However, a gross lesion of any description on the external or internal female genitals is suspicious, and with rare exceptions, a biopsy should be taken for histologic analysis.

A histologic specimen encompassing pathologic as well as normal squamous epithelium is obtained from the vulva.

**Physiologic Changes.** None.

**Points of Caution.** The biopsy should provide reliable pathologic specimens; tangential cutting may lead to misinterpretation.

## Technique

**1** The patient is placed in the dorsal lithotomy position. The area of pathologic abnormality is cleansed with aseptic solution, and the proposed biopsy site is selected.

**2** A Keys punch, commonly used by dermatologists, is excellent for this purpose. The 5–7-mm size allows appropriate pathologic specimens to be taken without leaving a defect large enough to require sutures.

**3** The area is anesthetized with 1 mL of 1% Xylocaine injected subcutaneously. The biopsy is then taken by rotating the Keys punch over the skin in 180° arches.

**4** A delicate forceps is used to elevate one margin of the biopsy, and a small cuticle scissors is used to dissect the biopsy off its bed. A suture is rarely required, and no dressing is applied.

**5** The biopsy is oriented on a piece of saline-soaked gauze, enabling the pathologist to perform ideal sections.

**6** If necessary, a plug can be cut from an Avitene or Gelfoam wafer by using the sharp edge of the Keys punch.

**7** This plug can be placed in the biopsy defect to provide hemostasis. It will act as an excellent dressing for the wound and, in most cases, omit the need for suturing. The patient is instructed to keep the site clean with ordinary soap and water and to wear a perineal pad as required.

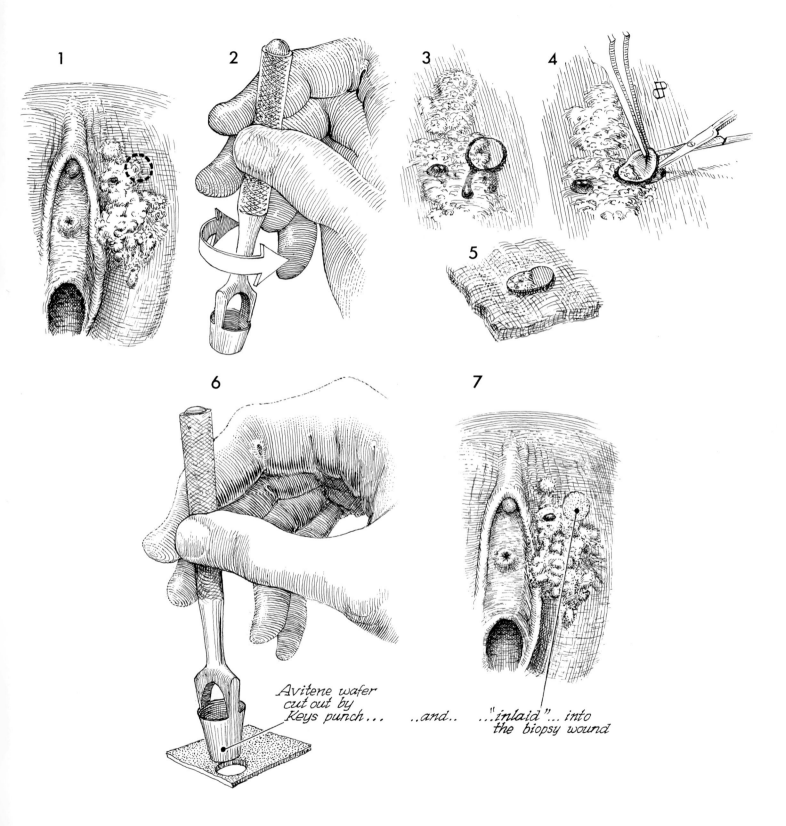

1

2

3

4

5

6

7

Avitene wafer
cut out by
Keys punch...   ..and..   ..."inlaid"...into
the biopsy wound

# Excision of Urethral Caruncle

Urethral caruncles are frequently associated with atrophic genital epithelium in elderly patients. They can become a source of chronic hematuria, infection, and urethritis. When medical therapy with estrogen suppositories and cream does not adequately clear the lesion, surgical excision is indicated.

The lesion is excised, and normal urethral mucosa is sutured to the epithelium of the vestibule.

**Physiologic Changes.** The removal of the inflamed granulation tissue eliminates a cause of chronic infection and bleeding.

**Points of Caution.** The operation can frequently be bloody and, in general, should be performed in an operating room rather than in an office or clinic.

The need for Foley catheter drainage following removal of the lesion may be necessary. The application of estrogen cream reduces the risk of recurrent caruncles.

## Technique

**1** The patient is placed in the dorsal lithotomy position, and appropriate anesthesia is administered (general, regional, or local). The vulva and perineum are prepped.

**2** The caruncle is grasped with an Allis clamp and retracted slightly forward. A scalpel is used to excise some of the vestibular epithelium and to transect the urethra proximal to the caruncle.

**3** The specimen is removed, and the urethral mucosa as well as the vestibular epithelium is exposed.

**4** The urethral mucosa is closed to the vestibular epithelium with interrupted 3-0 synthetic absorbable sutures.

**5** The urethral mucosa is sutured to the epithelium of the vestibule.

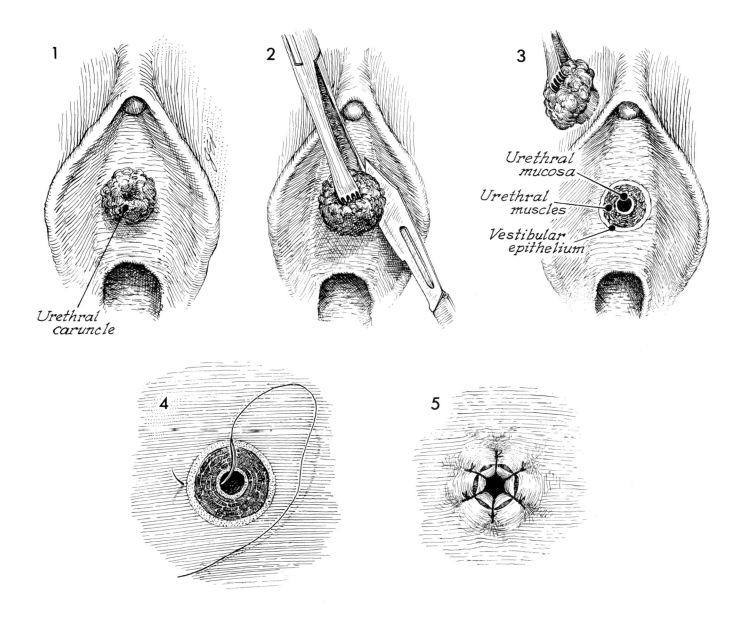

1

Urethral
caruncle

2

3

Urethral
mucosa

Urethral
muscles

Vestibular
epithelium

4

5

5

# Bartholin's Gland Cyst Marsupialization

Marsupialization of the Bartholin's gland is generally indicated when there is a large abscess that makes surgical excision of the gland difficult. In this operation, the surgeon opens wide the wall of the abscess and allows the purulent exudate to drain. The membrane of the abscess is then sutured to the vaginal mucosa and to the skin of the introitus in order to effect granulation and reepithelialization of the wound from the bottom of the abscess to the top.

The operation is fast. Hemostasis is not difficult and can be performed under local anesthesia.

The purpose of marsupialization of the Bartholin's gland is to exteriorize the abscess in such a fashion that it will become epithelialized from the base.

**Physiologic Changes.** If marsupialization is successful, the epithelium within the gland will be epithelialized with squamous epithelium.

**Points of Caution.** The opening into the gland must be sufficient to promote adequate drainage.

## Technique

**1** A thorough bimanual examination should be performed to determine the extent of the abscess.

**2** The labia are retracted with interrupted 3-0 sutures, and the introitus of the vagina is exposed. An incision is made over the mucosa of the vagina at its junction with the introitus down to the wall of the gland.

**3 & 4** The wall of the gland is incised. The entire length of the superficial incision is shown.

**5** The contents of the abscess are evacuated.

**6** A culture is taken of the abscess. The walls of the abscess are grasped with Allis clamps.

**7** The wall of the abscess is sutured with interrupted 3-0 synthetic absorbable suture to the skin of the introitus laterally and to the vaginal mucosa medially.

**8** The marsupialization is complete. Generally, no packing or drain is necessary. The patient is placed on a regimen of hot sitz baths on the second postoperative day. A laxative and stool softener are given on the third postoperative day. Antibiotic therapy should be directed by the results of the culture. Sexual intercourse can usually be resumed in 4 weeks.

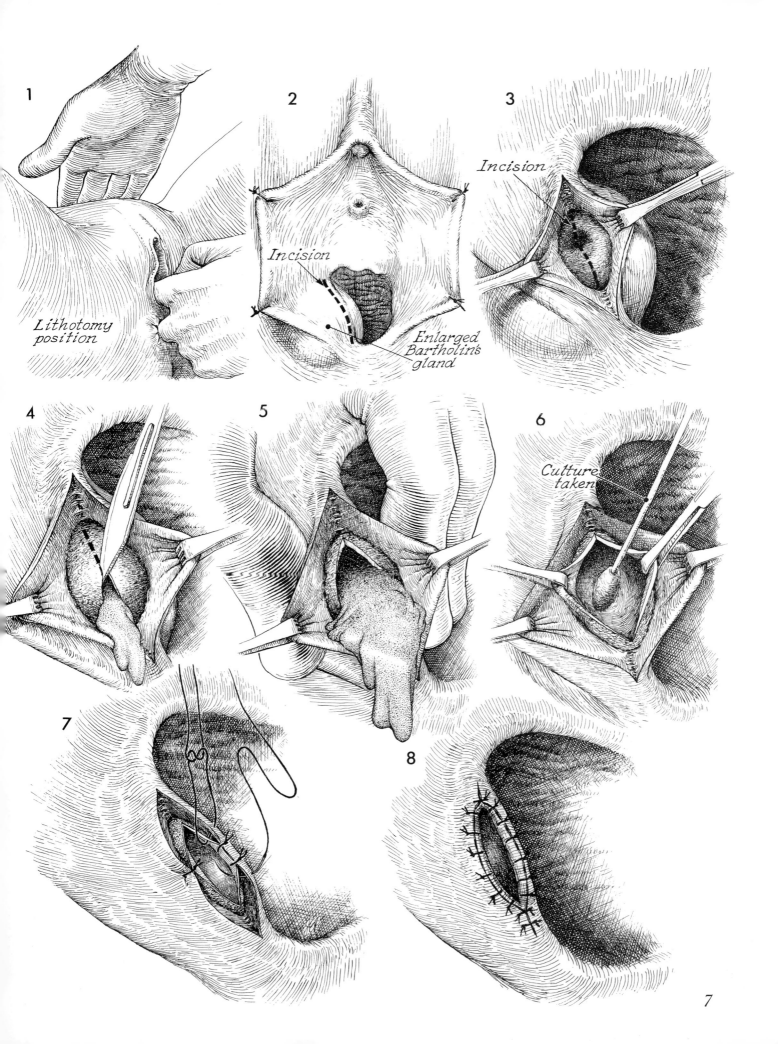

**1**

Lithotomy position

**2**

Incision

Enlarged Bartholin's gland

**3**

Incision

**4**

**5**

**6**

Culture taken

**7**

**8**

7

# Excision of Vulvar Skin,
# With Split-Thickness Skin Graft

A cutaneous vulvectomy is indicated for young women with extensive in situ carcinoma of the vulva. The goal in such an operation is to remove the in situ carcinoma but to leave a functional vulva that is psychologically as well as physically satisfactory to the patient. To accomplish this, the surgeon removes the cancerous vulvar epithelium and replaces it with a split-thickness skin graft of normal epithelium from a selected donor site.

**Physiologic Changes.** The in situ cancer is removed.

**Points of Caution.** Meticulous hemostasis should be complete in the wound prior to applying the split-thickness skin graft. This aids essential nutrition through transudation during the first 48–72 hours, until microcapillary neoangiogenesis connects the graft with the general circulation within the recipient site.

## Technique

**1** The patient is placed in the dorsal lithotomy position. The perineum is prepped and draped. The skin to be removed is carefully outlined with brilliant green solution.

**2** An incision is made down to the dermis. An Allis clamp is placed on the skin, and a scalpel is used to carefully dissect the skin off of the dermis.

**3** The dissection follows the outline of the incision around the external genitalia, removing the involved skin. Note that noninvolved structures may be left intact.

**4** A split-thickness skin graft is taken as shown in Section 2, page 93. The graft is tailored to fit the wound. Edges of the graft are sutured to the edges of the epithelium of the labia with interrupted 3-0 nylon suture, the ends of which are left long and tagged with small hemostats.

**5** The skin has been placed on the vulva and sutured to the remaining skin of the vulva and vagina. A Graftac stapler is used to staple through the split-thickness skin graft into the bed to hold the graft in place for the required number of days.

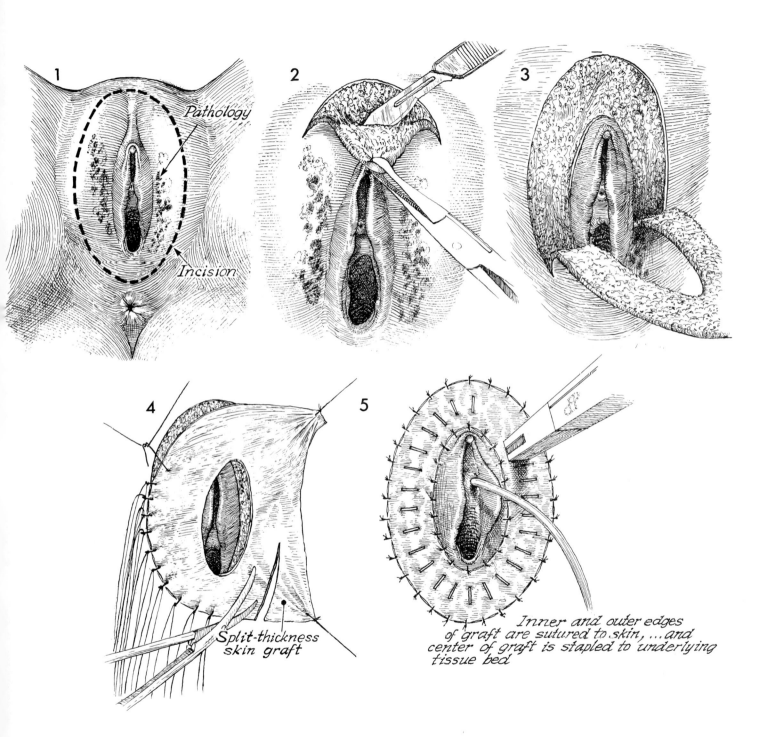

**1** *Pathology* *Incision*

**2**

**3**

**4** Split-thickness skin graft

**5** *Inner and outer edges of graft are sutured to skin, ...and center of graft is stapled to underlying tissue bed*

9

# Bartholin's Gland Excision

Excision of the Bartholin's gland has been called the "bloodiest little operation in gynecology." It is indicated for persistent and recurrent Bartholin's gland abscess and cyst. The key to successful excision is hemostatic control of the copious blood supply to the gland.

The purpose of the operation is to remove the entire Bartholin's gland.

**Physiologic Changes.** Bilateral removal of Bartholin's gland eliminates the secretion of fluid from the gland that is useful as a vaginal lubricant. In the well-estrogenized vagina, however, this is generally not a clinical problem.

**Points of Caution.** Meticulous hemostasis is essential. The branches of the pudendal artery are frequently lacerated during excision of the Bartholin's gland. They must be carefully identified, clamped, and tied, or postoperative vulvar hematoma will result.

---

## Technique

**1** The patient is placed in the dorsal lithotomy position, and the perineum is prepped and draped.

**2** Careful rectovaginal examination is performed to outline the entire Bartholin's gland cyst or abscess.

**3** To control bleeding, it is essential that the surgeon understand the vascular supply to the labia and vagina.

**4** The labia are retracted laterally with several Allis clamps. For resection of the Bartholin's gland, it is preferable to make the incision over the vaginal mucosa, directly over the meatus of the gland, rather than over the labia majora. Healing in this area appears to be faster and less painful for the patient than does healing to an incision in the skin of the labia.

**5** The vaginal mucosa is retracted medially, and the skin of the introitus is retracted laterally to expose the wall of the gland. Its meatus may be seen if not distorted by old infection and scarring.

**6** A small Metzenbaum scissors is used to lyse the filmy adhesions between the wall of the abscess or cyst and the overlying vaginal mucosa and subcutaneous tissue of the labia majora. Either forceps or an Allis clamp is placed on the wall of the cyst. The wall is retracted to allow adequate dissection and identification of the blood supply to the gland from branches of the pudendal artery.

**7** It is important to excise the entire gland. Incomplete removal may lead to a recurrence of the cyst or abscess.

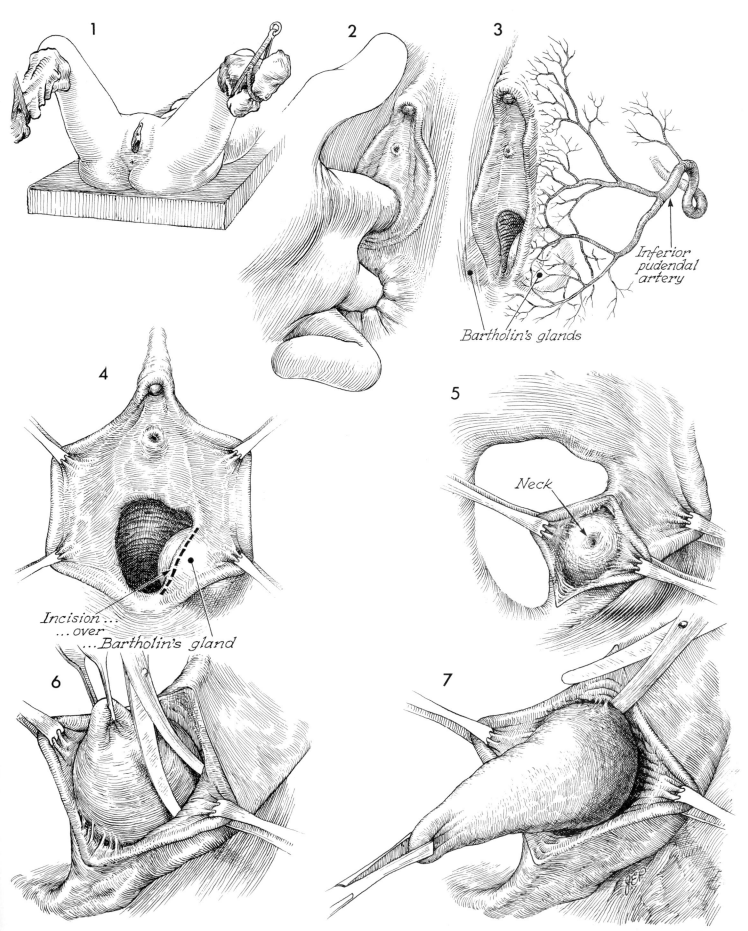

1

2

3

Inferior
pudendal
artery

Bartholin's glands

4

5

Neck

Incision...
...over
...Bartholin's gland

6

7

# Bartholin's Gland Excision

## (Continued)

**8** The last few filmy adhesions to the gland are incised with Metzenbaum scissors, and the gland is removed.

**9** After removal of the gland, there is frequently bleeding from the wound.

**10** Care must be taken that meticulous hemostasis is carried out throughout the bed of the gland. Hemostasis frequently requires electrocoagulation and suture ligation.

**11** The bed of the gland should be closed with interrupted 3-0 absorbable suture to eliminate dead space.

**12** A small closed suction drain is inserted into the wound and sutured into place with interrupted 5-0 absorbable suture. This prevents the drain from being prematurely dislodged but allows for easy removal.

**13** The closure of the vaginal mucosa to the skin of the introitus is completed with interrupted 3-0 Dexon suture.

The closed suction drain is removed on the third or fourth day when there is no further drainage.

Cultures of the abscess should be made. Frequently, gonococci, streptococci, or other organisms are found; therefore, preoperative antibiotics are used in most cases.

On the third postoperative day, the patient is placed on a regimen of hot sitz baths and is given a stool softener and laxative

Sexual intercourse can usually be resumed in 4 weeks.

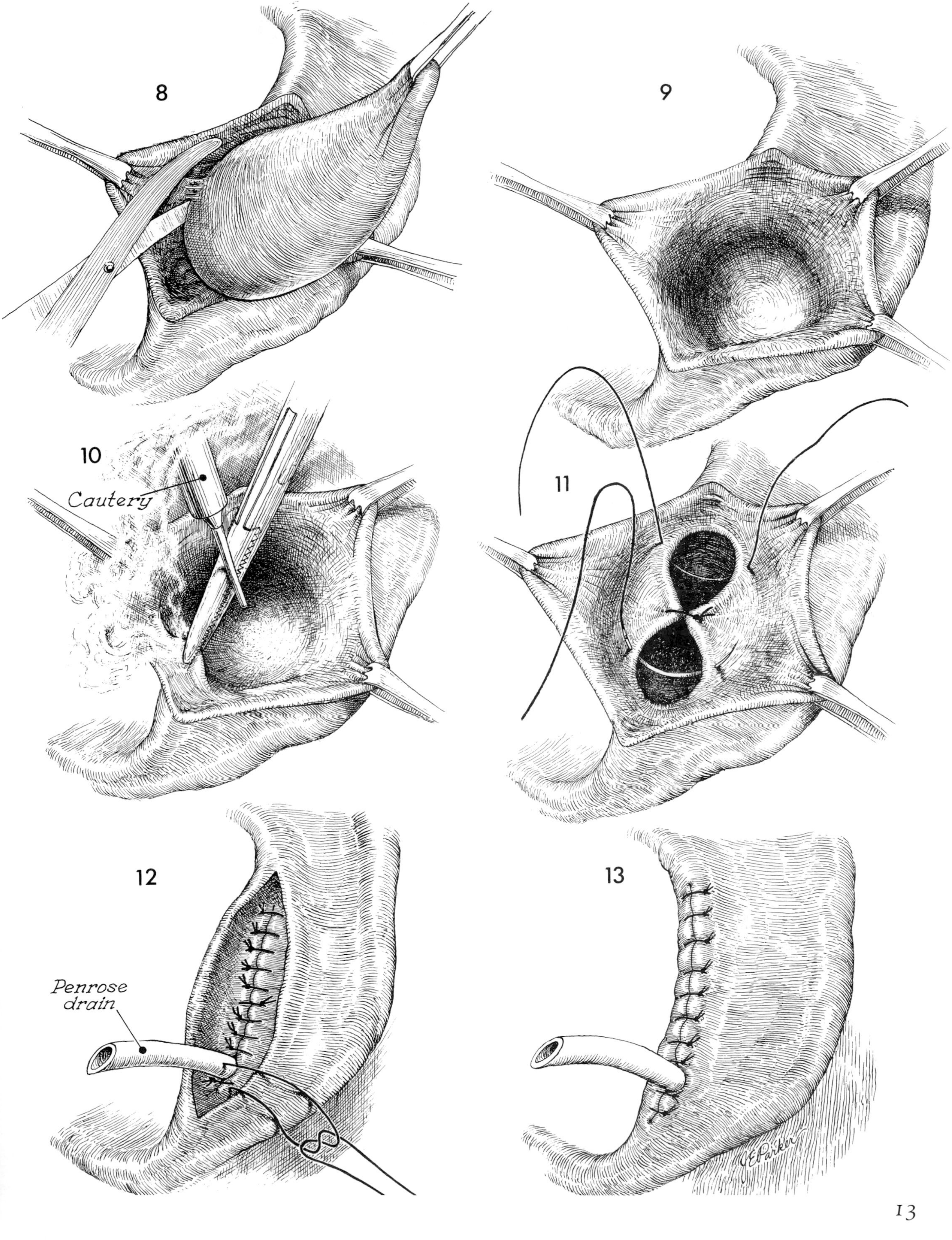
8
9
10
Cautery
11
12
Penrose drain
13
J.E. Parker

# Vaginal Outlet Stenosis Repair

Vaginal outlet stenosis is sometimes seen in virgins, but it appears most often in a woman who has undergone repair of an episiotomy or posterior repair. In relieving this condition, which is obviously associated with extreme dyspareunia, the surgeon opens the posterior outlet and pulls the mobilized vaginal mucosa onto the posterior fourchette and the peritoneal body.

Postoperatively, the vaginal mucosa is treated with estrogen so that it becomes well cornified.

**Physiologic Changes.** The vaginal outlet is opened sufficiently to allow pain-free sexual intercourse.

**Points of Caution.** Adequate mobilization of the posterior vaginal wall is extremely important in order that it may be pulled over the peritoneal body.

## Technique

**1** In a standard case of vaginal outlet stenosis, Allis clamps are applied at the 7 and 5 o'clock positions, respectively, and an incision is made at the posterior fourchette.

**2** Dissection is carried up under the posterior vaginal wall for a distance of approximately 7–8 cm. A triangle of skin is removed from the perineal body, from the posterior fourchette down toward the anus.

**3** The superficial transverse peritoneal (*STP*) muscle is exposed. Small incisions are made into this muscle in order to relax the vaginal outlet. An Allis clamp is used to keep the posterior vaginal wall on traction.

**4** The posterior vaginal mucosa is pulled over the denuded superficial transverse peritoneal muscle onto the peritoneal body.

**5** If insufficient posterior vaginal wall mucosa is not available to cover the perineal defect, the vaginal mucosa can be split in the midline, thereby enlarging the flap to allow adequate coverage.

**6** The posterior vaginal mucosa is sutured to the skin of the perineal body with interrupted 4-0 synthetic absorbable sutures.

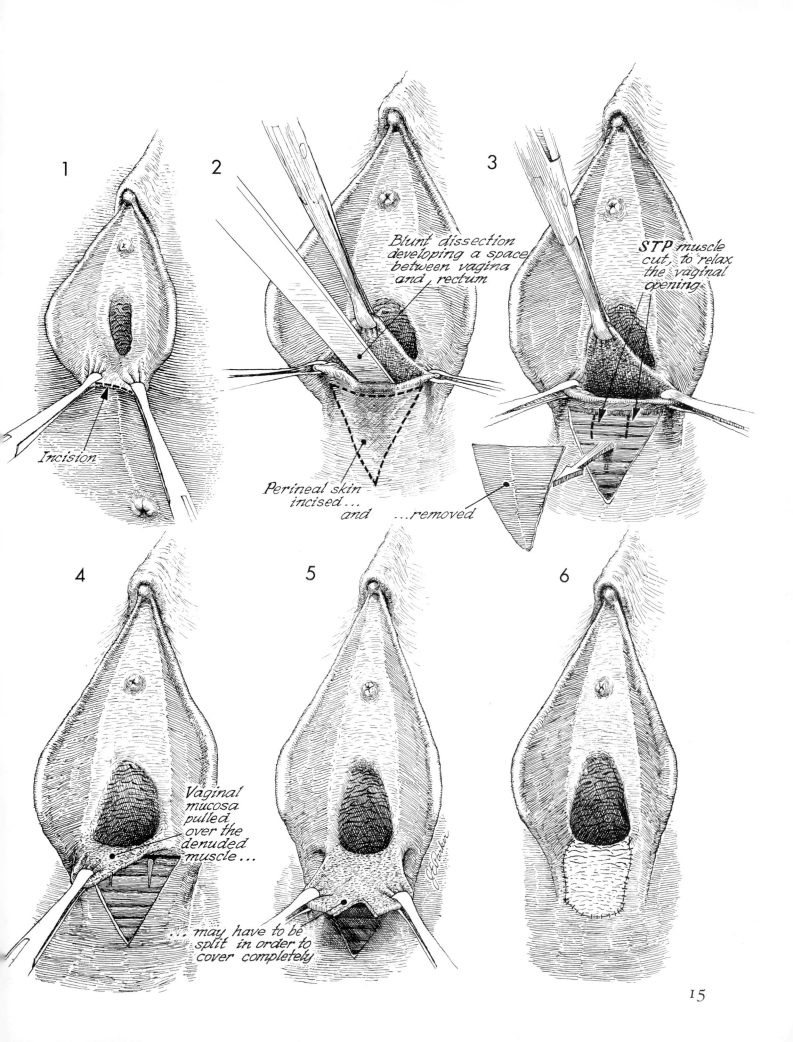

**1**

*Incision*

**2**

*Blunt dissection
developing a space
between vagina
and rectum*

*Perineal skin
incised...
and      ...removed*

**3**

*STP muscle
cut, to relax
the vaginal
opening.*

**4**

*Vaginal
mucosa
pulled
over the
denuded
muscle...*

**5**

*...may have to be
split in order to
cover completely*

**6**

# Closure of Wide Local Excision of the Vulva

Early intraepithelial neoplasias of the vulva frequently have multicentric foci of disease. To adequately excise these lesions with an appropriate surgical margin of 2 cm, wide local excision of the vulva may be required. This kind of excision can be closed by mobilizing the skin lateral to the incision and creating a relaxing incision at an appropriate place to allow coverage of the vulvar defect. This technique provides a skin flap with the blood supply coming from both the mons pubis femoral area and the skin covering the buttocks.

**Physiologic Changes.** The neoplastic lesion is excised, and primary closure of the wound is made without distortion of the vulva or stricture of the vaginal orifice.

**Points of Caution.** Prior to excision of the lesion, the margin of normal skin to be removed is measured with a centimeter ruler and outlined with a marking pen. This will ensure adequate margins around the neoplastic lesion.

The skin flap must be adequately mobilized in order to move it easily. Hemostasis is essential.

Suction drainage should be utilized.

## Technique

**1** A wide local excision of the vulva is made. The incision is carried down both sides of the vulva to points parallel to the anus. This permits closure of the perineal body without tension.

The tissue lateral to the excised area is sufficiently undermined to provide adequate coverage. The site is selected for the second incision, either at the crural fold or on the leg.

**2** The relaxing incision on the leg has been made, and the skin flap has been moved medially and sutured to the margin of the vulvar skin. Note the two angle lines of incision parallel to the anus and how they connect with the U-shaped incision of the skin flap.

The skin lateral to the second incision is undermined and mobilized for primary closure of the relaxing incision.

**3** The lesions on the vulva have been adequately excised; the defect in the vulva is now closed with a skin flap that is brought medially from the tissue lateral to the vulva out onto the skin of the leg.

It is important that suction drains are placed under the skin flap and, when they no longer produce fluid, are removed.

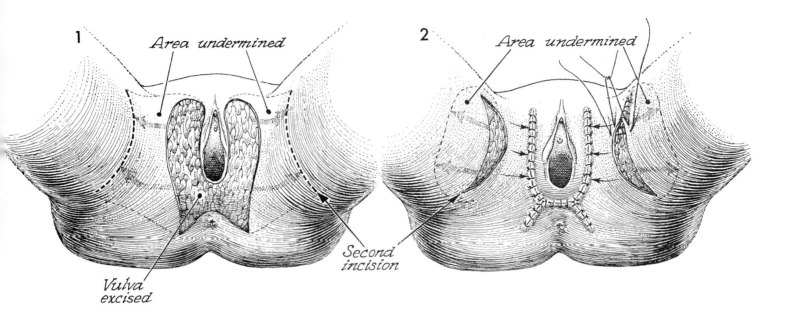

**1** *Area undermined*

*Vulva excised*

*Second incision*

**2** *Area undermined*

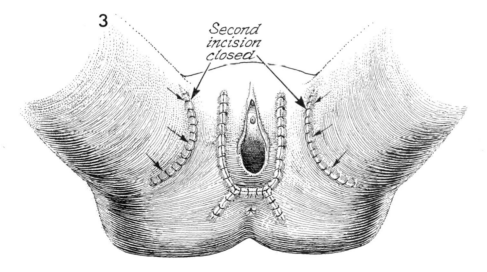

**3** *Second incision closed*

# Wide Local Excision of the Vulva, With Primary Closure or Z-plasty Flap

A wide local excision is indicated for women with in situ or microinvasive carcinoma of the vulva. The goal of this operation is to remove the carcinoma and a 2-cm margin of normal skin surrounding the gross lesion. It is imperative that prior to making the incision the surgeon measure the margin with a centimeter rule and outline it with a marking pen to ensure that the specimen is adequate.

If the 2-cm margin is not measured and the skin is not marked prior to the incision, all too often the specimen sent to the pathologist will not have an adequate margin.

In most cases, adjacent vulvar skin can be mobilized and used to effect a primary closure of the vulva. This is done in two layers after adequate hemostasis has been achieved.

In cases where extensive lesions are removed and the defect is too large for primary closure, a Z-plasty flap may be used to cover the wound without resorting to a split-thickness skin graft.

**Physiologic Changes.** The in situ carcinoma is removed without significant alteration of the physiology of the vulva.

**Points of Caution.** Preoperative measurement and marking of the diseased areas are mandatory. The Z-plasty flap or primary closure should be completed, as large defects should not be left in the vulvar area to simply granulate in and epithelialize. If primary closure is to be performed, adjacent vulvar skin should be adequately mobilized so that the suture line enclosing the vulva is not under tension.

If the excised defect is too large for primary closure, as demonstrated by tension on the suture line, the Z-plasty flap procedure should be performed. In this case, care should be taken to ensure that (1) the distance from *point* A to *point* B on the Z-plasty flap is shorter than the distance from *point* B to the margin of the excised defect and (2) there is an adequate blood supply entering the base of the flap. It is essential that all tissues be adequately mobilized to avoid any tension on any suture line within the flap area.

Patients who have undergone a Z-plasty flap procedure recover best with complete bed rest for 7 days. Intermittent pressure cuffs are applied to the legs for thromboembolic prophylaxis. Defecation should be postponed by a low-residue diet and the administration of Lomotil, 1 tablet q.i.d. for 7 days.

Patients having primary closure for relatively small vulvar defects do not require bed rest or bowel restriction.

# Wide Local Excision of the Vulva, With Primary Closure or Z-plasty Flap

## (Continued)

## Technique

### WIDE LOCAL EXCISION

**1** The patient is placed in the dorsal lithotomy position. The perineum is prepped and draped. With a centimeter ruler, a 2-cm margin is measured around the lesion and marked with brilliant green solution. Frequently, the labia minora have to be sacrificed.

**2** The margin of the lesion is excised down to the subcutaneous tissue, and the tissue is elevated with forceps. The entire lesion with its 2-cm margin and its subcutaneous tissue is excised.

Meticulous hemostasis is achieved at this point with fine pickups and electrocautery. Larger vessels are delicately tied with 4-0 or 5-0 delayed synthetic absorbable suture. At this point the defect is measured, and the surgeon decides whether to proceed with primary closure of the wound or with a Z-plasty flap operation.

### PRIMARY CLOSURE

**3** Adequate mobilization of adjacent vulvar skin is made by sharp and blunt dissection. It is essential that the wound be closed without tension. Sutures should merely hold the tissue that has been adequately mobilized and approximated.

**4** A continuous layer of 4-0 synthetic absorbable sutures stitched with an intestinal needle is used to close the subcutaneous space.

**5** A subcuticular technique can be used to approximate the skin, using 4-0 synthetic absorbable suture. Small stainless steel skin clips can also be used and can be removed on the seventh or eighth postoperative day. Fine nylon sutures can be used in either a mattress technique or the so-called flap stitch technique. These are removed on the seventh or eighth postoperative day.

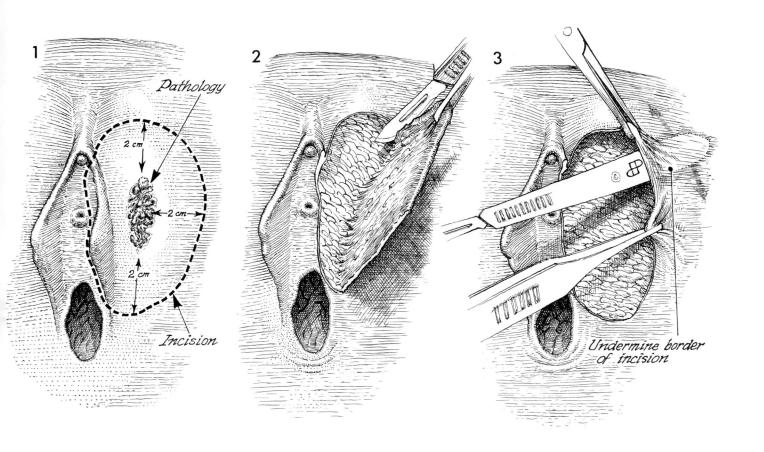

**1**

*Pathology*

2 cm

2 cm

2 cm

*Incision*

**2**

**3**

*Undermine border of incision*

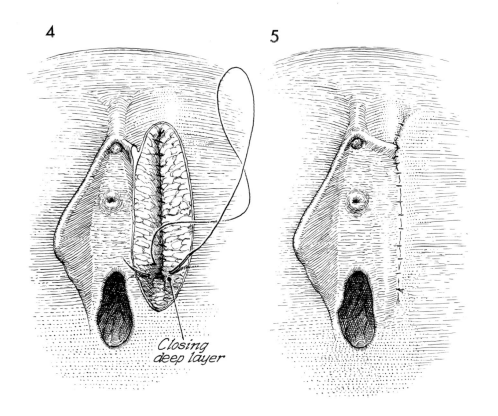

**4**

*Closing deep layer*

**5**

21

# Wide Local Excision of the Vulva, With Primary Closure or Z-plasty Flap

## (Continued)

Z-PLASTY FLAP

**6** If the lesion to be removed leaves an excessively large defect, primary closure may be impossible. In these cases, a Z-plasty flap may be the procedure of choice.

**7** The defect is measured with a ruler. The medial margin usually extends from the clitoral area to the posterior fourchette of the vagina and is equal to the distance on the proposed flap by the line marked A–D. It is essential that the base of the flap from B to the lateral edge of the defect be wider than the length of the flap. The blood supply to the flap will enter through this area, and if the length of the flap is longer than the width of the base, the flap will have insufficient blood supply, and its tip may necrose. A scalpel is used to incise the border of the flap through a full thickness of skin and subcutaneous fat. Meticulous hemostasis must be achieved at this point.

**8** The portion of the flap marked *a* should be stitched with fine synthetic absorbable suture to the ventral margin of the defect. This suture should be in the form of a flap stitch that enters the full thickness of the skin of the margin of the defect and is brought through the flap with a subcuticular technique. The needle reenters the subcuticular layer of the flap skin adjacent to the first suture, then reenters the full thickness of the margins of the defect from the subcutaneous layer and exits the cutaneous layer adjacent to the first suture. This flap stitch aids healing by less con-

striction of the blood supply in the flap. The second suture should be placed in the posterior fourchette of the vagina and be brought to the angle of the flap marked D with the same stitch described above. At this point, the part of the flap marked C should be sutured with the flap stitch to the angle (ABC) created by the entire Z-plasty. After the margins of the flap have been sutured, the surgeon can make adjustments if necessary. If undue tension is noted at any particular point, it can be released by greater mobilization of adjacent skin.

**9** Several techniques are acceptable for suturing the flap to the adjacent recipient skin and vaginal wall. The new stainless steel skin clips have the advantage of being inert and causing little tissue reaction. They can be left in for long periods of time to allow for complete closure and healing of the wound. Synthetic absorbable suture material can be utilized and, in general, gives improved cosmetic result. Sutures of fine nylon, in the flap stitch technique, can be used throughout the closure. These require removal after the margins of the wound have completely healed. Patients who have undergone large perineal Z-plasty flaps should remain in bed for a minimum of 6–7 days.

Thromboembolic prophylaxis utilizing the contemporary technique of intermittent pressure cuffs is essential. Defecation should be delayed for 6–8 days until the margin of the flap has sealed. This is achieved by a low-residue diet and the administration of Lomotil tablets q.i.d.

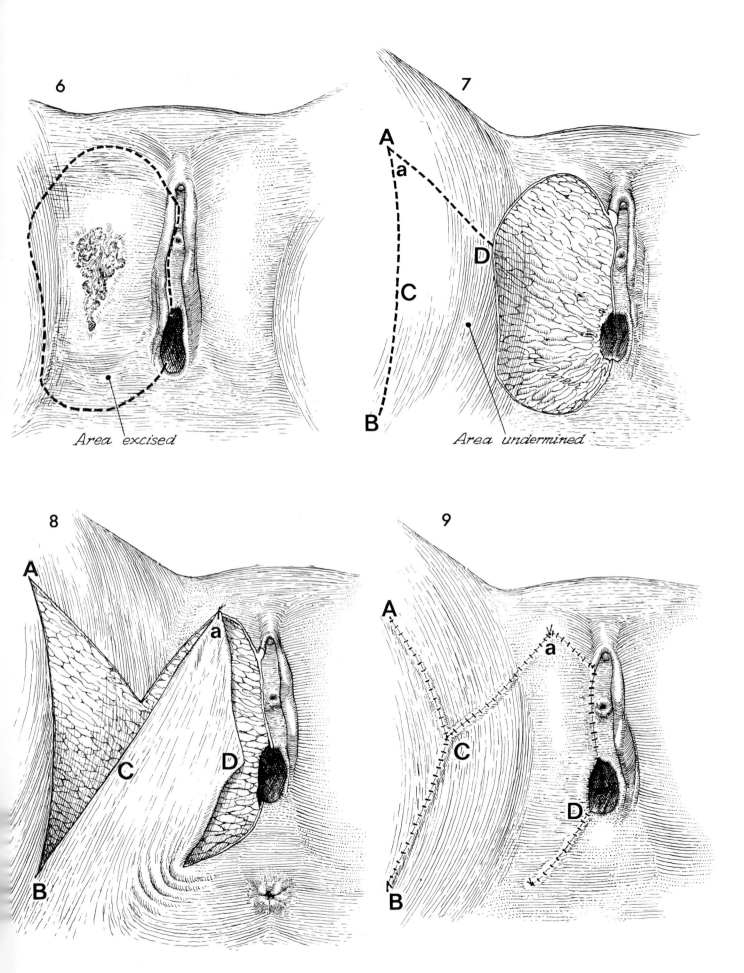

6

Area excised

7

Area undermined

8

9

23

# Alcohol Injection of the Vulva

In patients with chronic and severe pruritus of the vulva not amenable to steroid cream therapy, denervation of the vulva is often needed to break the vicious cycle of itching, scratching, excoriation, microlacerations, and irritation of cutaneous nerves. Alcohol injection of the vulva gives the patient a temporary period of denervation. Surgical denervation should be reserved for those patients in whom medical therapy and alcohol injection have failed.

Denervation by alcohol injection requires an understanding of the innervation of the vulva.

To prevent microulcerations and infection, care must be taken to inject the 95% alcohol into the subcutaneous space and not the intradermal space.

The purpose of this operation is to temporarily denervate the vulva by injecting alcohol in a systematic fashion that will denervate each of the cutaneous branches of the ilioinguinal, genitofemoral, posterior femoral, and pudendal nerves. This denervation generally lasts 4–6 months.

**Physiologic Changes.** Denervation of the perineum blocks the awareness of itching, thereby eliminating the need for scratching. Scratching produces microlacerations that become infected, producing more itching and, thus, the vicious cycle. By stopping the itching and eliminating the scratching, this procedure allows the perineum to heal during the 4–6 months of denervation.

**Points of Caution.** The alcohol must be injected subcutaneously, not subcuticularly, or sloughing of the epidermis will occur.

## Technique

**1** Innervation of the vulva is shown. To inject each of the cutaneous branches of these nerves, it is necessary to have a system that will allow controlled injection.

**2** The procedure is carried out under general anesthesia. The patient is placed in the dorsal lithotomy position and prepped and draped. A 2-0 silk suture that has been dipped in a medicine glass of brilliant green is used to mark off a grid on the vulva. Using the silk suture, vertical lines extending from the mons pubis to the anus are made 1 cm apart across the entire vulva. To complete the grid, the same technique is used to make horizontal lines 1 cm apart.

**3** A tuberculin syringe and several 25-gauge needles are needed to inject systematically 0.1 mL of 95% alcohol at each point of intersection on the grid. It is important to use several needles so that one needle can be left in the last row to identify the last point of injection as one moves to a new row. Without a marker, it is possible to get confused and skip one or more rows, leaving an area of the vulva innervated.

Cessation of itching is immediate. It is not unusual for the patient to develop cellulitis in the perineal area following the procedure; this can be treated with antibiotics.

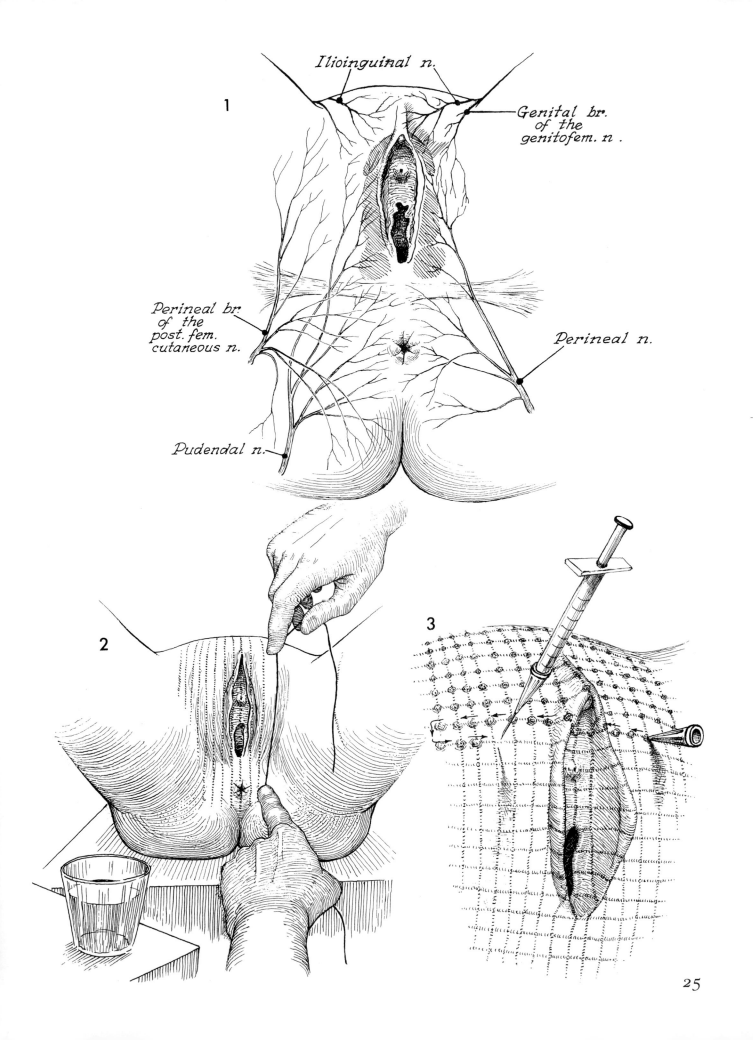

1

*Ilioinguinal n.*

*Genital br. of the genitofem. n .*

*Perineal br. of the post. fem. cutaneous n.*

*Perineal n.*

*Pudendal n.*

2

3

# Cortisone Injection of the Vulva

In patients with chronic pruritus of the vulva, subcutaneous injection of the vulva with a fluorinated cortisone preparation will often relieve the patient and break the vicious cycle of itching, scratching, excoriation, and irritation of cutaneous nerves. Pruritus of the vulva is often associated with parakeratosis that does not allow steroid cream to penetrate the skin and reach the important subdermal area. The injection must cover the entire vulva. Particular attention must be given to those areas that the patient designates as especially troublesome.

**Physiologic Changes.** Pruritus of the vulva is eliminated. Cortisone reduces the inflammatory reaction and improves the vascular supply and thus improves the nutrition of the vulvar skin.

**Points of Caution.** Care must be exercised to inject the entire vulva and to avoid penetration of the perineal branches of the pudendal artery and vein.

## Technique

With the patient under general or local anesthesia in the lithotomy position, the surgeon outlines the inflamed areas of the vulva.

**1** Innervation of the vulva including the ilioinguinal nerves, the genital branch of the genitofemoral nerve, the perineal branch of the posterior femoral cutaneous nerve, and the perineal branches of the pudendal nerve is shown.

**2** Forty mg of a fluorinated steroid solution in a 20-mL syringe mixed with 1 mL of Xylocaine are injected in a radial design underneath the squamous epithelium. The entire area affected is covered.

The injection can be repeated 1–2 times/week for up to 4 weeks.

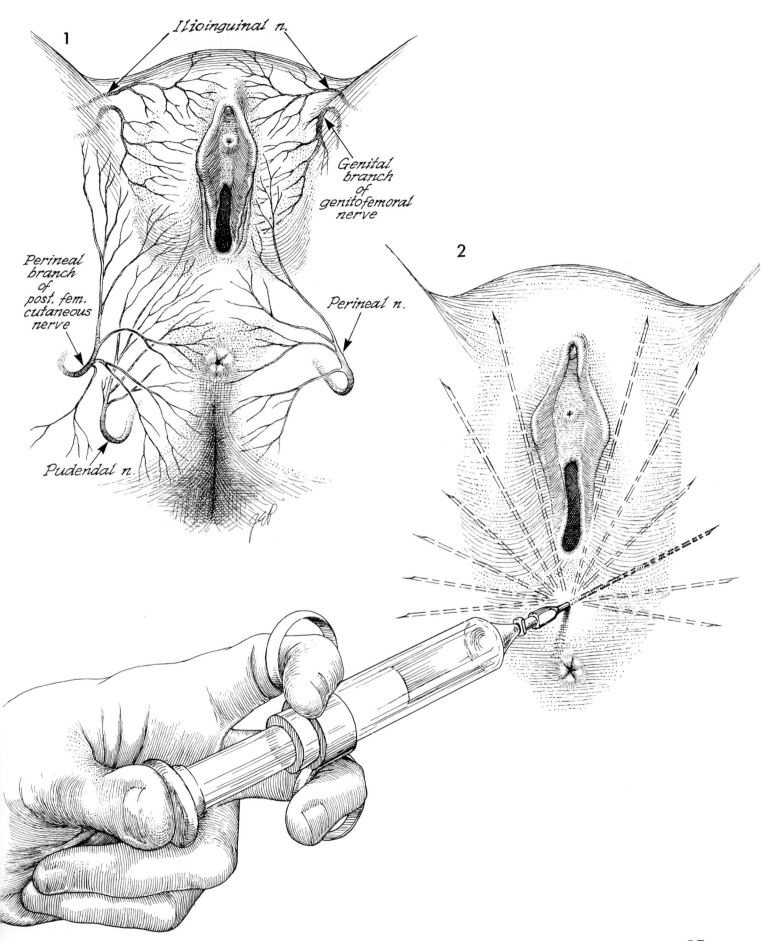

1

*Ilioinguinal n.*

*Genital
branch
of
genitofemoral
nerve*

*Perineal
branch
of
post. fem.
cutaneous
nerve*

*Perineal n.*

*Pudendal n.*

2

27

# Simple Vulvectomy

Simple vulvectomy is indicated for severe lesions of the vulva that are not amenable to local excision or other forms of conservative therapy. These conditions include extensive in situ or microinvasive carcinoma of the vulva, Paget's disease, and severe leukoplakia.

Unlike radical vulvectomy, this simpler procedure does not require an incision all the way to the perineal fascia. With adequate preoperative counseling, the patient usually experiences few psychologic problems with regard to her sexual functioning.

**Physiologic Changes.** The skin and subcutaneous tissues of the vulva are removed.

**Points of Caution.** To avoid complications, particular attention must be paid to the control of hemorrhage around the urethra and the lateral pudendal vessels.

## Technique

**1** The patient is placed in the dorsal lithotomy position with her buttocks at least 3 inches off the end of the table.

**2** An outline of the lesion is made with a brilliant green ink preparation. An elliptical incision is made down to the subcutaneous fat. The incision starts from above the labial folds on the mons pubis and is extended down the lateral fold of the labia majora and across the posterior fourchette. A dry pack is used to occlude the small bleeding vessels in the skin until this incision is completed.

**3** As the 3 and 9 o'clock positions on the vulva are approached, the pudendal artery and vein are encountered. These vessels, before being incised, should be clamped to avoid major blood loss. For maximum exposure, the specimen should be kept on tension by placing multiple Allis clamps around the edges of the skin.

**4** The pudendal vessels are securely tied, and the incision is continued around the entire circumference of the lesion, as shown in Figure 2.

**5** Exposure to the vaginal orifice and urethra is made by retracting the labia laterally. The line of incision around the urethra and vaginal orifice has been marked with brilliant green surgical ink. The incision is started above the urethral meatus and carried around the vaginal introitus with an adequate margin around the lesion.

**6** By palpating the incision above the urethral meatus with the finger and placing a small hemostat behind the suspensory ligaments of the clitoris, the surgeon makes an opening above the urethra to ensure that damage to the urethral meatus is avoided. A similar technique is used laterally to perforate the cutaneous tissue from the lateral incision to the vaginal incision.

This technique can also be used inferiorly to avoid damaging the rectum. The surgeon may place a finger in the rectum while retracting the specimen superiorly and perforating the dermis tissue between the inferior skin margin and the vagina along the lines of the incision made in both structures. After the dermis has been permeated, one blade of curved Mayo scissors may be inserted to cut between the perforations.

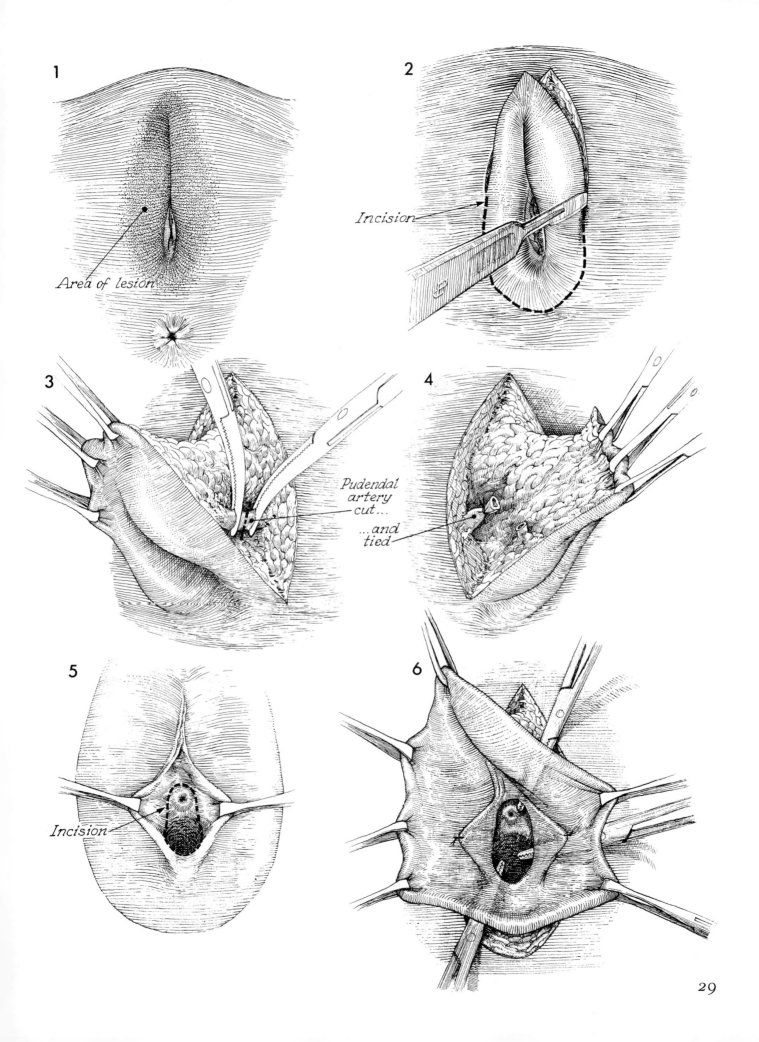

**1**

Area of lesion

**2**

Incision

**3**

Pudendal
artery
cut...

...and
tied

**4**

**5**

Incision

**6**

29

# Simple Vulvectomy

## (Continued)

---

**7** The specimen has been transected between the perforations made in the vaginal mucosa, leaving the specimen attached only to the fat pad in the mons pubis and to the vascular plexus surrounding the suspensory ligaments of the clitoris. This area should be clamped and tied before it is transected with scissors.

**8** Primary closure of the wound is begun. First, the posterior wall of the vaginal mucosa is undermined and brought out to the posterior fourchette so that contracture of the vaginal introitus is avoided. After hemostasis is achieved, closure of the wound is continued superiorly in the mons pubis by closing the subcutaneous tissue with interrupted 2-0 synthetic absorbable suture.

**9** Three or four 2-0 synthetic absorbable sutures are placed in the levator ani muscles, which are plicated in the midline after the posterior vaginal mucosa has been mobilized. Note that the subcutaneous tissue of the mons pubis has been closed almost down to the urethral meatus.

**10** A close-up of the plicated levators, the pudendal vessels, and the mobilized posterior wall of the vagina is shown.

**11** Closure of the subcutaneous tissue of the perineal body is begun with interrupted 2-0 synthetic absorbable sutures. The subcutaneous tissue remaining superiorly is then closed.

**12** A catheter is inserted into the urethral meatus, and the periurethral mucosa is sutured to the skin with interrupted 3-0 synthetic absorbable sutures. The vaginal mucosa is likewise sutured to the skin with interrupted 3-0 synthetic absorbable sutures.

**13** Skin closure is begun in a subcuticular fashion over the mons and the perineal body, respectively, with interrupted 3-0 synthetic absorbable sutures. The remaining vaginal mucosa is sutured to the skin with interrupted 3-0 synthetic absorbable sutures.

**14** Final closure of the simple vulvectomy is made by using synthetic absorbable sutures, making permanent sutures unnecessary. During closure of this incision, it is most important to eliminate tension on the suture line. The surgeon should mobilize the perineal tissues until the margins of the wound come together without tension. The Foley catheter is left in place for 24 hours and then removed. The patient is ambulated immediately. Laxatives and stool softeners are administered on the third postoperative day.

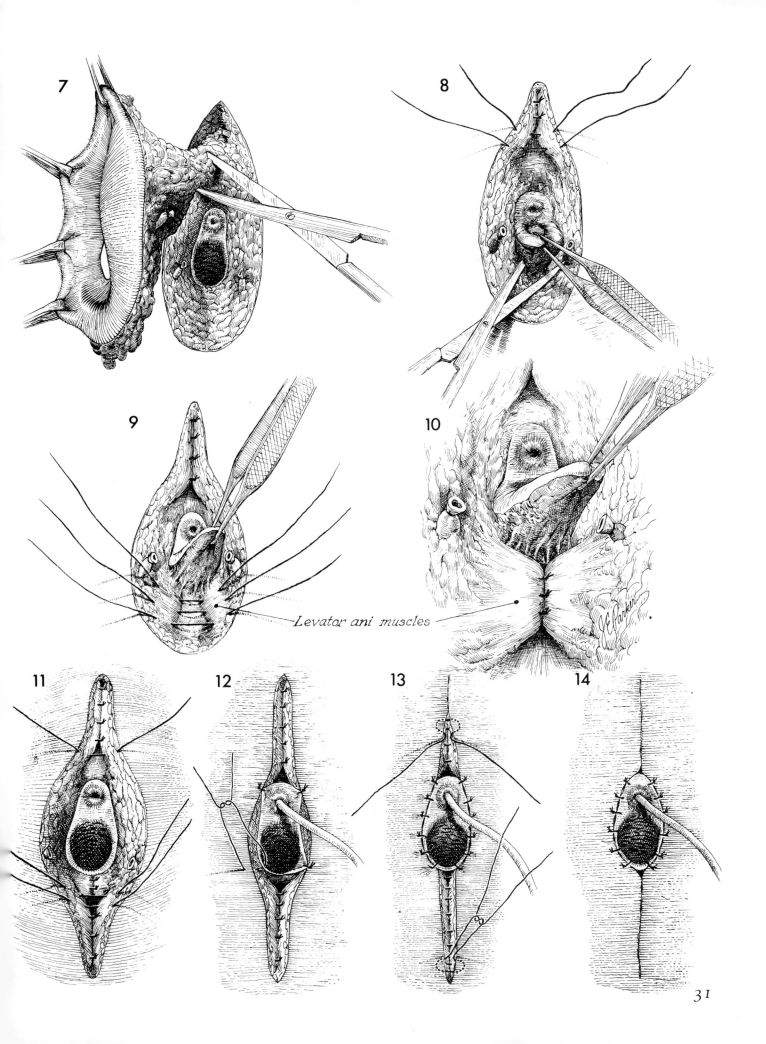

*Levator ani muscles*

31

# Excision of the Vulva by the Loop Electrical Excision Procedure (LEEP)

The technique for removal of small lesions from the vulva, e.g., condyloma acuminatum and in situ carcinomas, has varied over time with the technologic facilities available to the surgeon. The techniques have ranged from sharp knife, to laser vaporization, to the currently popular electrosurgical excision. Electrosurgical excision has the advantage of being inexpensive and available as an office or outpatient clinic procedure. Local anesthesia is adequate and should be performed 5–6 minutes prior to the excision. Smoke evacuation is important for two reasons: (1) The human papilloma virus (HPV) has been shown to survive flumen of the electrosurgical and laser procedure; and (2) smoke seen arising from the vulva might incite anxiety and reduce the patient's ability to cooperate.

With the advent of laser vaporization, many of these excised lesions of the vulva were left open to epithe-lialize over 4–6 weeks by second intention. We always close laser vaporization and electrosurgical wounds.

**Physiologic Changes.** The excision of in situ carcinoma reduces the breakdown and excoriation of the vulva, with constant drainage of these lesions. Untreated condylomata can break down, become infected, and cause undesirable drainage from the vulva.

**Points of Caution.** The electrosurgical instrument should be set on a blend between the cutting and coagulation current. The predominate wattage should be used for cutting, and the smaller wattage should be devoted to coagulation in order to reduce thermal injury to the tissue. For most standard electrosurgical machines, we prefer a wattage of 60 for cutting to 10–20 for coagulation. Small areas of bleeding can be lightly touched with the ball cautery on coagulation.

---

## Technique

**1** The vulva is shown with the left labia minora retracted and a lesion surrounding the left vestibule.

**2** The electrosurgical excision instrument is set on 60 watts for cutting and 20 watts for coagulation and is used to excise the lesion.

**3** The lesion is removed with a full thickness of skin down to the subcutaneous fat.

**4** The completed resection of the lesion is shown with additional excised areas if they are suspicious for disease.

**5** Fine 4-0 rapid synthetic absorbable suture is placed in the subcutaneous fat.

**6** A subcuticular suture is placed, closing the skin.

**1**

Lesion

**2**

Lesion
excised by
cautery loop

**3**

**4**

Additional
tissue may
be excised
as necessary

**5**

Wound is
closed in
two layers

**6**

Buried
subcuticular
sutures

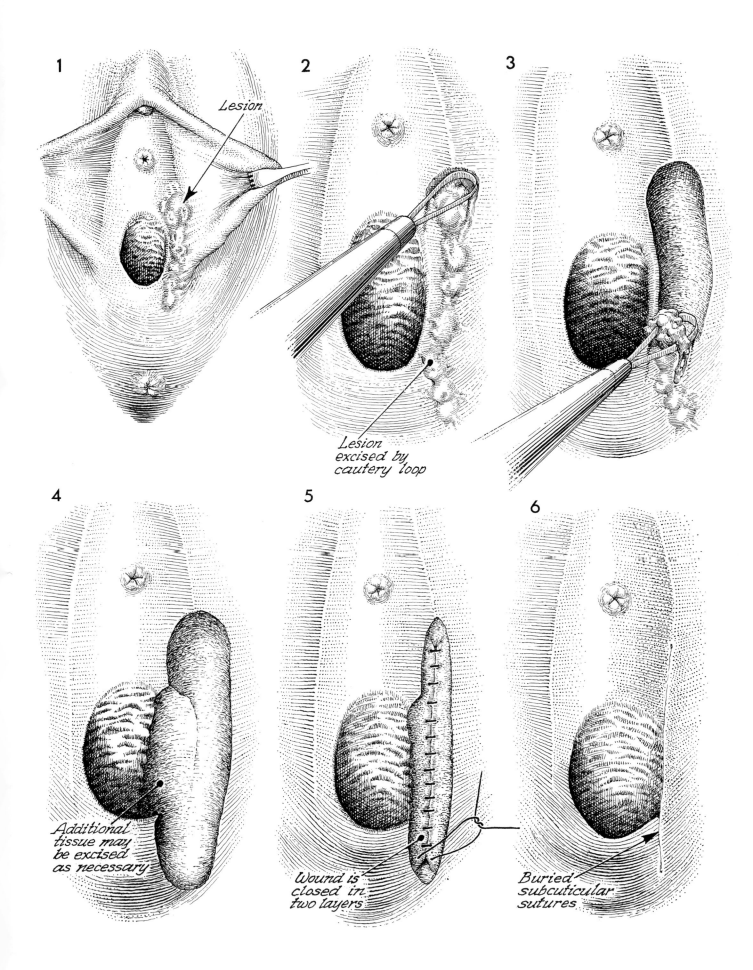

33

# Excision of Vestibular Adenitis

Nonspecific inflammation in the glands in the vestibule of the vulva, termed vulvodynia by the International Society for the Study of Vulva Disease, has been broken down into three categories: (1) vestibulitis, (2) squamous papillomatosis (vulvar dermatoses, cyclic candidiasis, squamous papillomatosis), and (3) essential vulvodynia. All too often these patients have a 6-month or greater history of being treated with anti-inflammatory, antifungal, and antibacterial agents prescribed by numerous physicians. All to often these patients undergo laser vaporization that results in more constriction and dyspareunia to the vaginal outlet.

Excision of the hymen along with the adjacent inflamed glands has produced relief of symptoms in about 75–90% of cases. Where there is diagnostic uncertainty, every effort should be made to treat these patients with conservative therapy prior to surgical resection.

Once surgical resection has been chosen, it is important that the entire vestibular glandular area involved in the process be surgically removed.

**Physiologic Changes.** The predominate physiologic change in resection of vestibular adenitis is removal of the inflamed vestibular glands that cause severe pain and dyspareunia. The absence of this tissue produces little change in the physiology of the functioning vagina and vulva.

**Points of Caution.** The involved area of the vestibule should be carefully marked out under superior light and, if possible, with optical magnification to ensure that an adequate excision of the vestibular adenitis is made.

Thorough mobilization and advancement of the posterior and lateral vaginal wall sufficient to come out on the posterior fourchette without tension should be performed. If the posterior vaginal wall is brought out under tension, it will retract, and contracture of the vaginal outlet with its sequela will occur.

---

## Technique

**1** The involved vestibule of the vulva and vagina is shown. The punctated area needs to be carefully marked off, and the incision should encompass the entire lesion. Crosscutting will result in recurrence of the problem.

**2** The vestibule is removed along the marked off lines.

**3** One of the most important aspects of the operation is thorough mobilization of the posterior vaginal wall from the posterior fourchette to the top of the vagina. All to often, insufficient mobilization is made. This is performed by elevating the posterior vaginal wall and dissecting under the vaginal mucosa with scissors.

**4** The posterior vaginal wall is gently pulled out onto the posterior fourchette. It should lie in place without traction. The purpose of sutures is not to retract the posterior wall out of the vagina but to hold it adjacent to the skin of the vulva for proper wound healing.

**5** The edges of the vaginal mucosa are sutured to the edge of the skin. The new rapid synthetic absorbable suture is superior for this purpose if adequate mobilization has occurred. If inadequate mobilization occurs, a longer acting suture is needed that may require removal of the suture in the office in 2 weeks.

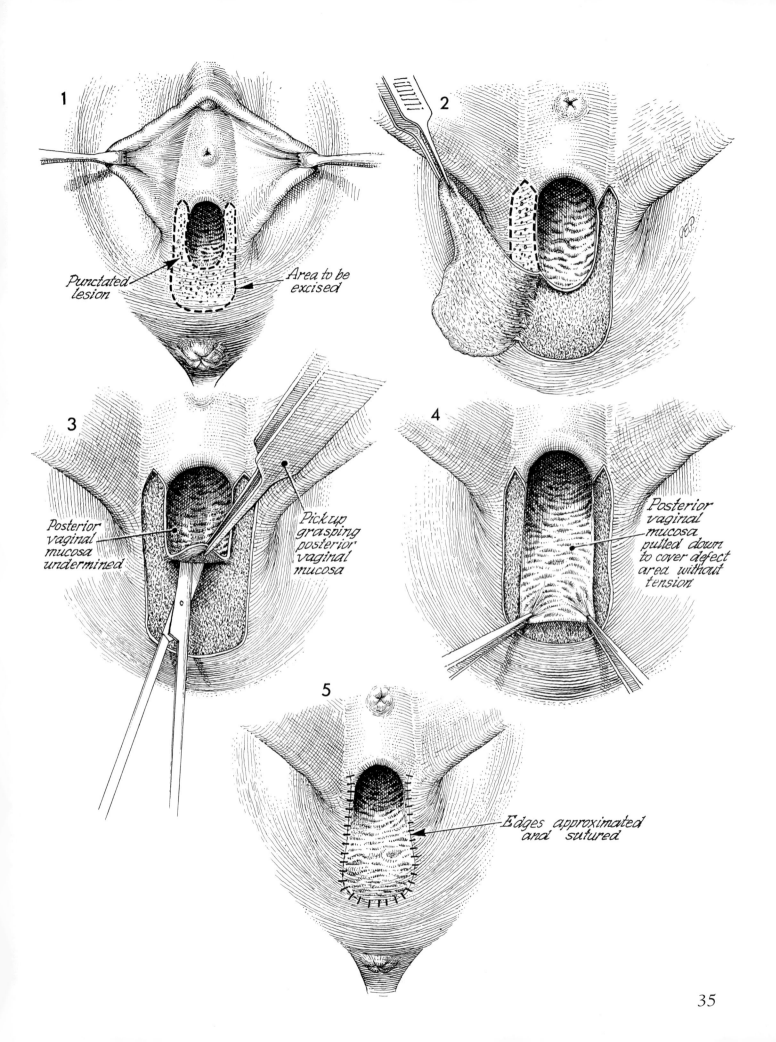

**1**

*Punctated lesion*

*Area to be excised*

**2**

**3**

*Posterior vaginal mucosa undermined*

*Pickup grasping posterior vaginal mucosa*

**4**

*Posterior vaginal mucosa pulled down to cover defect area without tension*

**5**

*Edges approximated and sutured*

# Release of Labial Fusion

Labial fusion is secondary to a urogenital sinus deformity, and in the majority of cases the labia separate on their own or with applications of estrogen cream. There are, however, some cases where the fusion is not amenable to conservative management and surgical intervention is required.

The importance of preoperative evaluation prior to surgical management is vital to the success of the procedure. The gender of some patients may be unclear. The clitoris is mistaken for a micropenis, and the fused folds of the labia may be mistaken for a scrotum with undescended testes. Appropriate cytogenetic studies are indicated. An examination under anesthesia with careful probing of all openings under the clitoris/penis should be performed.

Only after the patient has been adequately evaluated should surgical management be started.

**Physiologic Changes.** The fused labia are opened, resulting in a normal vaginal canal.

**Points of Caution.** Care should be taken to identify all genital canals within the pelvis. A silver wire probe and uterine sound should be gently inserted into the various canals under general anesthesia in order to identify each opening prior to making an incision into the labia.

## Technique

1. With the patient under general anesthesia in the dorsal lithotomy position, the external genitalia should be carefully examined, and a search should be made for the opening of the orifice of the urogenital sinus.

2. A pediatric cystoscope is used to visualize the urethral meatus and vagina.

3. A large sound is passed into the orifice of the urogenital sinus, and a scalpel is used to open the median raphe.

4. The squamous epithelium of the labia majora is sutured to the mucous membrane of the vestibule with interrupted 4-0 synthetic absorbable sutures.

5. When the last suture has been placed, the normal female anatomy is essentially restored. Bladder catheterization and vaginal packs are not required.

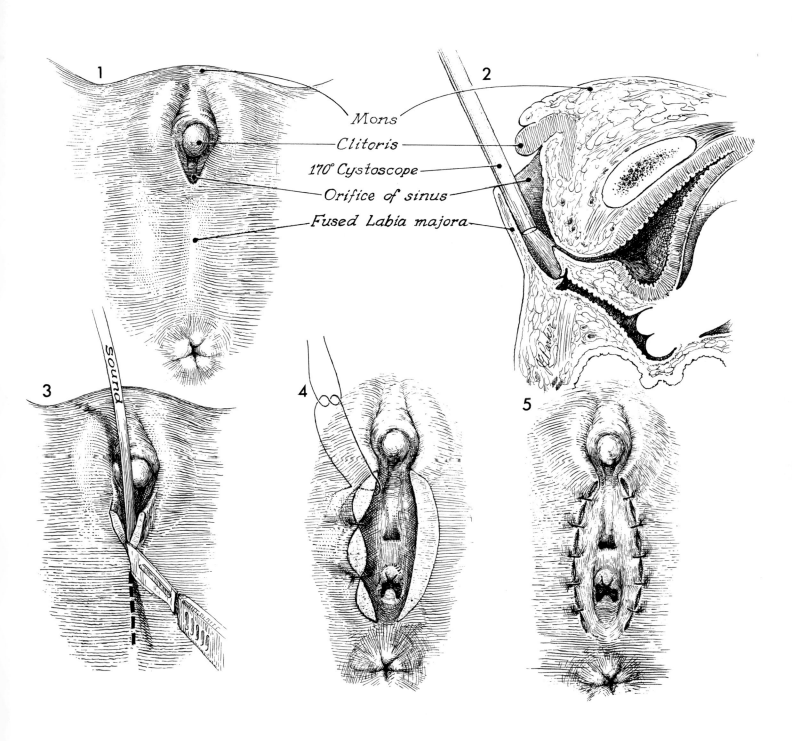

1

2

Mons

Clitoris

170° Cystoscope

Orifice of sinus

Fused Labia majora

Sound

3

4

5

# Hymenectomy

Hymenectomy may be indicated in the presence of (1) an imperforate hymen creating a mucocolpos, a hematocolpos, or hematometra at menarche or (2) a perforated hymen with hymenal hypertrophy obstructing intercourse. The latter can be frightening and can be associated with major hemorrhage if the lateral pudendal artery is lacerated along with the hymen during initial attempted intercourse.

Hymenectomy is performed to open the hymen without hemorrhage and to leave a patent introitus.

**Physiologic Changes.** The procedure allows proper drainage of the vagina and permits vaginal intercourse.

**Points of Caution.** If a mucocolpos or hematocolpos is present, the hymen should be incised as the initial procedure but not removed in order to allow adequate drainage and to restore normal anatomy prior to reconstruction.

Caution should be observed in performing this operation in a clinic, office, or other outpatient facility where adequate resources are not available for control of hemorrhage.

## Technique

**1** The patient is placed in the dorsal lithotomy position. The perineum is prepped and draped. The labia are retracted.

**2** The hymenal tags are grasped by tissue forceps, and a small Metzenbaum scissors is inserted through the opening. Stellate incisions are made to open the vaginal canal. If mucus is present, it is gently irrigated away with saline solution.

**3** As each stellate tag is elevated with tissue forceps, it is excised at the introital level, and its base is sutured with interrupted 3-0 synthetic absorbable suture.

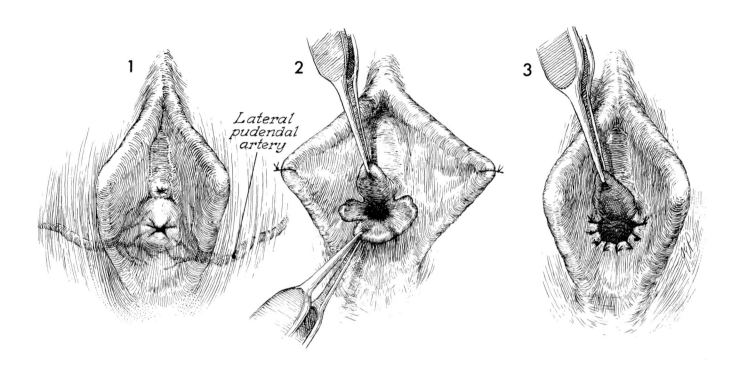

1

2

*Lateral
pudendal
artery*

3

# 2

---

# Vagina and Urethra

# Anterior Repair and Kelly Plication

Anterior repair is used for correction of a cystourethrocele. It can be combined with Kelly plication of the urethra when, in addition to a cystourethrocele, the patient is experiencing stress incontinence of urine.

The purpose of the anterior repair is to reduce the cystourethrocele and reinforce the pubovesical cervical fascia support of the bladder and urethra. The purpose of the Kelly plication of the urethra is to reduce the diameter of the urethra.

**Physiologic Changes.** In the Kelly plication, the surgeon increases the intraurethral pressure to a level higher than the intravesical pressure in the resting and stress state, i.e., with a Valsalva maneuver. When the patient tries to void, however, the detrusor contractions reverse the pressure relationship so that the intravesical pressure exceeds the intraurethral pressure.

**Points of Caution.** Care must be taken to dissect the anterior vaginal mucosa off the pubovesical cervical fascia without carrying the dissection beneath the fascia. The depth of penetration of the plication suture must be controlled; the purpose is to plicate the fascia, not the urethra. Excessive amounts of mucosa should not be removed to avoid unduly reducing the volume of the vagina.

## Technique

**1** The patient is placed in the dorsal lithotomy position. The perineum, vulva, and vagina are surgically prepared. The anterior repair can be performed with the uterus in place or after it has been removed. The technique is the same. The urethrocele and cystocele are shown. A transverse incision is made at the junction of the vaginal mucosa and cervix. This incision should be carried down to the pubovesical cervical fascia while the cervix is held on traction with a Jacobs tenaculum.

**2** The uterus has been removed. The lateral edges of the vaginal cuff are held with Allis clamps on tension. Several Allis clamps are placed 3–4 cm apart up the midline of the anterior vaginal wall. The vaginal mucosa itself is held with thumb forceps and, with curved Mayo scissors, is undermined for approximately 3–4 cm up to the first of the Allis clamps placed in the midline. It is important for the assistant to hold the three Allis clamps in the immediate area of dissection on tension, creating a triangle. This will assist the surgeon in keeping the dissection in the proper plane between vaginal mucosa and pubovesical cervical fascia.

**3** When the vaginal mucosa has been dissected off the pubovesical cervical (PVC) fascia, it is opened with scissors in the midline.

**4** The procedure in Step 3 is repeated after wide Allis clamps have been applied to the edges of the vaginal mucosa.

**5** The vaginal mucosa is opened in the midline up to the next Allis clamp. This is continued until the vagina is opened to within 1 cm of the urethral meatus. As the vagina is opened, the edges of the mucosa are grasped with wide Allis clamps and held in the lateral position by the assistants.

**6** The pubovesical cervical (PVC) fascia is separated from the vaginal mucosa. The surgical assistants maintain tension on the wide Allis clamps to form an opening like a "Chinese fan." Scalpel, scissors, or blunt dissection can be used to remove the fascia from the vaginal mucosa. It is helpful to start the dissection with a scalpel, cutting the pubovesical cervical fascia at the edge of the vaginal mucosa and dissecting it downward with the finger or the handle of the scalpel. This dissection should be continued until the bladder and urethra are separated from the vaginal mucosa and are clearly identified and the urethral vesical angle has been ascertained.

**7** If the patient has stress incontinence of urine and needs a Kelly plication, the first mattress suture is placed in the wall of the urethra approximately 1 cm below the urethral meatus. Traditionally, a nonabsorbable suture has been used for the plication. The suture, 1 cm in length, should be placed along the lateral margin of the urethra. When the suture is completed, a curved Kelly clamp is held in position to invert the urethral tissue as the suture is tied.

**8** Additional Kelly plication sutures are placed.

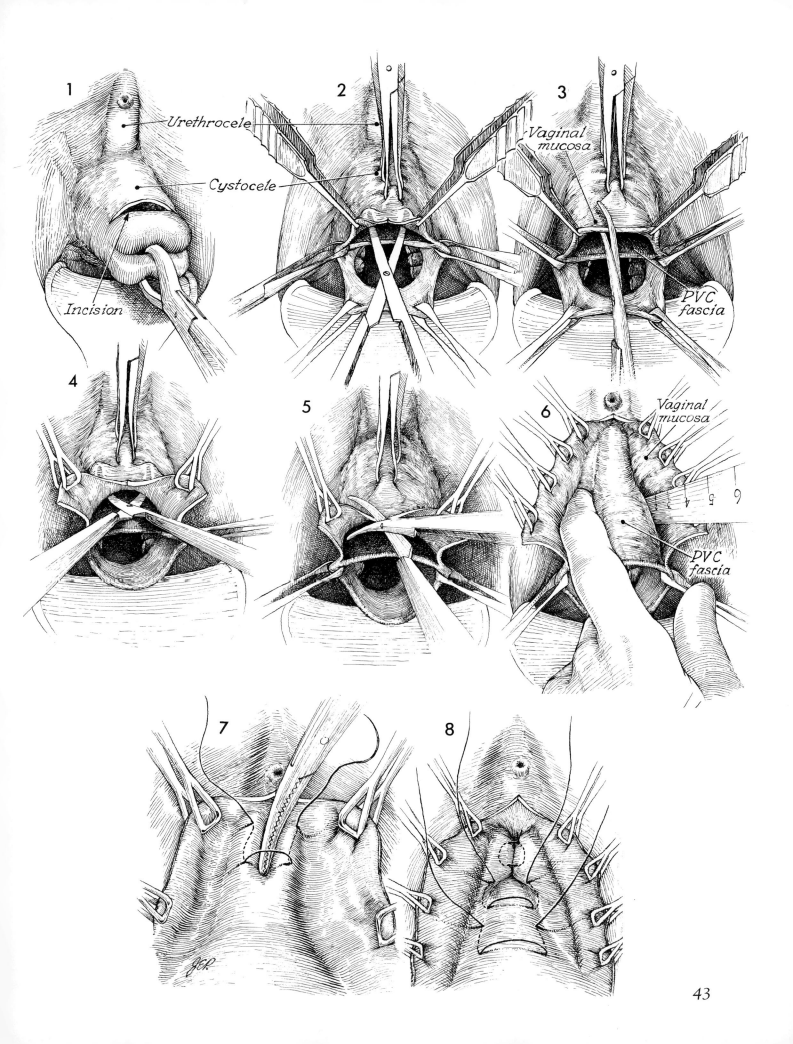

1

Urethrocele

Cystocele

Incision

2

3

Vaginal
mucosa

PVC
fascia

4

5

6

Vaginal
mucosa

PVC
fascia

7

8

43

# Anterior Repair and Kelly Plication

## (Continued)

**9** The last Kelly plication suture is placed approximately 2 cm beyond the urethral vesical angle.

**10** The anterior repair is started by placing 0 synthetic absorbable sutures in the pubovesical cervical (PVC) fascia, starting at the level of the first Kelly plication suture or 1 cm below the urethral meatus. This suture should be placed only in the pubovesical cervical fascia, not in the bladder wall.

**11** The edges of the vaginal mucosa are retracted laterally with Allis clamps. The remaining pubovesical cervical fascia is plicated in the midline with multiple interrupted 0 absorbable mattress sutures.

**12** The plication of the pubovesical cervical fascia should continue until the entire cystourethrocele has been reduced.

**13** The edges of the vaginal mucosa are held on tension. The excessive vaginal mucosa is trimmed away. The lower portion of the drawing shows a cross section of vaginal cuff and plicated pubovesical cervical fascia.

**14** The vaginal mucosa is sutured in the midline with interrupted 0 synthetic absorbable suture down to the vaginal cuff. The edge of the vaginal cuff is sutured with a running 0 absorbable suture and left open.

**15** The completed anterior repair and Kelly plication with the sutured anterior vaginal mucosa is shown. The sutured but open vaginal cuff is seen. A Foley catheter is inserted transurethrally.

**16** An alternative method of bladder drainage is the suprapubic insertion of a Foley catheter (see Section 3, page 136).

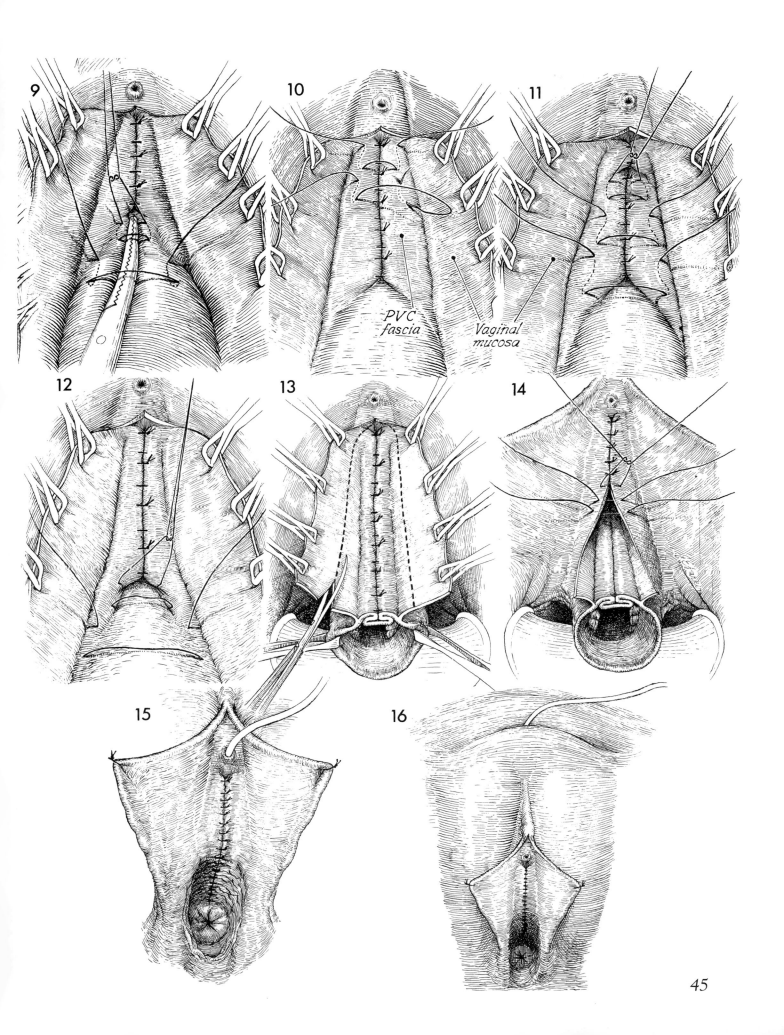

9

10

11

*PVC fascia*    *Vaginal mucosa*

12

13

14

15

16

45

# Posterior Repair

Posterior repair is performed in conjunction with perineorrhaphy to correct a rectocele and to reconstruct the peritoneal body. A rectocele is a hernia that develops when the perirectal fascia is insufficient to support the anterior rectal wall and the rectum prolapses through the levator sling. The strength of the posterior vaginal mucosa is insufficient to prevent prolapse of the anterior rectal wall.

The purpose of posterior repair is to plicate the perirectal fascia and levator ani muscles over the anterior rectal wall and provide a two-layer closure of this hernia.

**Physiologic Changes.** The anterior rectal wall is reduced to its normal anatomic position and is prevented from prolapsing into the vagina. In severe cases, this prolapse can be of such magnitude that defecation becomes incomplete and difficult.

**Points of Caution.** The preoperative diagnosis should be precise. A rectocele should be differentiated from an enterocele. The surgeon must be careful not to enter the rectum during dissection.

## Technique

**1** The patient is placed in the dorsal lithotomy position. The pelvis and large intestine are prepared for surgery.

A bimanual examination under general anesthesia is performed to differentiate between an enterocele and a rectocele. Observation of the perineal body is made to determine the extent of reconstruction needed.

**2** The labia are retracted with interrupted sutures. The upper extent of the rectocele is identified. Allis clamps are applied to the posterior vaginal mucosa over this area. The clamps are elevated, creating a triangle.

**3** Allis clamps are placed at the margins of the original hymen. An additional Allis clamp is placed in the midline at the top of the rectocele. A transverse incision is made at the posterior fourchette. A Kelly clamp is inserted under the posterior vaginal mucosa, dissecting the posterior vaginal mucosa off the perirectal fascia. An additional incision is made in the perineal body, removing a triangular piece of skin, outlined by the *dotted line*. This will expose the insertion of the bulbocavernosus muscle. Only the skin of the perineal body should be removed, and care should be taken not to remove the underlying superficial transverse perineal muscles.

**4** The vertical incision in the posterior vaginal mucosa has been made, and the edges are held with Allis clamps. The perirectal fascia is dissected off the posterior vaginal mucosa. The apex of the rectocele is held in an Allis clamp. The dissection of perirectal fascia off the vaginal mucosa is started with a scalpel but is completed with the handle of the scalpel or with scissors.

**5** A finger is placed over the rectocele, pushing it into the rectum, thus revealing the margins of the levator ani muscles. A heavy, number 1 synthetic absorbable suture is passed through the margin of the levator ani from the apex down to the posterior fourchette. Frequently, 5–6 sutures are required to completely approximate the levator ani. By depressing the anterior rectal wall downward with one finger and elevating the previously placed suture, the surgeon sees the margin of the levator ani more clearly, and placement of sutures becomes easier.

**6** After all levator ani sutures have been placed, they are progressively tied.

**7** The excessive posterior vaginal mucosa has been trimmed away; the triangular defect in the perineal body can be seen. The insertion of the bulbocavernosus muscle is adjacent to the triangular defect in the perineal body.

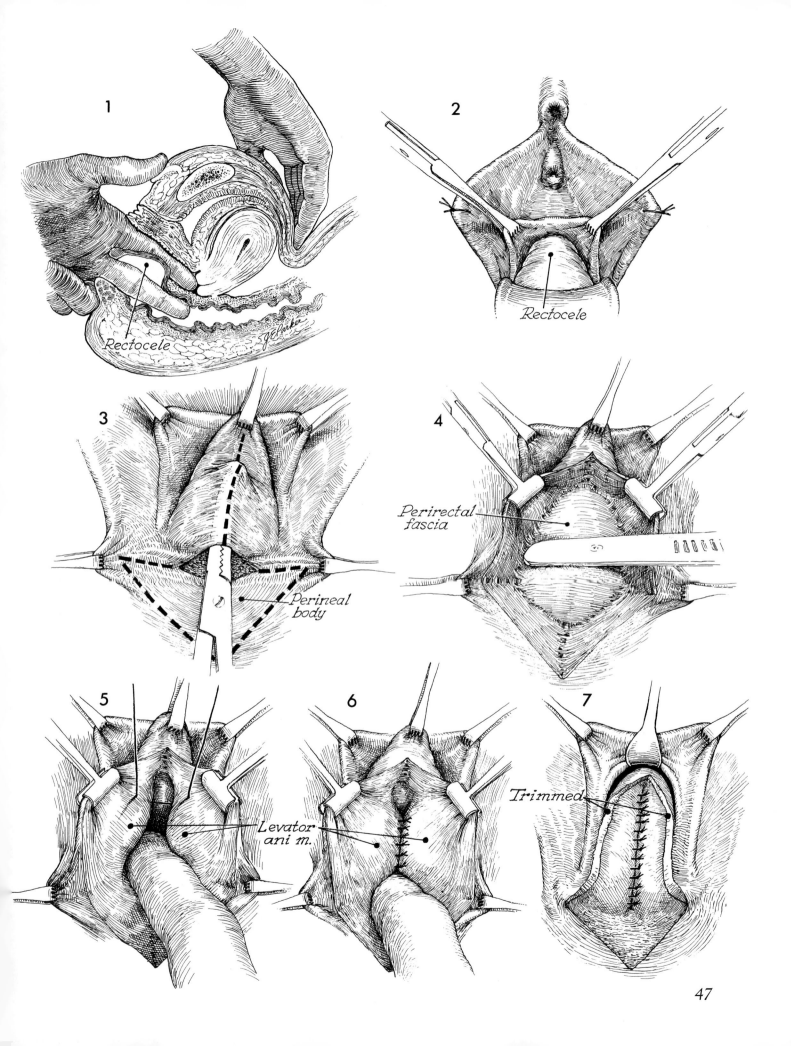

**1**

Rectocele

**2**

Rectocele

**3**

Perineal body

**4**

Perirectal fascia

**5**

Levator ani m.

**6**

Levator ani m.

**7**

Trimmed

47

# Posterior Repair

## (Continued)

**8** The perirectal fascia is closed with interrupted 0 synthetic absorbable suture in the midline.

**9** A 0 synthetic absorbable suture is placed at the apex of the vaginal mucosa and tied (a). The tail of the suture is left for a length of 20 cm. The suture (b) is placed superficial to the tail of the suture (a).

**10** The closure of the posterior vaginal wall is completed to the posterior fourchette. The former hymenal ring is reconstructed. The suture (b) is tied to the tail of the first suture (a) placed at the apex. The vaginal mucosa is approximated to the perirectal fascia to eliminate dead space.

**11** The same suture completes the closure of the peritoneal body. Several interrupted 0 synthetic absorbable sutures are placed in the insertions of the bulbocavernosus muscles to reconstruct the perineal body.

**12** The posterior vaginal mucosa suture (b) is placed in the subcutaneous tissue of the perineal body. Note that the suture marked a is still left long for eventual tying.

**13** The same suture (b) that completed the closure of the posterior vaginal wall is used to close the subcutaneous tissue and the insertions of the bulbocavernosus muscles. The suture marked a is the long end of the tie at the apex of the posterior vaginal mucosa incision.

**14** The subcuticular suture (b) is placed in the skin of the perineal body from the apex of the wound immediately above the anus to the posterior fourchette. At the posterior fourchette it is tied to suture a.

**15** The completed operation is shown, with the rectocele reduced and the perineal body reconstructed. Vaginal packs are not required. Bladder catheterization is rarely indicated.

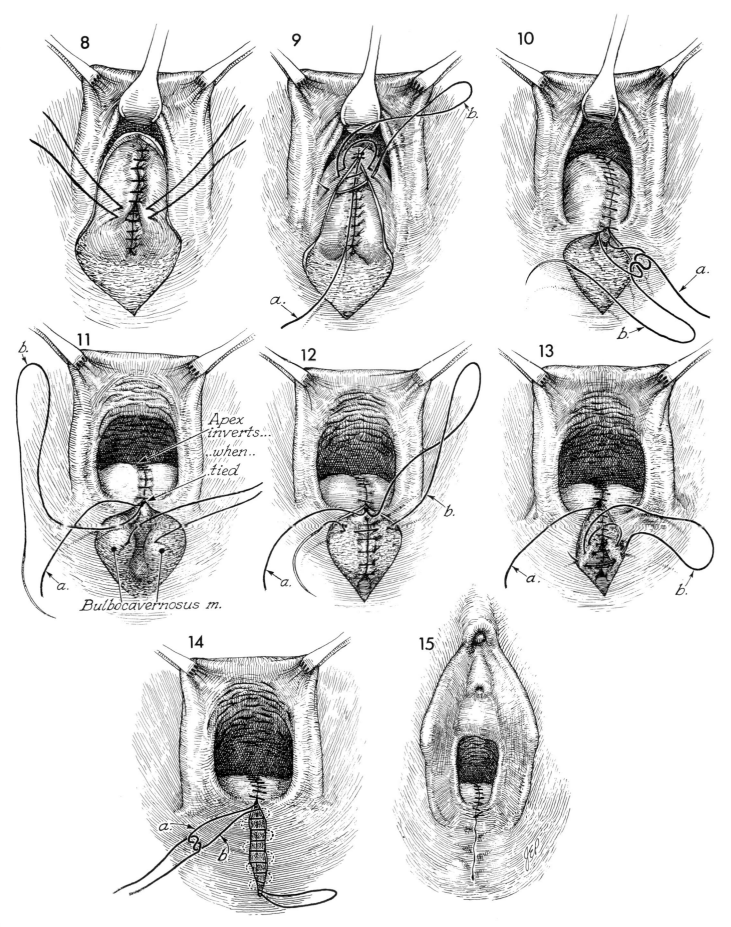

8

9

10

11

*Apex inverts... ..when.. .tied*

*Bulbocavernosus m.*

12

13

14

15

49

# Sacrospinous Ligament Suspension of the Vagina

Sacrospinous ligament suspension of a prolapsed vagina is an ideal procedure for a sexually active woman who has a complete prolapse of the vaginal canal. Prolapse of the vagina can occur following a hysterectomy or can evolve with the uterus in place. If the uterus is still in place, it is best to remove it by vaginal hysterectomy, as shown in Section 5, page 232. The sacrospinous ligament suspension operation has the advantage of retaining an adequate length and width of the vaginal canal.

**Physiologic Changes.** Total prolapse of the vagina may interfere with bladder function, defecation, and sexual intercourse. Some women with total prolapse of the vagina have no evidence of urinary incontinence. There are, however, some women who after correction of the prolapse may experience urinary incontinence unless certain surgical techniques are employed to ensure that the intravesical pressure does not exceed the intraurethral pressure, other than in the act of micturition. After suspension of the prolapsed vagina, rectal function should improve, and the patient should be able to defecate without digital manipulation of the rectum. Comfortable sexual intercourse can be achieved if the vagina is of adequate length and diameter and if the vaginal outlet has not been constricted.

**Points of Caution.** To achieve a safe and permanent sacrospinous ligament suspension of the vagina, there must be appropriate attention to detail. The rectovaginal space must be entered and dissected prior to entering the pararectal space through the vagina. If the lateral extent of the cardinal ligament is inadvertently entered, copious hemorrhage can occur from the hypogastric venous plexus that resides in the upper two-thirds of this area (the web).

The sacrospinous ligament must be visualized and identified. Failure to place sutures directly into the ligament is the most common cause of recurrent prolapse. Care must be taken to avoid the pudendal artery and nerve, since these are immediately posterior and inferior to the ischial spine. The sutures must be placed at least 2 cm medial to the ischial spine to avoid injury to the pudendal nerve, which could result in chronic pain. The type of suture material used must be carefully chosen to avoid recurrence. We prefer a synthetic nylon suture mounted on a small Mayo needle or a Deschamps ligature carrier for placement.

# Sacrospinous Ligament Suspension of the Vagina

## (Continued)

---

*Technique*

**1** The patient is placed in the dorsal lithotomy position and is prepped and draped in the usual manner.

If the patient has not had a hysterectomy, the procedure is started by circumscribing the vaginal mucosa at the junction of the cervix and vagina in the routine manner for starting a vaginal hysterectomy.

**2** A sagittal view of total prolapse of the urethra, bladder, uterus, and rectum is shown. The vaginal hysterectomy is completed at this point according to the technique shown in Section 5, page 232.

**3** A perineal view of total prolapse of the vagina following the vaginal hysterectomy and anterior repair is shown.

**4** The prolapsed vagina is returned to its original position.

**5** The suture line can be seen in the anterior vaginal mucosa following the anterior repair. The posterior vaginal mucosa is opened in the routine fashion as described in Section 2, page 46. A finger is inserted through the incision in the posterior vaginal mucosa, dissecting out the rectovaginal space (*RVS*). The rectal pillars on both sides can be immediately identified. The right rectal pillar (*RRP*) is identified. The rectal pillar can be bluntly perforated either with the finger or with the tip of a long Kelly clamp.

**6** A Breisky-Navratil retractor is ideal for exposing the rectovaginal space in order to enter the pararectal space. The narrow Deaver retractor may also be used, but the curve of the Deaver retractor is less effective than that of the Breisky-Navratil retractors. Adequate retraction of the cardinal ligament, vagina, and rectum is essential for safe operative exposure. Visualization and illumination can be achieved by a bright fiberoptic head lamp focused onto the pararectal space.

**7** With long thin retractors, the surgeon displaces the rectum to the left and the cardinal ligament and ureter anteriorly. A narrow right-angle retractor is used to displace the side walls of the pelvis and perineum. The superior surface of the pelvic diaphragm is exposed. A sponge dissector is used to bluntly dissect the sacrospinous ligament. It is important for the surgeon to remove the areolar tissue from the surface of the right sacrospinous ligament in order to visualize it directly.

The ischial spine should be palpated directly, and a zone approximately 2 cm medial to the spine should be selected for insertion of the suture needle.

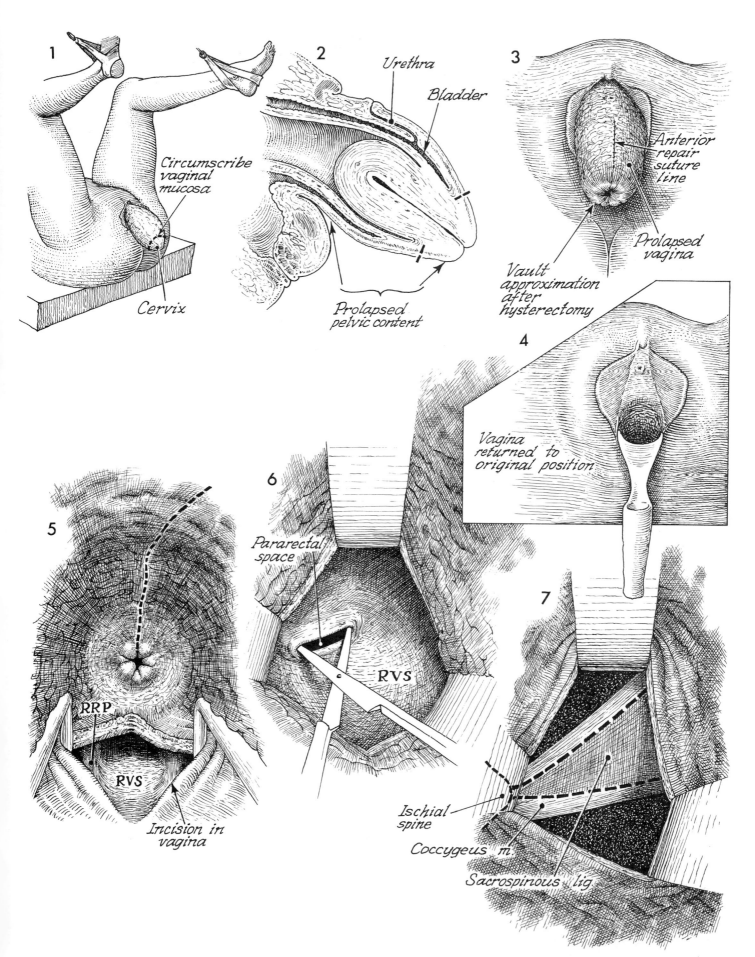

**1**

Circumscribe vaginal mucosa

Cervix

**2**

Urethra

Bladder

Prolapsed pelvic content

**3**

Anterior repair suture line

Prolapsed vagina

Vault approximation after hysterectomy

**4**

Vagina returned to original position

**5**

RRP

RVS

Incision in vagina

**6**

Pararectal space

RVS

**7**

Ischial spine

Coccygeus m.

Sacrospinous lig.

53

# Sacrospinous Ligament Suspension
## of the Vagina
### (Continued)

**8** The Deschamps ligature carrier, loaded with a 0 monofilament nylon suture, can be inserted directly into the ligament. The suture is grasped with a skin hook and held while the Deschamps carrier is removed. If the suture is placed too close to the ischial spine, it may entrap the pudendal nerve.

**9** A second suture is loaded into the Deschamps ligature carrier and passed through the sacrospinous ligament in a similar manner.

**10** One end of the suture previously inserted through the sacrospinous ligament is placed through the muscular layer of the vagina. In a similar manner, the second suture is placed. The opposite end of the suture in the sacrospinous ligament is left free and held on a small hemostat. Traction on this suture will draw the vaginal vault directly to the ligament, where a square knot will promptly affix it to the sacrospinous ligament.

**11** The pulley stitch has been tied, and the ends of the suture have been cut. The safety stitch is then tied.

**12** A posterior colporrhaphy is carried out in the routine fashion, and the vaginal mucosa is closed.

**13** The completed sacrospinous ligament suspension with the apex of the vagina suspended from the sacrospinous ligament approximately 2 cm from the ischial spine is shown.

A Foley catheter is inserted into the bladder and left for a minimum of 4 days. Thereafter, management of bladder function is similar to that following surgery for urinary incontinence. No vaginal packs or drains are used.

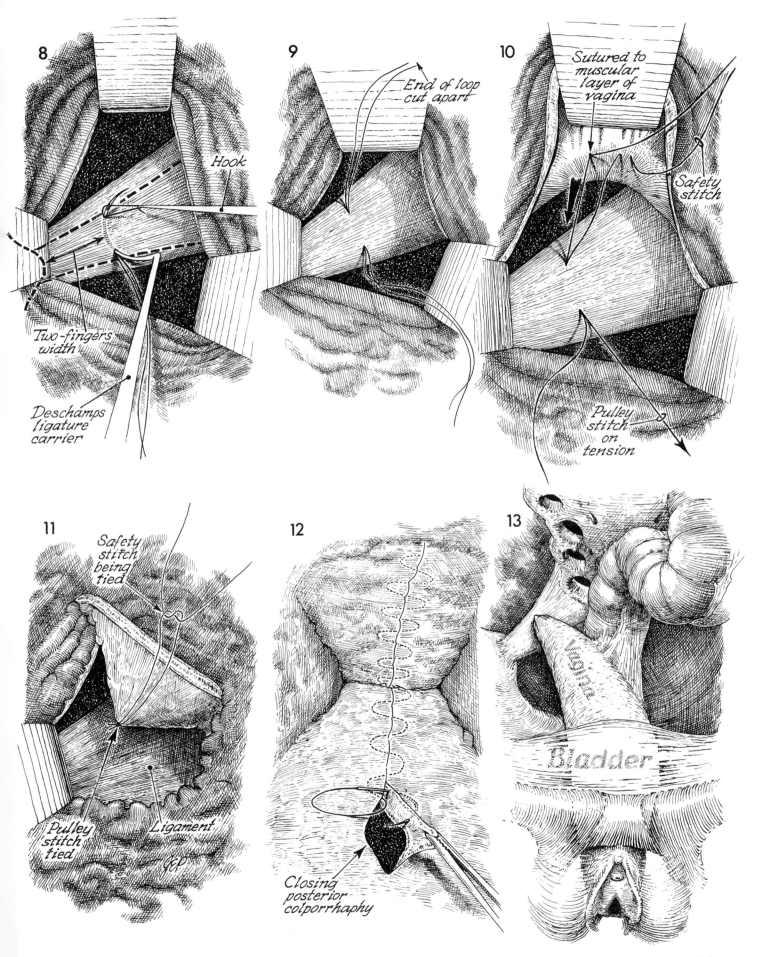

**8**

Hook

Two-fingers width

Deschamps ligature carrier

**9**

End of loop cut apart

**10**

Sutured to muscular layer of vagina

Safety stitch

Pulley stitch on tension

**11**

Safety stitch being tied

Pulley stitch tied

Ligament

**12**

Closing posterior colporrhaphy

**13**

Bladder

# Vaginal Repair of Enterocele

Enterocele is a hernia of the lining of the peritoneal cavity with or without abdominal viscera. The enterocele can occur posteriorly with or without inversion of the vagina. The enterocele should be distinguished from a rectocele, for the procedure for surgical correction is different.

**Physiologic Changes.** Repair of the hernia changes the physiology that produces the pain and possible incarceration of the intestine.

**Points of Caution.** The sac of the enterocele must be entered with care to avoid damage to possible intestinal contents.

The proximity of the ureter to the uterosacral ligaments must be noted, and care must be taken not to include it when approximating the uterosacral ligaments. Finally, care must be taken to depress the rectum so that it is not incorporated into the plication of the levator muscles.

## Technique

1 The patient should be placed in the dorsal lithotomy position and prepped and draped in the usual manner for pelvic surgery. At this point, an accurate diagnosis should be made as to whether the patient has an enterocele alone or an enterocele associated with a rectocele. *STP* identifies the superficial transverse perineal muscle.

2 By excising an edge of perineal body skin at the fourchette, the surgeon carries the triangle up over the posterior fourchette into the posterior vaginal mucosa and converts the triangle to a diamond-shaped defect. The Allis clamps on the vaginal mucosa over the rectocele are elevated by an assistant.

3 The posterior vaginal mucosa is undermined by curved Mayo scissors and opened in the midline. The edges of the vaginal mucosa are grasped with T-clamps and held on traction. It is essential that the assistant create a triangle for the surgeon by elevating the Allis clamps on the posterior vaginal mucosa upward and the T-clamps on the edge of the vaginal mucosa downward. The incision in the posterior vaginal mucosa should be carried up to the vaginal apex and should expose the sac of the enterocele.

4 When the entire posterior vaginal mucosa has been opened, the sac of the enterocele is identified and grasped with an Allis clamp. Blunt dissection is carried out to remove the perirectal fascia from the posterior vaginal mucosa so that the sac of the enterocele can be clearly identified. A small incision is made into the sac.

5 A finger is immediately inserted into the opening of the sac, and the intestinal contents are identified and displaced back into the abdomen. A pursestring suture of 0 synthetic absorbable suture is placed around the neck of the enterocele sac.

6 A second pursestring suture of 0 synthetic absorbable suture is placed around the neck of the enterocele sac.

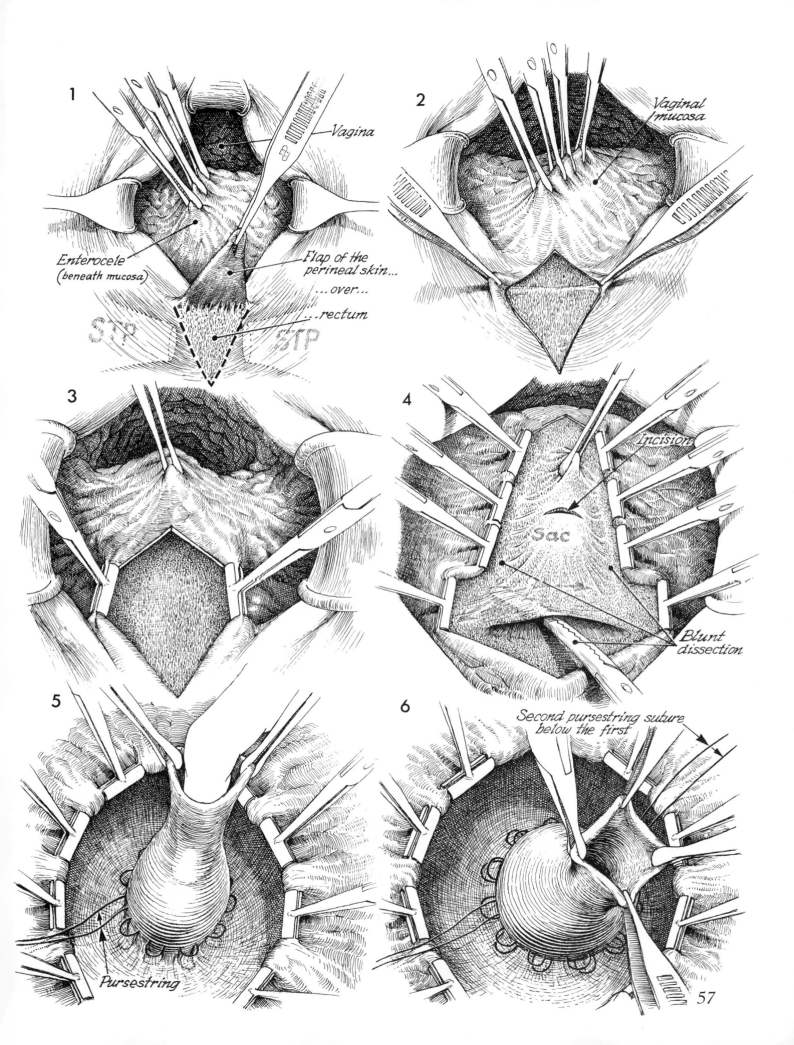

**1**

Vagina

Enterocele
(beneath mucosa)

Flap of the
perineal skin...

...over...

...rectum

STP

STP

**2**

Vaginal
mucosa

**3**

**4**

Incision

Sac

Blunt
dissection

**5**

Pursestring

**6**

Second pursestring suture
below the first

57

# Vaginal Repair of Enterocele

## (Continued)

**7** Before either of these sutures is tied, a finger should again be inserted into the sac to displace any intestinal contents back into the abdomen. The rear pursestring suture should be tied first; then the front pursestring suture should be tied.

**8** High ligation of the sac has been completed, and the sac can now be removed.

**9** The stump of the sac is seen. The uterosacral ligaments and the anterior rectal wall are identified. Three sets of 0 synthetic absorbable sutures should be placed between the anterior rectal wall, the stump of the enterocele sac, and the uterosacral ligaments. Each suture is placed progressively lower in the genital canal than the previous one. Each suture is held on hemostats until all are placed; then each is progressively tied.

**10** Uterosacral ligaments, the stump of the amputated sac of the enterocele, and the anterior rectal wall have all been plicated. The development of any future enterocele is unlikely.

**11** Attention can now be directed toward repair of the rectocele if present. A finger is inserted in the midline, depressing the rectum and exposing the levator muscles. Zero synthetic absorbable sutures should be placed in the levators and held prior to tying. After all sutures have been progressively placed in the levators, they should be tied from the lowest suture in the genital canal, placed first, to the uppermost suture, placed last.

**12** Excessive vaginal mucosa is trimmed away.

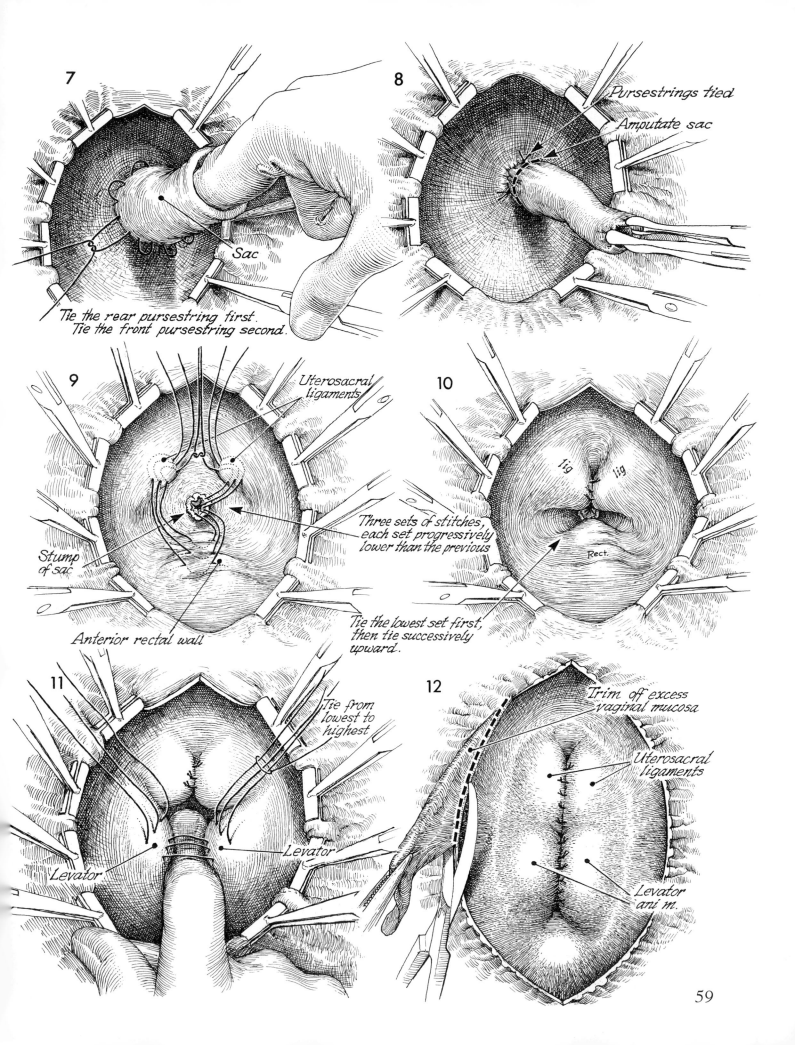

**7**

Sac

Tie the rear pursestring first.
Tie the front pursestring second.

**8**

Pursestrings tied

Amputate sac

**9**

Uterosacral
ligaments

Stump
of sac

Anterior rectal wall

**10**

lig   lig

Rect.

Three sets of stitches,
each set progressively
lower than the previous

Tie the lowest set first,
then tie successively
upward.

**11**

Tie from
lowest to
highest

Levator

Levator

**12**

Trim off excess
vaginal mucosa

Uterosacral
ligaments

Levator
ani m.

# Vaginal Repair of Enterocele

## (Continued)

**13** A 0 synthetic absorbable suture is used in a running fashion to close the posterior vaginal mucosa. Notehow the long end of this suture is left in place from the apex of the closure. Each suture is carefully placed above this suture; care is taken not to entrap the suture with another bite of the running stitch. *STP* identifies the superficial transverse perineal muscle.

**14** The entire posterior vaginal wall down to the hymenal ring has been closed. At this point, the suture is tied. Note that the free end of the original suture placed at the apex remains. By tying the free end of the suture left after the vaginal mucosa has been closed down to the hymenal ring, the surgeon draws the apex of the posterior vaginal mucosa against the levator muscles and eliminates dead space. After tying the running suture in the posterior vaginal mucosa at the hymenal ring, the surgeon inserts the needle behind the hymen into the vagina and brings it out through the insertion of the bulbocavernosus muscle.

At this point, plication of the superficial transverse perineal muscle (*STP*) is made by several interrupted 0 synthetic absorbable sutures. The insertion of the bulbocavernosus muscle is plicated in the midline, incorporating a suture into the superficial transverse perineal muscle to completely reconstruct the perineal body.

**15** The bulbocavernosi muscles are approximated in the midline by the running suture. The skin of the perineal body is approximated by a subcuticular suture.

**16** The reconstructed vaginal vault and perineal body are shown.

**17** A sagittal view shows how the direction of intra-abdominal pressure is now applied to the anterior vaginal wall. Note how the cul-de-sac has been obliterated by the suturing together of the posterior vaginal wall, pelvic peritoneum (*P*), anterior rectal wall, and uterosacral ligaments. This line of pressure is directed away from the genital hiatus in the levator plate, reducing the possibility of recurrent prolapse. *B*, bladder; and *R*, rectum.

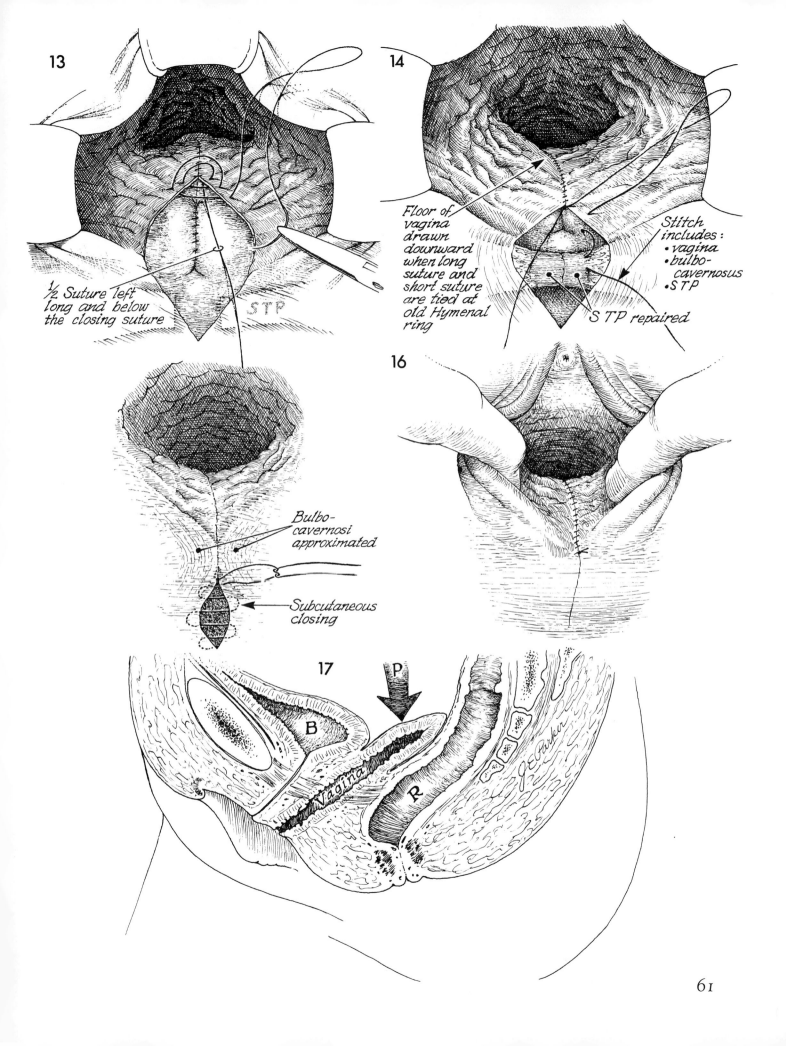

**13**

½ Suture left long and below the closing suture

STP

**14**

Floor of vagina drawn downward when long suture and short suture are tied at old Hymenal ring

Stitch includes:
• vagina
• bulbo-cavernosus
• STP

STP repaired

Bulbo-cavernosi approximated

Subcutaneous closing

**16**

**17**

B

Vagina

P

R

J.E.Parker

# Vaginal Evisceration

Although vaginal evisceration of the intestine is rare and usually follows hysterectomy within the immediate postoperative period, some cases have been reported years after surgery. The problem can arise after abdominal as well as vaginal hysterectomy and also as a sequela of the rupture of large enteroceles, with or without previous hysterectomy.

A contemporary source of vaginal evisceration has been suction curettage for termination of pregnancy. During this procedure, if the uterine wall is perforated, the small intestine can be sucked into the eye of the vacuum curet and pulled through the perforation in the uterus and out into the vagina.

The etiology of vaginal evisceration, except for that associated with suction for termination of pregnancy, is not associated with any specific pattern of events.

**Physiologic Changes.** The anatomy of the small bowel and the length of its mesentery make vaginal evisceration difficult. If a laceration occurs in the mesentery of the small bowel, evisceration is more likely. All patients with vaginal evisceration must undergo an exploratory laparotomy with extensive inspection of the small bowel and its mesentery. Because of the unique blood supply to the small bowel, an undiagnosed laceration in its mesentery may result in necrosis. This may explain why the overall mortality from vaginal evisceration is as high as approximately 10%.

**Points of Caution.** No attempt should be made to simply replace the bowel through the vaginal cuff and close it. All patients should be treated with an abdominoperineal approach. The entire length of the small bowel should be carefully inspected for areas of devascularization.

A classic repair for obliteration of the cul-de-sac through use of the vaginal cuff, the uterosacral ligaments, and the anterior rectal wall should be made to reduce the chance of recurrence.

---

## Technique

**1** A sagittal view of the evisceration is shown. In this particular case, the evisceration has occurred through an open vaginal cuff after a hysterectomy. B identifies the bladder; and R, the rectum. The *insert* to Figure 1 shows the perineal view with the anatomical location of the cecum and other loops of small bowel.

**2** An exploratory laparotomy has been performed, and the loops of the eviscerated small bowel are carefully withdrawn into the peritoneal cavity.

**3** The entire small bowel is carefully inspected from the ileocecal junction to the ligament of Treitz.

In **a** are areas of devascularization and laceration in the mesentery that cause acute loss of blood to the small bowel. In **b,** a potential enterotomy with laceration of the serosa and muscularis is causing the intestinal mucosa to balloon through a crack in the bowel serosa. Contusions and necrosis are depicted in **c.**

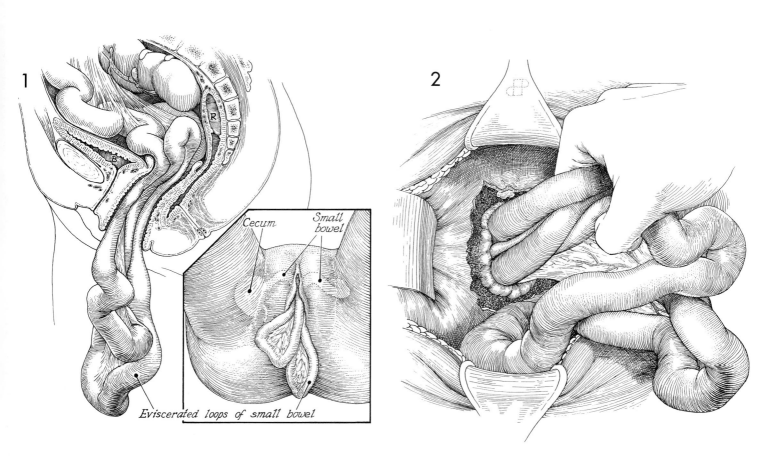

**1**

Cecum

Small bowel

Eviscerated loops of small bowel

**2**

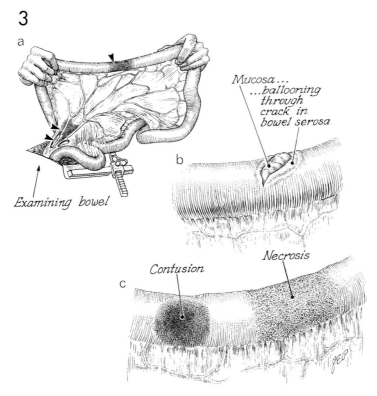

**3**

a

Examining bowel

Mucosa...

...ballooning through crack in bowel serosa

b

Contusion

Necrosis

c

63

# Vaginal Evisceration

## (Continued)

**4** It is wise for the surgeon to resect all areas of contusion, necrosis, and enterotomy and to carefully inspect the vasculature in the small bowel mesentery. Linen-shod clamps are placed in an oblique fashion away from the defect to ensure that the antimesenteric border of the small bowel used in the anastomosis will have an excellent blood supply.

The anastomosis is performed according to the Gambee or stapler technique as indicated in Section 8, page 349. The *insert* shows the mesentery plicated with interrupted absorbable suture.

**5** The opening in the vagina through which the evisceration occurred is shown. After the small bowel has been adequately inspected and cared for, the defect in the pelvis must be repaired. The important structures shown here are the cardinal ligaments, uterosacral ligaments, anterior rectum, and vagina. The cardinal ligaments should be reapproximated to the angles of the vagina. The vaginal defect itself should be closed with 0 synthetic absorbable suture.

The cul-de-sac should be obliterated by several 0 synthetic absorbable sutures placed in the posterior vaginal wall through the uterosacral ligaments, the anterior wall of the rectum, the uterosacral ligament on the opposite side, and back to the posterior vaginal wall. After all of these sutures have been placed, they should be progressively tied from the deepest to the most superficial.

The pelvic peritoneum should be reconstructed. If there has been any contamination from intestinal contents, a suction drain should be placed in the pelvis.

**4**

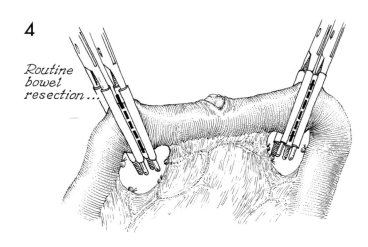

*Routine bowel resection...*

*...and reanastomosis*

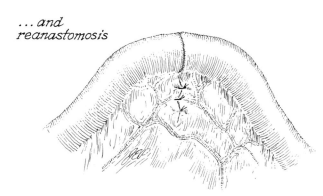

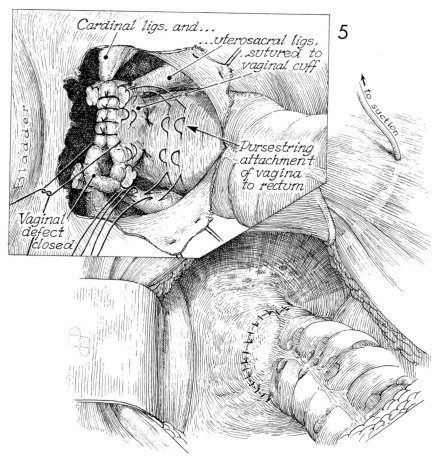

**5**

Cardinal ligs. and...

...uterosacral ligs. ...sutured to vaginal cuff

Bladder

Pursestring attachment of vagina to rectum

Vaginal defect closed

to suction

# Excision of Transverse Vaginal Septum

Transverse vaginal septum generally occurs between the upper one-third and lower two-thirds of the vaginal canal. This is additional evidence that the upper one-third of the vagina is of Müllerian origin and that the lower two-thirds of the vagina is embryologically developed via the urogenital sinus.

The septum can be either complete or partial. If it is complete, the symptoms of vaginal obstruction occur at the time of menarche, since menstrual blood is entrapped above the septum and has no egress from the vagina. If the septum is partial, it may be discovered on a routine gynecologic examination, or the patient may present with dyspareunia.

The operation is performed to remove the transverse vaginal septum without significantly shortening the vaginal canal.

**Physiologic Changes.** The physiologic changes desired are (1) the egress of menstrual blood from the vaginal canal without obstruction and (2) the normal functioning of the vagina.

**Points of Caution.** If the septum is complete and hematometra or hematocolpos is present, it is unwise to attempt surgical correction of the septum at the time the obstruction is relieved. The procedure of choice is incision and drainage of the hematometra or hematocolpos, with reconstruction delayed 6–8 weeks until the tissues have completely healed.

To avoid unduly shortening the vagina, excessive vaginal mucosa should not be removed.

---

## Technique

**1** The typical position of most transverse vaginal septa at the junction of the upper one-third and the lower two-thirds of the vagina is shown. B, bladder.

**2** With the patient in the dorsal lithotomy position, the perineum is prepped and draped, and adequate vaginal retraction is applied to allow exposure of the septum, which is incomplete here. Initially, the septum is grasped with Allis clamps, and a vertical incision is made through the septum to divide it in half.

**3** The septum is picked up with tissue forceps, traction is applied, and with a scalpel the septum is separated from the vaginal mucosa.

**4** The vaginal mucosa is then approximated with interrupted 3-0 synthetic absorbable suture throughout its circumference.

**5** A sagittal view illustrates closure of the defect in the vaginal mucosa.

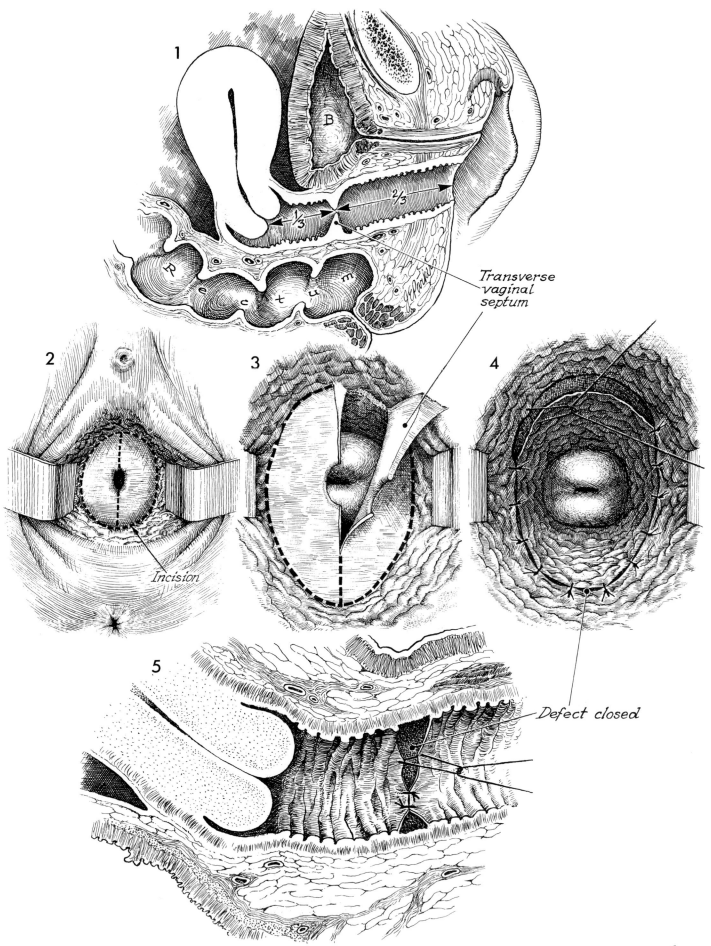

**1**

B

2/3  1/3

R e c t u m

*Transverse vaginal septum*

**2**

*Incision*

**3**

**4**

*Defect closed*

**5**

67

# Correction of Double-Barreled Vagina

The Müllerian ducts are said to account for the upper one-third of the vagina. Their failure to fuse can leave the vaginal canal with a longitudinal horizontal septum that may extend from the upper vagina as far as the vaginal outlet. This condition, known as a "double-barreled vagina," is frequently unnoticed by the patient until an initial gynecologic examination or delivery of the first baby. It requires the surgeon to perform an appropriate workup for failure of the other structures derived from the Müllerian ducts, such as the cervix and the uterus. In addition, some patients with Müllerian duct abnormalities have concomitant urinary tract abnormalities and, therefore, an intravenous pyelogram (IVP) may be indicated. The best procedure for correcting the longitudinal septum is excision.

The purpose of the operation is to create a single-barreled vagina and, at the same time, avoid dyspareunia.

**Physiologic Changes.** A normal vagina is created.

**Points of Caution.** In creating a single-barreled vagina, the surgeon must be careful not to remove excessive vaginal mucosa.

## Technique

**1** The longitudinal septum is demonstrated in this cutaway section of the vagina.

**2** With the patient in the dorsal lithotomy position, the vulva and vagina are prepped, the patient is draped, and the bladder is emptied by catheterization. Adequate exposure to each vaginal canal is made by lateral retractors. The longitudinal septum is grasped with a clamp or tissue forceps, and slight traction is applied. Extreme traction should be avoided in order not to tent the underlying urethra and bladder tissue into the area to be excised. The junction of the longitudinal septum and vaginal mucosa should be excised with scissors. The same procedure is carried out at the junction of the longitudinal septum on the posterior vaginal wall. A defect is made in the anterior and posterior vaginal walls that should extend no deeper than the pubovesical cervical fascia anteriorly and the perirectal fascia posteriorly.

**3** Primary repair can be carried out by closing the defect with interrupted 2-0 synthetic absorbable suture.

**4** The same technique is used to repair the posterior vaginal wall.

**5** The repair is completed. No vaginal pack is left in the vagina, and no catheter is needed for drainage of the bladder. The patient can usually be discharged within 1–2 days after the operation and can resume sexual intercourse 1 month after closure of the vaginal incision.

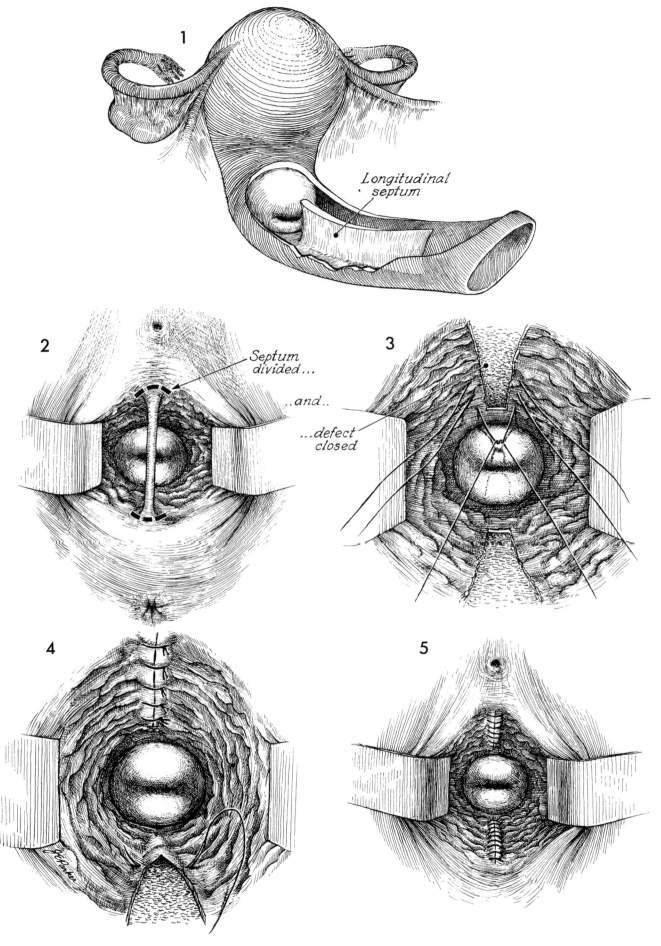

1

Longitudinal septum

2

Septum divided...

..and..

...defect closed

3

4

5

69

# Incision and Drainage of Pelvic Abscess via the Vaginal Route

A pelvic abscess can be drained through the vagina if three conditions are present. The abscess must (1) be fluctuant, (2) dissect the rectovaginal septum, and (3) be in the midline. If any of these three criteria is absent, complications are increased significantly. If the abscess is not fluctuant, adequate drainage cannot be achieved. If the abscess has not dissected the rectovaginal septum, the vaginal incision may enter the rectum. If the abscess is not in the midline, incision and drainage will result in peritoneal spread of purulent material.

The purpose of the operation is to drain the abscess and thereby allow reversal of the septic process.

**Physiologic Changes.** The physiologic changes associated with incision and drainage of any abscess are release of the purulent material to the outside and relief of the septic condition associated with the abscess.

**Points of Caution.** In addition to the above-mentioned criteria essential for drainage, the abscess must remain open 4–6 days to allow complete drainage and granulation of the abscess cavity.

## Technique

**1** The patient is placed in the dorsal lithotomy position and is prepped and draped.

**2** A sagittal view illustrates one of the three criteria necessary for drainage, i.e., dissection of the rectovaginal septum by the abscess. *B*, bladder; *R*, rectum; and *V*, vagina.

**3** The posterior lip of the cervix is grasped with a Jacobs tenaculum, and traction is applied. A scalpel is used to incise the vaginal mucosa.

**4** With the posterior lip of the cervix under traction, a Kelly clamp is used to puncture the abscess, allowing the egress of pus.

**5** A finger is inserted into the abscess cavity to break up adhesions and drain any additional small loculated abscesses.

**6 & 7** A convenient drain for pelvic abscess is a T-tube. We prefer a 16-French size, with the arm of the T cut off approximately 3 cm from the shaft of the tube. In addition, small holes are made along the arms of the T. The arms of the T are then folded back on the shaft of the tube, which is grasped with a Kelly clamp and inserted up into the pelvic abscess. When the Kelly clamp is removed, the arms of the T return to their original position, thereby holding the drain in place.

**8** A sagittal section shows the drain in place in the pelvic abscess. Suction on the T-tube is not necessary and may inadvertently result in its removal. The shaft of the T-tube should be trimmed behind the introitus so that it does not protrude through the labia minora and hymenal ring.

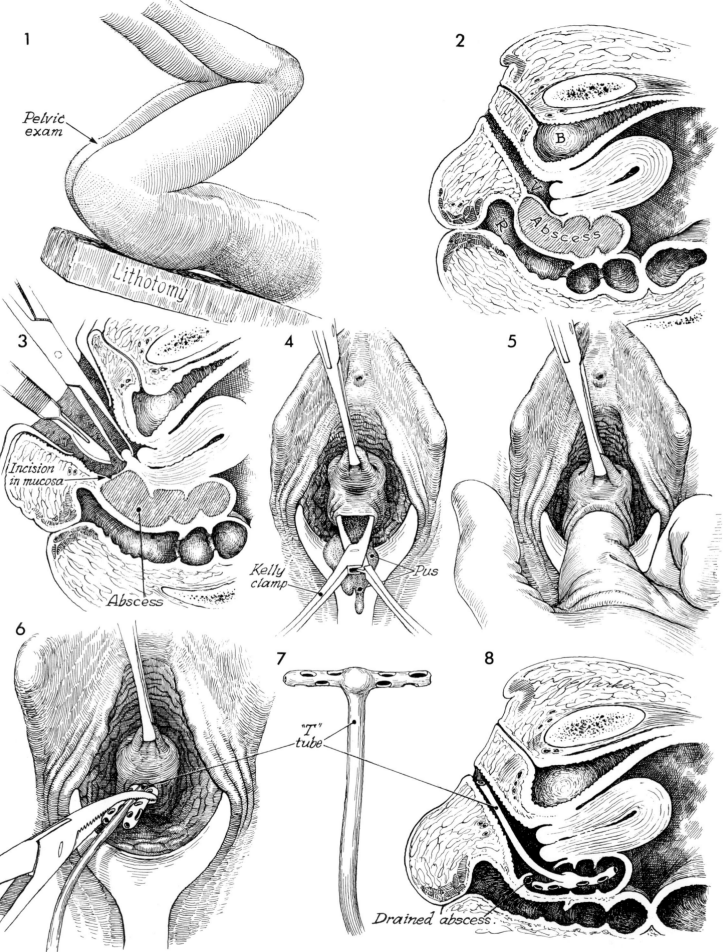

1

*Pelvic exam*

*Lithotomy*

2

B

V

R

*Abscess*

3

*Incision in mucosa*

*Abscess*

4

*Kelly clamp*

*Pus*

5

6

7

*"T" tube*

8

J. F. Parker

*Drained abscess.*

71

# Sacral Colpopexy

Sacral colpopexy is a surgical procedure designed for correction of prolapse of the vagina. It is an ideal procedure for those women who are sexually active but who have total prolapse of the vaginal canal. Prolapse of the vagina can occur following a hysterectomy or with the uterus in place. If the uterus is still in place and the patient is menopausal, it is best to remove it by a hysterectomy (Section 5, page 235) prior to performing sacral colpopexy, unless there are compelling reasons to leave it in situ. Sacral colpopexy is an alternative procedure to sacrospinous ligament suspension of the vagina (see Section 2, page 51). In some clinics, sacral colpopexy is reserved for those patients who have recurrent prolapse following sacrospinous ligament suspension of the vagina, since sacral colpopexy involves a pelvic laparotomy, whereas the sacrospinous ligament suspension of the vagina can be performed through the vagina. To date, there are no prospective, randomized studies showing that one procedure is more efficacious the other. Both procedures have their advocates.

The strap material used in the sacral colpopexy varies. There are some who prefer synthetic permanent mesh material made from Prolene (Marlex and Mersilene). We prefer the patient's own fascia. Our preference for the patient's own fascia (rectus fascia or fascia lata) stems from our desire to avoid the sequelae of putting a foreign body into or around the bacteria-contaminated vagina. The additional effort to obtain fascia lata or rectus fascia is small compared to the long-term sequelae of an infected foreign body.

**Physiologic Changes.** Vaginal prolapse is an incapacitating and debilitating problem for women. The exposed vaginal mucosa can become ulcerated with associated bleeding and infections.

Replacing the vagina back into the pelvis in its proper anatomical configuration is important. The normal vagina is shaped somewhat like a backward hockey stick. The upper one-half to one-third of the vagina should tilt posteriorly back upon the rectum. If the surgeon creates a situation for the apex of the vagina to be in the midplane of the pelvis, intra-abdominal pressure will produce recurrent prolapse.

**Points of Caution.** Sacral colpopexy is not a difficult operation to perform. Several points need to be emphasized, however, if the procedure is to be done successfully.

First, after entering the abdomen, identification of the right ureter is vital. It should be mobilized and retracted laterally. The rectosigmoid colon should also be mobilized and retracted laterally.

The vascular plexus on the periosteum of the sacrum can be associated with copious bleeding if it is not properly managed.

The material used for the strap (natural fascia or synthetic mesh) should be of the proper length and width to support the apex of the vagina. The strap must be retroperitonealized and not cross the pelvis like a "clothesline." Such a situation is an invitation to internal herniation and incarceration of the small bowel, leading to obstruction and necrosis.

# Sacral Colpopexy

## (Continued)

*Technique*

**1** For the surgeon to harvest the fascia lata, the patient is placed in the lateral decubitus position with flexion of both the hips and knees at approximately 60°. A pillow should be placed between the knees to abduct the thigh until it is level. Two large pieces of tape are used to stabilize the patient and prevent her from moving to either side. The lateral thigh is prepped and draped. The *solid line* marks the site of the initial incision, and the *dotted line* marks the direction of the tunneled Masson fascia stripper.

**2** The Masson fascia stripper consists of two hollow metal tubes—one inside, one outside. The inner tube has a narrow opening,"the eye," near one end; the edge of the outer tube is sharpened to allow cutting of the fascia strip at the desired level.

**3** The incision is open; the base of the fascia strap is started by hand with a scalpel. The handle of the scalpel is used to perform blunt dissection of the fascia strap off its bed. The finger is used to tunnel underneath the subcutaneous fat on top of the fascia. The base of the strap should be 4 cm wide. At least 6 cm of the strap should be taken by the knife before applying the Masson stripper.

**4** The Masson fascia stripper is moved into position. The strap that has been formed by sharp dissection is placed through the opening of the fascia stripper. Two straight Kocher clamps are placed across the strap, and a suture is placed adjacent to the Kocher clamps as a safety suture to retrieve the strap if it breaks and retracts up the thigh.

**5** The surgeon retracts the Kocher clamps caudally as the Masson fascia stripper is advanced cephalad. A point is reached where the Masson fascia stripper will advance no farther. At that point the surgeon unscrews the handle of the Masson fascia stripper and evulses the strap. The strap is brought out through the leg wound.

**6** The fascia strap is shown. The suture at the end of the strap is removed.

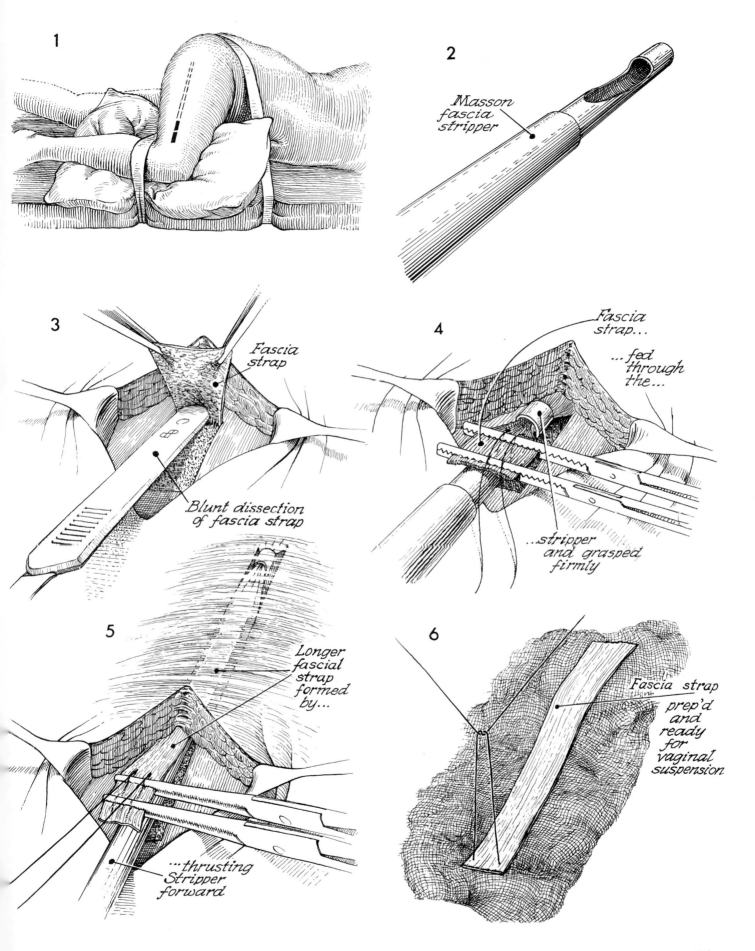

**1**

**2**

Masson
fascia
stripper

**3**

Fascia
strap

Blunt dissection
of fascia strap

**4**

Fascia
strap...

...fed
through
the...

...stripper
and grasped
firmly

**5**

Longer
fascial
strap
formed
by...

...thrusting
Stripper
forward

**6**

Fascia strap
prep'd
and
ready
for
vaginal
suspension

# Sacral Colpopexy
## (Continued)

**7** The patient is changed to the dorsal lithotomy position. The prolapsed vagina is noted. Two Allis clamps are placed on the vaginal apex. If a hysterectomy has previously been performed, the suture line will be noted in the vaginal apex.

**8** A midline incision—Pfannenstiel or midline—is made. The peritoneal cavity is entered.

**9** After packing the bowel away with moist gauze, the surgeon identifies the right ureter and the rectosigmoid colon. An incision is made in the posterior peritoneum from the sacral promontory (*P*). This incision is carried down over the cul-de-sac and the vaginal apex. The vagina is replaced into the abdominal cavity by either a 4-cm obturator or a sponge stick held in an ovum forceps.

**10 & 11** The fascia strap is sutured to the periosteum of the sacrum. Sutures should be placed into the periosteum of the sacrum and then brought through the fascia as shown here. Three to four

sutures are placed. The distal end of the strap is sutured to the apex of the vagina. Three sutures are placed in the anterior vaginal wall with interrupted synthetic permanent sutures. The strap is placed over the dome of the vagina, and additional sutures are applied if needed. The cul-de-sac is obliterated by suturing the uterosacral ligaments in the midline.

**12** The peritoneum is sutured over the strap to reperitonealize the pelvis and prevent the "clothesline" effect.

**13** A sagittal view shows the suspension covered by the peritoneum. The strap is sutured to the periosteum of the sacrum and ultimately over the dome of the vaginal apex. The vagina should lie posteriorly over the rectosigmoid colon.

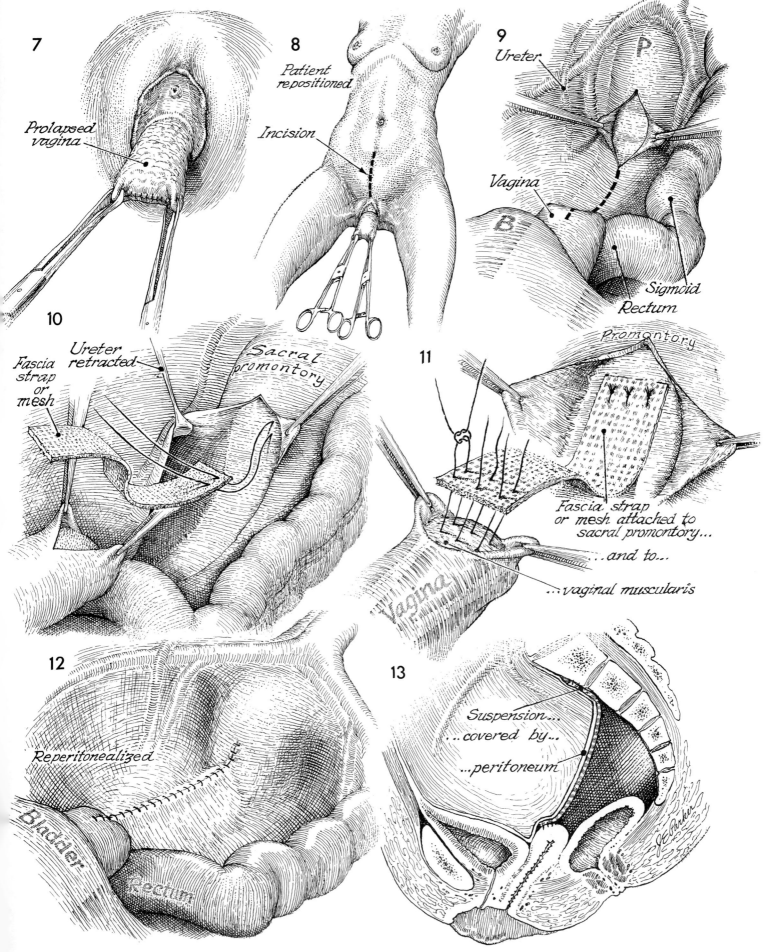

**7**

Prolapsed vagina

**8**

Patient repositioned

Incision

**9**

Ureter

Vagina

P

B

Sigmoid

Rectum

**10**

Fascia strap or mesh

Ureter retracted

Sacral promontory

**11**

Promontory

Fascia strap or mesh attached to sacral promontory...

...and to...

...vaginal muscularis

Vagina

**12**

Reperitonealized

Bladder

Rectum

**13**

Suspension...

...covered by...

...peritoneum

J.E.Parker

# Le Fort Operation

The Le Fort operation is an excellent procedure for complete prolapse in elderly women who have had adequate sexual counseling and who under no circumstances expect to have intercourse in the future. Failure or recurrent prolapse after the procedure is extremely rare. If the procedure removes excessive anterior vaginal wall, however, the urethrovesical angle may be brought down to the posterior fourchette, and some patients will have either stress or overflow incontinence of urine. To avoid this problem, we have modified the operation to include the upper two-thirds of the vagina but not the lower third of the anterior vaginal wall. Although a slight urethrocele may remain, this generally causes no discomfort to the patient and at the same time reduces the incidence of postoperative urinary incontinence.

**Physiologic Changes.** The vagina is obliterated except for two small drainage canals on the lateral side for discharge of vaginal mucus. Sexual intercourse is not possible after this operation.

**Points of Caution.** Possible pitfalls of the procedure include (1) failure to adequately dissect the anterior vaginal mucosa off the pubovesical cervical fascia and inadvertently entering the bladder or (2) penetrating the perirectal fascia and entering the rectum. Care must be exercised in placing the sutures in the pubovesical cervical fascia anteriorly and the perirectal fascia posteriorly in order not to penetrate the bladder or rectum.

## Technique

**1** The patient is placed in the dorsal lithotomy position and carefully examined under anesthesia. The vulva and perineum are prepped and draped.

**2** The labia are anchored laterally with interrupted 2-0 synthetic absorbable suture.

**3** The cervix is grasped with a Jacobs tenaculum and prolapsed from the vagina. A brilliant green marking pen is used to outline the area of the anterior vaginal mucosa that is to be undermined and removed.

**4** In a similar manner, a brilliant green marking pen is used to outline the posterior vaginal mucosa.

**5** With a scalpel, the posterior vaginal mucosa is incised transversely at its junction with the cervix.

**6** The blades of curved Mayo scissors are inserted underneath the posterior vaginal mucosa and on top of the perirectal fascia, and the vaginal mucosa is freed to the lateral margins of the marked area.

**7** The posterior vaginal mucosa is then cut along the prescribed marking lines with curved Mayo scissors and removed.

**8** A similar transverse incision is made in the anterior vaginal mucosa at its junction with the cervix. The blades of curved Mayo scissors are inserted underneath the anterior vaginal mucosa to dissect laterally and upward toward the urethral meatus until the limits of the marked area are reached. This procedure is facilitated if traction is held on the Jacobs tenaculum.

**9** The anterior vaginal mucosa is removed from the underlying pubovesical cervical fascia.

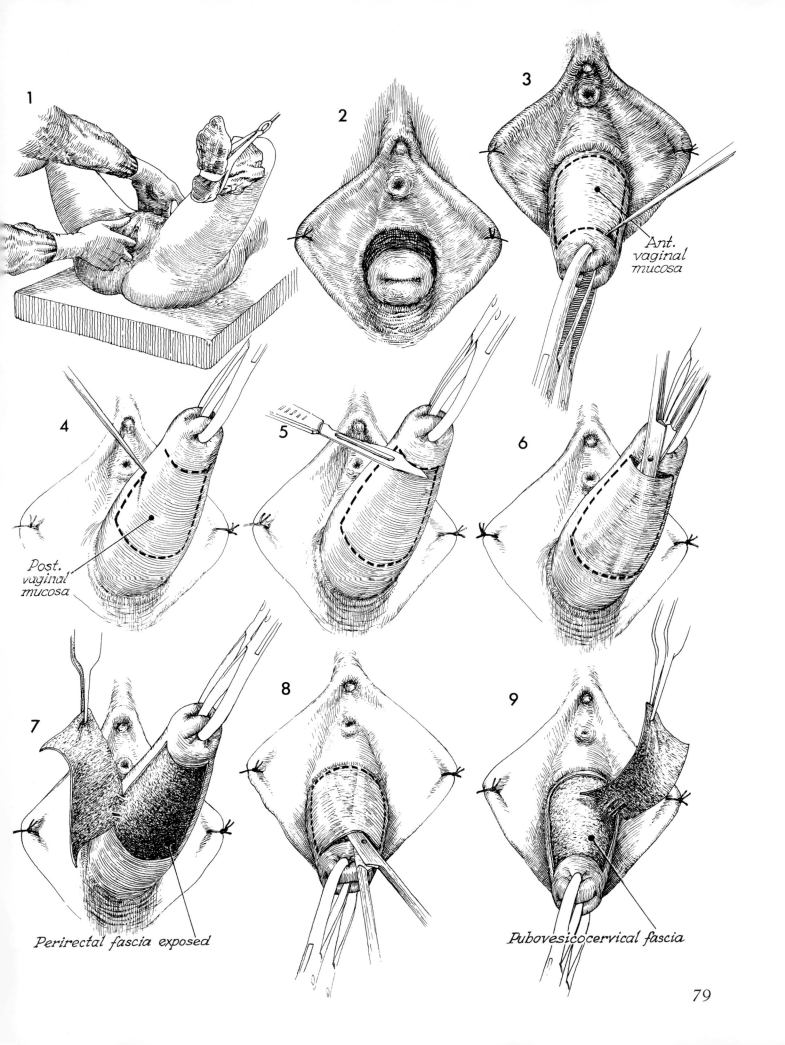

**1**

**2**

**3**

Ant.
vaginal
mucosa

**4**

Post.
vaginal
mucosa

**5**

**6**

**7**

Perirectal fascia exposed

**8**

**9**

Pubovesicocervical fascia

79

# Le Fort Operation

## (Continued)

---

**10** The surgeon progressively approximates the pubovesical cervical fascia anteriorly and the perirectal fascia posteriorly with Lembert inverting sutures.

**11** When this suture is tied, a tunnel is created along each lateral margin for drainage of cervical mucus, thereby preventing the formation of a mucocele. The cross section underneath Figure 11 demonstrates how this tunnel is formed.

**12** Several sutures are placed in a similar manner to complete the tunnel.

**13** Lembert 0 absorbable sutures are placed from the pubovesical cervical fascia anteriorly to the perirectal fascia posteriorly over the portio of the cervix.

**14** After several of these sutures have been placed, the surgeon inverts the portio of the cervix.

**15** After several rows of sutures have been completed, the cervix is totally inverted, and the pubovesical cervical fascia anteriorly and the perirectal fascia posteriorly are plicated.

**16** A final row of 0 synthetic absorbable sutures is placed between the remaining vaginal mucosa anteriorly and posteriorly. Note that a small wire probe can be inserted into the tunnel laterally on each side.

**17** The vaginal mucosal sutures are completed. Note that the urethra and the urethrovesical angle are not included in the procedure and are not sutured to the posterior fourchette. Such a procedure would distort the urethrovesical angle and in many cases lead to postoperative urinary incontinence.

**18** Although the finished operation leaves the patient with a slight urethrocele or bulge, the surgeon should make no attempt to close off the entire vagina.

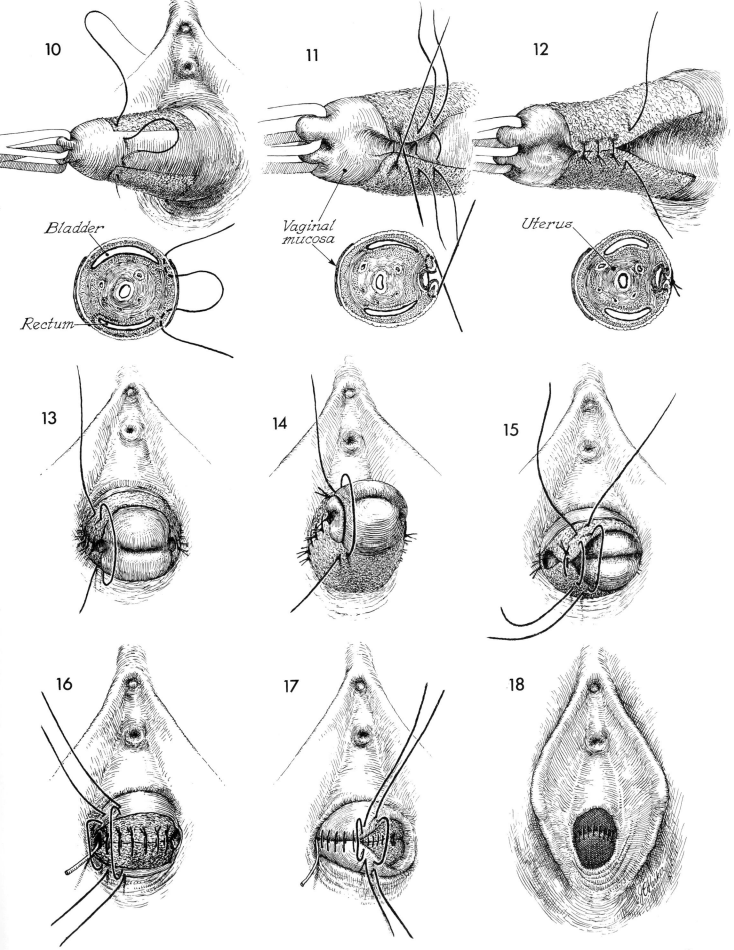

10

Bladder

Rectum

11

Vaginal
mucosa

12

Uterus

13

14

15

16

17

18

# Vesicovaginal Fistula Repair

Vesicovaginal fistulae are usually secondary to obstetrical trauma, pelvic surgery, advanced pelvic cancer, or radiation therapy for treatment of pelvic cancer.

The basic principles for treatment of vesicovaginal fistulae have changed little since the mid-19th century work of Marion Sims. The principles are (1) to ensure that there is no cellulitis, edema, or infection at the fistula site prior to closing the fistula and (2) to excise avascular scar tissue and approximate the various layers of tissue broadside to broadside without tension. A 20th century addition to these principles is that of using a transplanted blood supply from the vestibular fat pad, bulbocavernosus muscle, gracilis muscle, or the omentum.

The type of suture used appears less significant when the above principles are followed. In general, we have used the glycolic acid sutures such as Dexon or Vicryl because of their reabsorption and reduced tissue reaction. Many surgeons prefer, however, to use a nonabsorbable monofilament suture of nylon or Prolene on the vaginal mucosa. These sutures should not be placed into the bladder mucosa. If they are left in the bladder for long periods of time, urinary stone formation will occur.

The purpose of the operation is to close the vesicovaginal fistula permanently without encroaching on the ureter or the urethral orifices.

**Physiologic Changes.** The fistula is closed, and resumption of micturition via the urethra resumes.

**Points of Caution.** Adequate blood supply to the tissue surrounding the fistula must be provided. Excision of scar tissue is vital to closure. Recently, tissue transplants have been used to bring in an external blood supply to the fistula site. This is a vital point when the fistula is secondary to radiation therapy. In addition, when the fistula is secondary to radiation therapy, we have performed a temporary urinary diversion by ileal loop. This has dramatically improved our ability to permanently close radiation fistulae. At a subsequent operation, the ileal loop can be reimplanted in the dome of the bladder after the fistula has been closed and bladder function is adequate.

In all fistulae, the principle of dual drainage is vital for proper closure. A transurethral as well as a suprapubic Foley catheter is left in place until the fistula has closed. Generally, the transurethral catheter is removed after 2 weeks, but the suprapubic catheter is left in place for at least 3 weeks. Acidification of the urine with ascorbic acid or cranberry juice is helpful in reducing urinary tract infection. Frequent urine culture and appropriate antibiotic therapy are indicated, however.

If an alkaline urine is present with a vesicovaginal fistula, the urine will precipitate triple-sulfate crystals and deposit them on the opening of the vagina.

These are quite painful and must be completely removed prior to closure.

# Vesicovaginal Fistula Repair

## (Continued)

## Technique

**1** For vesicovaginal fistula closure the patient is placed in the dorsal lithotomy position. The vulva and vagina are prepped and draped.

**2** Adequate exposure of the fistula must be made. Many unsuccessful fistula closures have resulted from the failure to achieve adequate exposure of the fistula site, poor placement of the sutures, and closure of the fistula under tension. A large mediolateral episiotomy is frequently required and should be carried up to the area of the fistula.

**3** With adequate exposure the fistula tract can be excised with a scalpel. The incision is carried around the circumference of the fistula.

**4** The margin of the fistula tract is elevated with thumb forceps and excised with Metzenbaum scissors. The entire tract is dissected. Frequently, when dense scar tissue has been released, the fistula will be 2–3 times larger than noted preoperatively.

**5** The layers of the bladder wall and vagina should be adequately delineated, and each of these layers should be mobilized to allow the layers to be drawn together with fine sutures without tension.

**6** The bladder mucosa is identified and closed with interrupted 4-0 synthetic absorbable suture. An attempt should be made to keep the suture in the submucosal layer. We do not perform running locking sutures or continuous suture, since we feel this reduces the blood supply that is vital to proper closure.

**7** A second layer, the bladder muscle, is closed with 2-0 synthetic absorbable suture.

**8** The bladder muscle is completely closed over the fistula area with interrupted 2-0 synthetic absorbable suture.

**9** At this point, it is necessary in high-risk cases to seek an external blood supply for the fistula site. This can be the bulbocavernosus muscle from beneath the labia majora, or in cases where a large fistula exists or where the fistula is high in the vaginal canal, the gracilis muscle from the leg or the recrtus abdominis muscle can be brought in to cover the fistula site.

If the bulbocavernosus is selected, two incision sites are acceptable. One is on the inside of the labia minora as seen in Figure 9. The other is down the body of the labia majora. If the latter incision is selected, the bulbocavernosus muscle must be tunneled under the labia minora into the episiotomy wound.

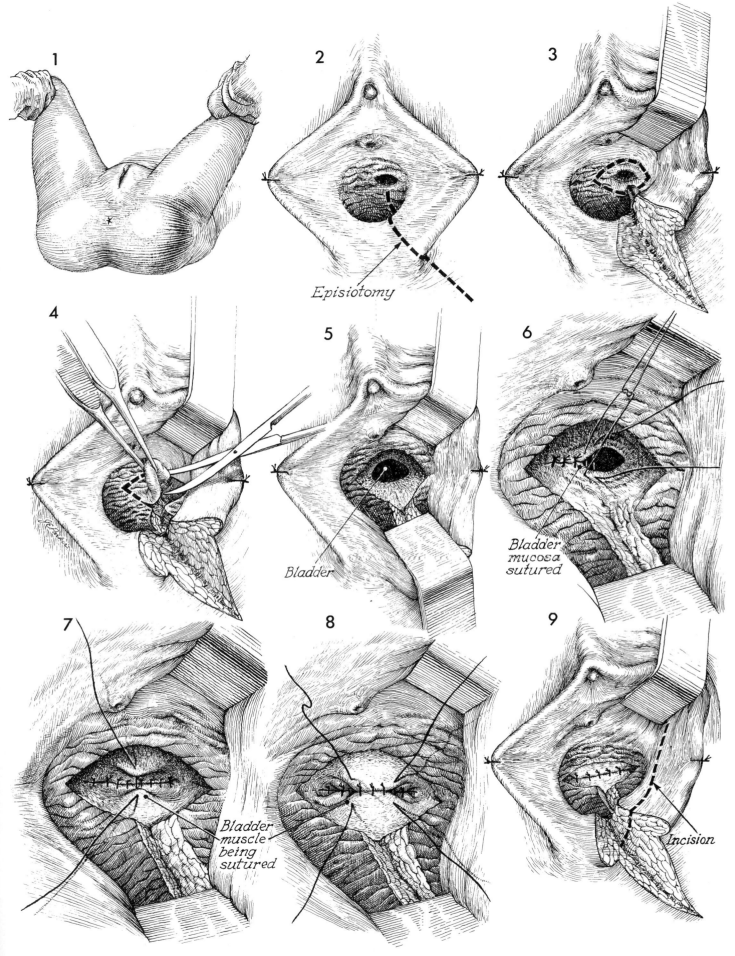

1

2

**Episiotomy**

3

4

5

**Bladder**

6

**Bladder mucosa sutured**

7

8

**Bladder muscle being sutured**

9

**Incision**

85

# Vesicovaginal Fistula Repair

## (Continued)

**10** Allis clamps are used for retraction of the labia, and a scalpel is used for dissection down to the bulbocavernosus muscle. It is important to enlarge the incision so that the entire muscle can be visualized.

**11** The bulbocavernosus muscle is identified and mobilized. Frequently, at the level indicated here, the branches of the pudendal artery and vein enter the muscle and may have to be clamped and ligated for hemostasis. The bulbocavernosus muscle should be mobilized by blunt and sharp dissection up to the level of the clitoris and transected at its insertion in the perineal body.

**12** If the initial incision has been made on the inside of the labia minora, no tunneling of the bulbocavernosus muscle is needed, and the muscle is swung into position, covering the fistula site. It is sutured to the perivesical tissue with interrupted 3-0 synthetic absorbable sutures. If the initial incision has been carried over the labia majora, a tunnel is created with a Kelly clamp under the labia minora into the episiotomy incision. The bulbocavernosus muscle is pulled through this tunnel, applied to the fistula site, and sutured into place with interrupted 3-0 synthetic absorbable suture.

**13** The vaginal mucosa must be mobilized for closure without tension. Generally, the wound is closed with interrupted 0 synthetic absorbable suture.

**14** The vaginal incision, the episiotomy incision, and the incision for the bulbocavernosus muscle transplant are closed.

**15** A Foley catheter is inserted through the urethra. The bladder is generally filled with approximately 200 mL of methylene blue or sterile milk solution to ascertain if the fistula is completely closed. We frequently perform this same procedure after Steps 7 and 8 to demonstrate complete closure of the fistula site.

In addition to the transurethral Foley catheter, a suprapubic Foley catheter is placed as demonstrated in Section 3, page 136. Dual drainage for the fistula closure is vital.

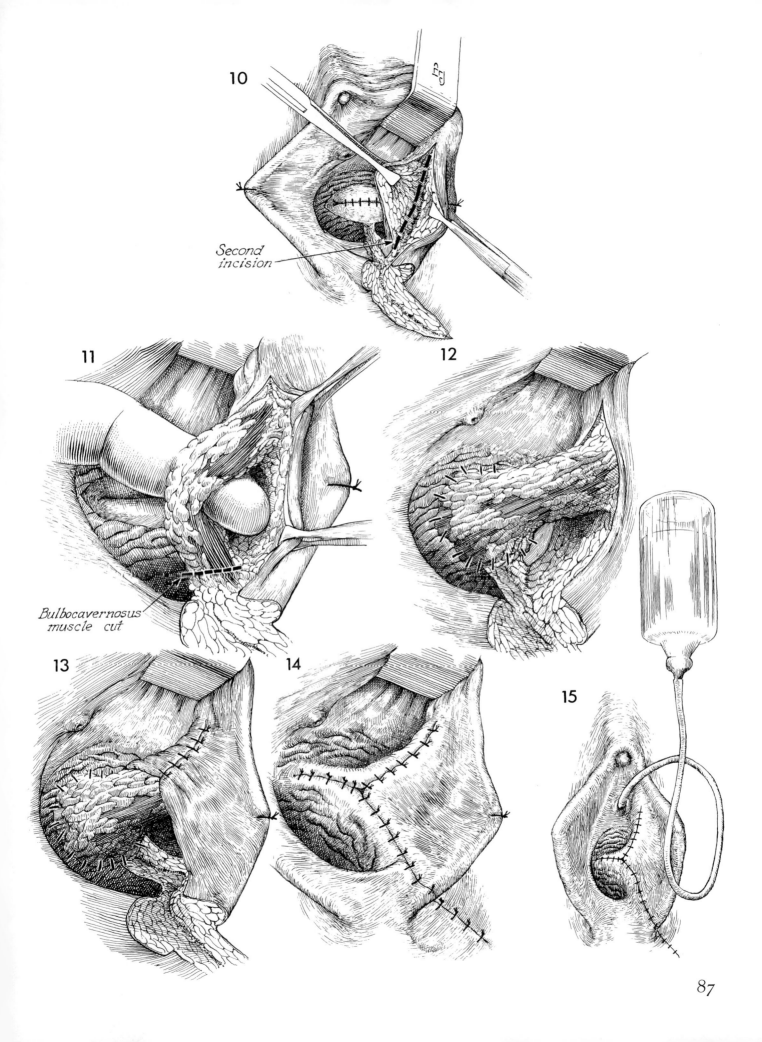

Second
incision

Bulbocavernosus
muscle cut

87

# Transposition of Island Skin Flap for Repair of Vesicovaginal Fistula

Vesicovaginal fistulae that have occurred secondary to irradiation and/or have recurred after repeated attempts to close them must be treated with procedures beyond the ordinary. In such cases, an island skin flap based on the bulbocavernosus muscle can be transposed to aid in the closure. This myocutaneous tissue, which in most patients with gynecologic malignancy is usually spared from heavy radiation, brings a nonirradiated blood supply to aid in wound healing.

**Physiologic Changes.** The vesicovaginal fistula is closed. The vulva is spared excoriation from constant urine leakage.

**Points of Caution.** The surgeon must ensure that the blood supply of the bulbocavernosus muscle is intact. If the patient has received radiation that has covered the vulva, the blood supply muscle and fat pad may be insufficient for proper nutrition to the island skin flap. In addition, the margins of the vesicovaginal fistula must be examined and found free of necrosis and cellulitis before closure is attempted.

## Technique

1 A vesicovaginal fistula is depicted slightly behind the trigone of the bladder. The surgeon has debrided the vesicovaginal fistula of all scarring and unhealthy tissue. Previous cystoscopy has shown that the ureteral orifices and ureters at the trigone are intact and not involved with the fistulae. If this is in doubt, however, catheters should be placed up the ureter to the kidney and left in for the entire operation.

2 A longitudinal incision is made from the top of the labia majora down to the point of the island myocutaneous flap. After measuring the diameter of the vesicovaginal fistula in the vagina, this island skin flap can be marked off and cut to appropriate size. It is always wise to cut the island skin flap a little larger than needed.

3 The island skin flap has been dissected out with its bulbocavernosus muscle and associated fat pad that ensures the blood supply to the skin flap through its small perforated vessels. A Kelly clamp is used to open a tunnel underneath the labia minora. The labia minora are retracted away from this area with Allis clamps.

4 The bulbocavernosus myocutaneous flap has been tunneled underneath the labia minora. It is placed into the defect of the vesicovaginal fistula.

5 The bulbocavernosus myocutaneous flap is sutured to the margins of the vaginal mucosa with interrupted 3-0 monofilament delayed synthetic absorbable suture. The bladder can be tested at this point by placing a catheter in the bladder and filling the bladder with a milk solution to note any leaks around the fistula. A cystoscope can be placed to ensure that the urethral orifices are intact and not compromised by the surgical procedure or the sutures used to place the flap.

6 The vesicovaginal fistula repair has been completed. The donor site incision is closed with interrupted monofilament synthetic absorbable suture.

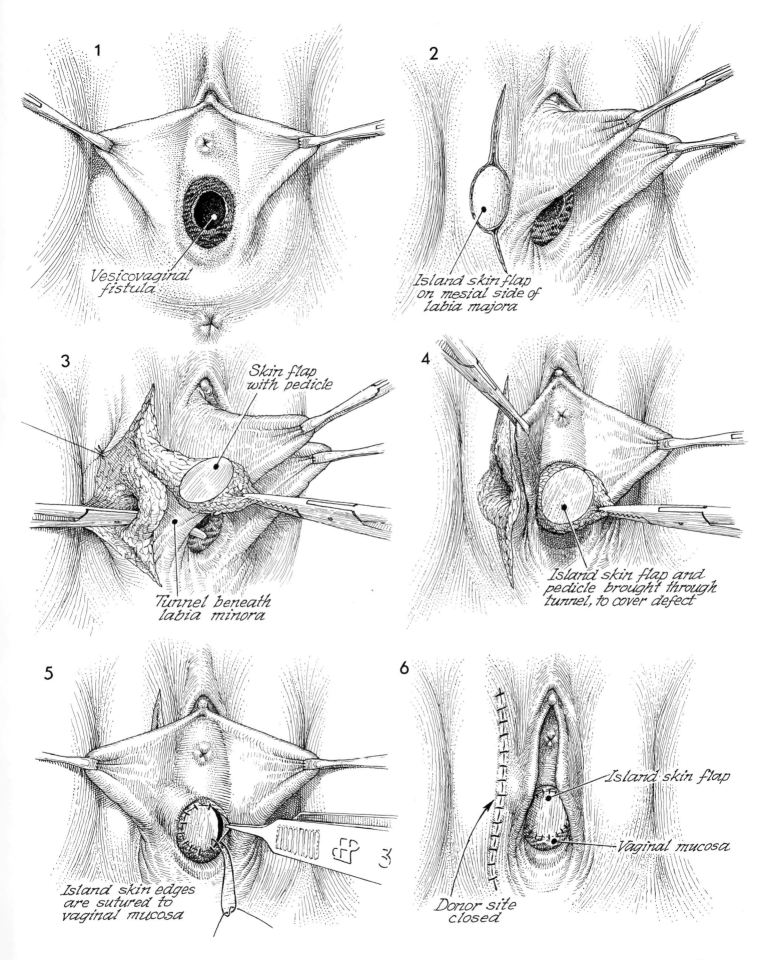

**1**

Vesicovaginal
fistula

**2**

Island skin flap
on mesial side of
labia majora

**3**

Skin flap
with pedicle

Tunnel beneath
labia minora

**4**

Island skin flap and
pedicle brought through
tunnel, to cover defect

**5**

Island skin edges
are sutured to
vaginal mucosa

**6**

Island skin flap

Vaginal mucosa

Donor site
closed

# McIndoe Vaginoplasty for Neovagina

The McIndoe vaginoplasty is indicated in patients with congenital absence of the vagina, in patients whose vagina must be removed, and in patients with severe stenosis following irradiation therapy. A split-thickness skin graft has traditionally been utilized with this operation, but we have changed to a full-thickness skin graft over an expandable foam rubber mold placed in the canal between the bladder and rectum. The use of the full-thickness skin graft reduces the postoperative contraction previously noted with the split-thickness skin graft requiring long-term utilization of a vaginal form, which is undesirable if unnecessary. Recently, it has been shown that a full-thickness skin graft takes as well as a split-thickness graft. Compared with a split-thickness skin graft, a full-thickness graft allows sufficient penetration of the transudate nutrients from the bed of the graft that are necessary for nutrition during the first 72 hours until microcapillary ingrowth has been completed. Full-thickness grafts do not have the same degree of contraction as the split-thickness grafts.

**Physiologic Changes.** One of the unique physiologic changes is the selection of thickness desired for the split-thickness skin graft. The split-thickness graft of 1/12,000ths of an inch has traditionally been used because it is thin enough to allow penetration of the transudate nutrients from the bed of the graft that are necessary for nutrition during the first 72 hours until microcapillary ingrowth has been completed. A split-thickness graft of 1/12,000ths of an inch is, however, associated with extensive contraction in the postoperative period unless a vaginal form is worn for many months. Currently, there has been greater utilization of thicker and thicker split-thickness skin grafts until, lately, full-thickness skin grafts have been utilized. Initially, it was thought that the blood supply to these full-thickness skin grafts would be insufficient and there would be excessive amounts of necrosis. The copious blood supply of the pelvis has demonstrated, however, that the full-thickness skin graft will survive. Thus with excellent survival of a full-thickness skin graft the patient is spared long-term vaginal form dilation.

**Points of Caution.** Careful dissection between the bladder and rectum is necessary to avoid cystotomy and enterotomy. Meticulous hemostasis is essential for the graft to adhere to the vaginal walls.

The skin grafts should be of uniform size and predominately of full thickness. The air-powered dermatome is preferred over the Reese or the electrical dermatome because it gives a uniform specimen of consistent thickness. The full-thickness grafts can be taken by the hand technique with a standard scalpel. We now prefer to take these from the skin covering the inguinal ligaments bilaterally. If there is tension on the suture line closing these donor site wounds, the new SureClosure skin-stretching system can be used to adequately close the wound. This has the advantage of leaving the patient with a cosmetic scar over the inguinal ligament versus a large scar over the buttocks or legs.

The vaginal mold should be soft and flexible. Foam rubber confined to a rubber condom has produced a soft vaginal mold that expands against the graft in a gentle manner without producing points of pressure. Excessive pressure could produce necrosis with possible vesicovaginal or rectovaginal fistula formation.

The vaginal form should be left in place for a minimum of 10 days. The form should then be removed, and the skin graft donor site should be inspected.

One of the most important criteria for this operation is the surgeon's conviction that the patient is mature enough to wear the vaginal form for at least 6 months, unless she is engaging in regular sexual intercourse. Failure to wear the vaginal form, especially with the split-thickness skin graft, is the major cause of failure in this operation. This generally occurs in adolescent girls who do not understand the importance of keeping the vaginal form in place even if it is inconvenient or uncomfortable.

# McIndoe Vaginoplasty for Neovagina

## (Continued)

### Technique

**1** A sagittal section through the pelvis demonstrates congenital absence of the vagina. The site of dissection will be in the areolar tissue between the bladder and rectum. The space is exaggerated here for illustration. The dissection should continue cephalad to 1–2 cm before the level of the peritoneum. Deeper dissection may allow the development of an enterocele.

**2** In this view of the introitus in congenital absence of the vagina, a slight indentation or dimple may exist where the urogenital sinus in the fetus failed to invaginate and fuse with the Müllerian duct to develop a normal vagina.

**3** A second cause of absence of the vagina is surgical removal for oncologic reasons.

**4** The air-powered dermatome is preferred because of the uniform thickness and size of the graft produced. The setting on the air-powered dermatome can be adjusted to 18/1,000ths or 24/1,000ths of an inch. *STSG* identifies the split-thickness skin graft.

**5** Two proposed paddle-shaped full-thickness skin grafts over the inguinal ligaments from the anterior superior iliac spine to the pubic tubercles are depicted. These paddles should be approximately 10 cm in length and 6 cm in width.

**6** Harvesting of the full-thickness skin graft is performed with the standard scalpel after marking the shape of the paddle in ink on the skin.

**7** The full-thickness skin grafts (*FTSG*)are placed in a graft pan and moistened with saline. The same is true for the split-thickness skin graft (*STSG*) if that is preferred to the full-thickness skin graft.

**8** After harvesting the full-thickness skin graft from the inguinal ligaments, if closure of the wound is on tension, the new SureClosure skin-stretching system can be utilized as shown. The stabilization needles are inserted in the subcutaneous space parallel to the line of the incision. Two, 4, or 6 of these can be utilized as necessary. Usually, no more than 2 are required. The skin-stretching device is anchored into the needle, and the ratchet on the skin-stretching device is activated until the skin is stretched to close the incision. Presently, a subcuticular suture of 3-0 delayed synthetic absorbable suture is utilized to close the wound.

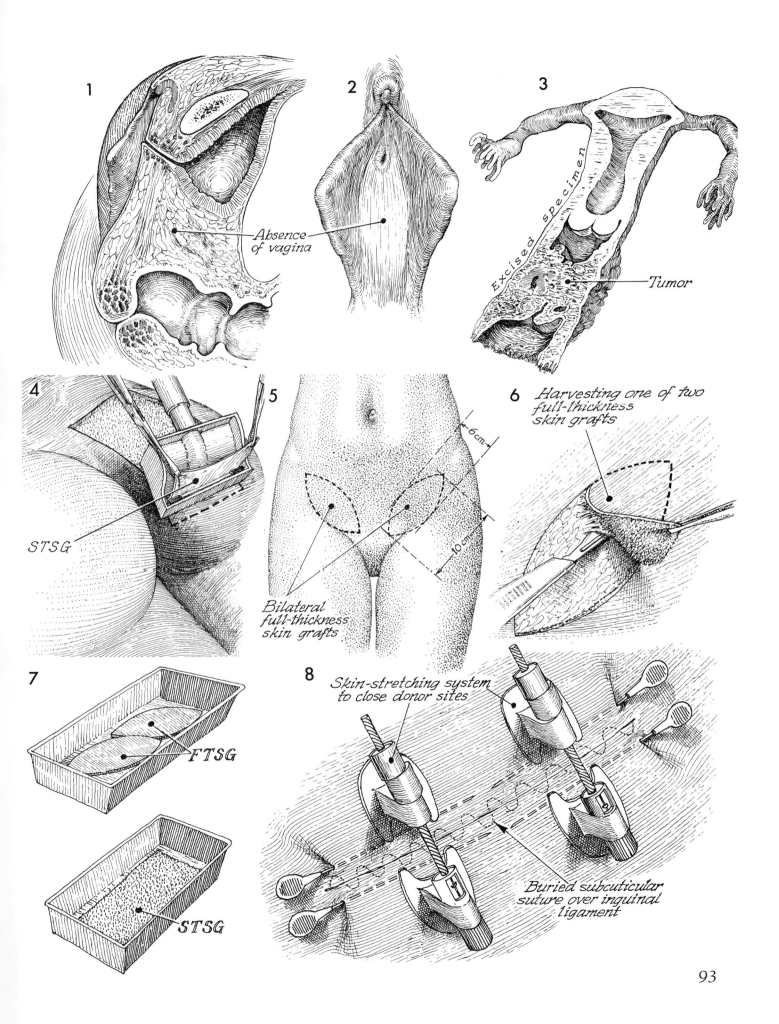

1

2

Absence
of vagina

3

Excised specimen

Tumor

4

STSG

5

6 cm

10 cm

Bilateral
full-thickness
skin grafts

6

Harvesting one of two
full-thickness
skin grafts

7

FTSG

STSG

8

Skin-stretching system
to close donor sites

Buried subcuticular
suture over inguinal
ligament

# McIndoe Vaginoplasty for Neovagina
## (Continued)

**9** A block of ordinary foam rubber, such as that used in the upholstery industry, is sterilized by gas autoclaving. The shape of the proposed vaginal form is outlined with brilliant green solution. The split-thickness skin graft is removed from the adhesive tape of the dermatome and placed in a sterile pan filled with saline solution. Ordinary contraceptive condoms that have been sterilized by gas autoclaving are used. Generally, two condoms are used to ensure against leakage of fluid into the foam rubber form.

**10** The foam rubber block is held in one hand and, with curved Mayo scissors, is shaped into the desired vaginal form.

**11** The condom is slipped over the foam rubber vaginal form. The condom can be removed partially or completely if the size of the vaginal form needs to be adjusted in diameter or length. When the size of the vaginal form is satisfactory, the end of the condom is tied with a 2-0 synthetic monofilament permanent suture.

**12** The vaginal form is laid on the epidermal side of the split- thickness skin graft. The split-thickness skin graft is folded over the vaginal form and sutured along its seam with interrupted 4-0 synthetic absorbable suture. Excess graft is trimmed away.

**13** The full-thickness, paddle-shaped skin grafts are placed over a foam rubber condom, and the margins are sutured together with synthetic absorbable suture.

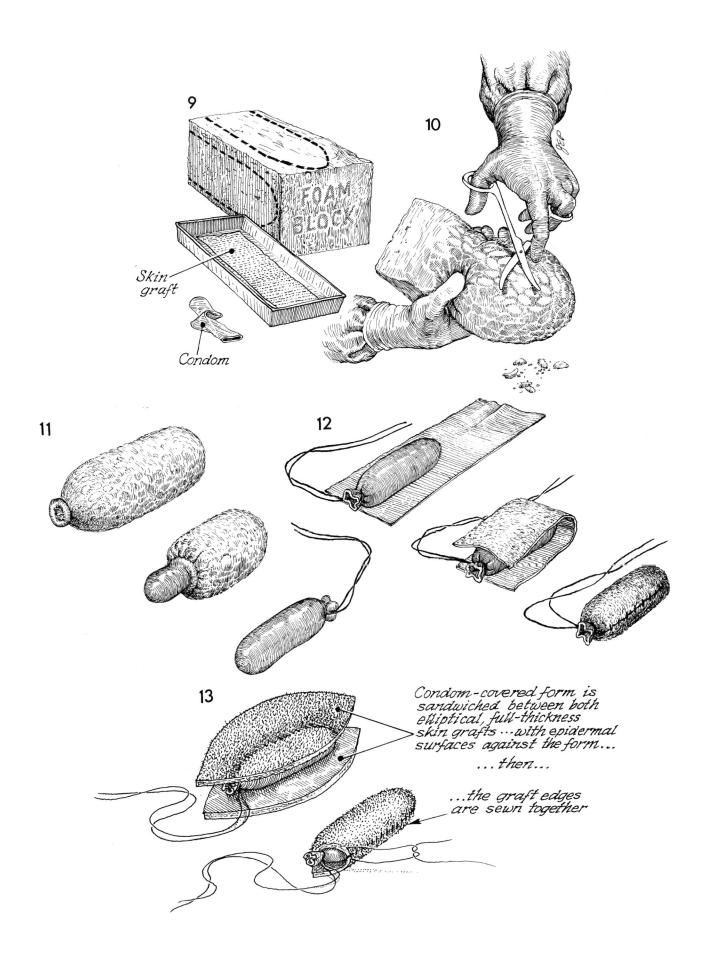

**9**

FOAM BLOCK

Skin graft

Condom

**10**

**11**

**12**

**13**

Condom-covered form is sandwiched between both elliptical, full-thickness skin grafts ...with epidermal surfaces against the form...

...then...

...the graft edges are sewn together

95

# McIndoe Vaginoplasty for Neovagina

## (Continued)

**14** The dimple in the introital area is identified. The labia are retracted with Allis clamps, and a transverse incision is made in the epithelium.

**15** Blunt dissection with the fingers opens the space between the bladder and rectum. Once the correct plane is reached, i.e., below the pubovesical cervical fascia under the bladder and superior to the perirectal fascia over the rectum, gentle blunt dissection is all that is needed to create an adequate cavity.

**16** A sagittal section shows the dissection carried approximately 2 cm from the peritoneum. This will reduce the incidence of enterocele in these patients.

**17** Meticulous hemostasis should be maintained throughout the cavity.

**18** The skin-covered form is inserted into the cavity.

**19** A sagittal view of the pelvis shows the skin-covered form inserted into the new vaginal canal.

**20** To hold the form in place for 12 days, the labia are sutured in the midline with interrupted 0 nylon sutures without tension.

**21** After the foam rubber vaginal form has been removed on the 12th postoperative day, the new vagina should be thoroughly inspected and irrigated with normal saline solution. A permanent vaginal form made of soft rubber or silicone should be fitted and inserted. Care should be taken that the new vaginal form does not protrude beyond the introitus. Protrusion will erode the introital area and cause pain, discouraging the patient from continuing to use the form.

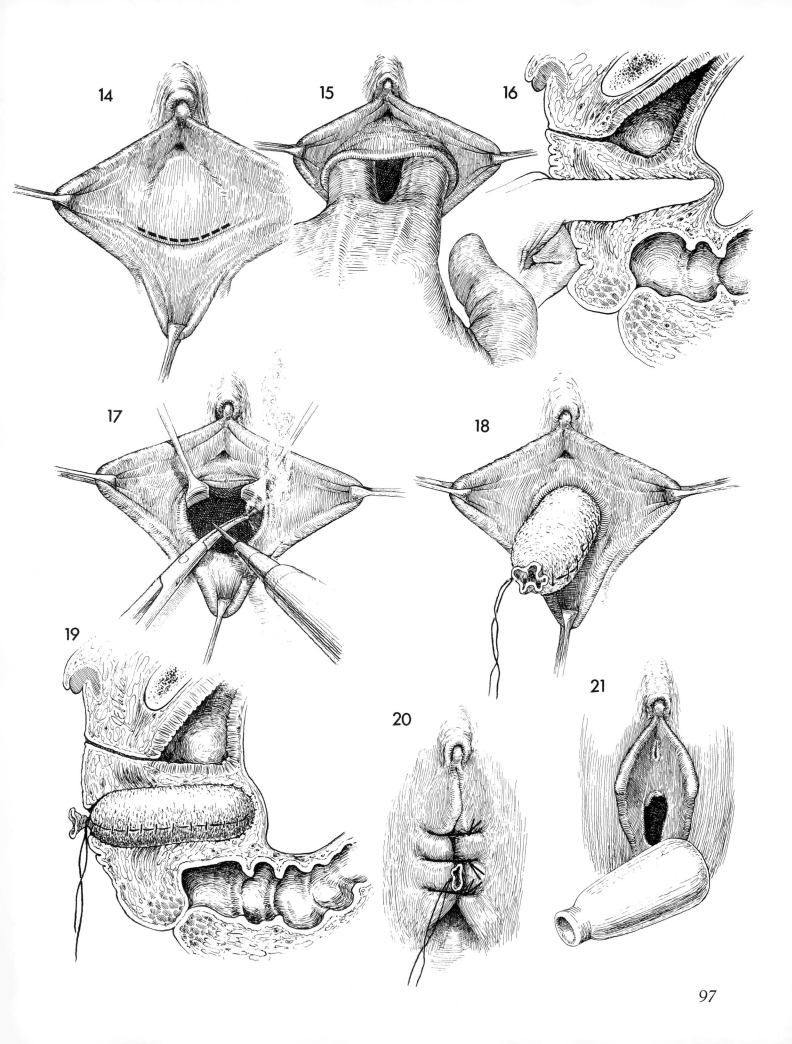

97

# Rectovaginal Fistula Repair

Rectovaginal fistulae must be divided into two groups. The first group consists of those that occur secondary to obstetric or gynecologic surgery for benign disease. The second group consists of those that are associated with radiation therapy for pelvic malignancy. Rarely is a diverting colostomy needed for fistulae from benign disease. A transverse colostomy is always needed, however, for pelvic cancer patients who have rectovaginal fistulae secondary to irradiation. An outside blood supply, such as a muscular flap, is not required for the repair of small rectovaginal fistulae secondary to obstetric or gynecologic surgery, unless there is excessive scarring or repeated attempts at closure have been unsuccessful. Patients with rectovaginal fistulae associated with pelvic irradiation, however, require a vascular flap to improve the blood supply to the irradiated tissues.

The bulbocavernosus muscle is the most convenient source of blood supply, but other sources include the omentum, gracilis muscle, and myocutaneous flaps.

The cardinal principles of repair of rectovaginal fistulae are (1) delay of repair until all inflammation has cleared at the fistula site, even if a preoperative perineotomy is required; (2) excision of all fibrotic and scar tissue surrounding the fistulous tract; (3) complete mobility of the rectum and colon to eliminate any tension on the rectal mucosa after excision of the scarred tissue; (4) use of delicate surgical technique to preserve as much vascularity as possible; (5) broad surface-to-surface closure; (6) improved vascularity using an outside blood supply; and (7) diverting colostomy, in cases of irradiation, until 3–4 months after the fistula has been confirmed closed by repeated examination.

**Physiologic Changes.** The rectovaginal fistula is closed, and normal defecation per anus is resumed.

The bulbocavernosus flap used to cover the rectovaginal fistula suture line improves vascularity and gives an additional layer to the closure, thus improving the chances of permanent fistula repair.

**Points of Caution.** The margins of the rectal mucosa must lie adjacent to each other without tension. Tension on the rectal mucosa suture line will invariably result in separation of the wound. Hemostasis is a vital factor. The hemorrhoidal plexus of veins can be difficult to control, but meticulous technique in clamping, tying, and/or electrocoagulating each of these vessels is imperative to fistula closure.

Dilation of the anus at operation produces temporary paralysis of the sphincter muscle and, thereby, temporary rectal incontinence, preventing the buildup of flatus and stool in the terminal rectum and avoiding tension on the suture line.

# Rectovaginal Fistula Repair

## (Continued)

## Technique

**1** Occasionally, a fistula high inside a narrow vagina is difficult to expose. Therefore, a mediolateral episiotomy should be performed without hesitation to allow maximum exposure to the operating site. The mediolateral episiotomy should be extended up the vaginal mucosa to the margin of the fistula. If adequate exposure cannot be obtained completely from the vaginal approach, the abdominal route should be considered, particularly in those cases where the fistula is high in a deep vagina.

**2** Extreme care should be taken that the bowel mucosa is adequately mobilized and that devitalized, scarred, or avascular portions of the mucosa have been excised. If the intestinal mucosa cannot be mobilized and it is apparent that the closure of the intestinal mucosa will be under tension, the surgeon should perform a laparotomy and totally mobilize the rectosigmoid colon from above. Many fistula repairs fail because this is not done. After adequate mobilization of the intestinal mucosa, the edges of the intestinal mucosa are closed in an inverting fashion with interrupted 3-0 Dexon suture with a Lembert stitch.

**3** The perirectal fascia and even some levator ani muscle may be drawn into a second layer of closure using 0 Dexon.

**4** If an outside blood supply is desirable, the margin of the excised fistula tract is connected with the incision of the episiotomy. The bulbocavernosus muscle is palpated under the labia majora, and a longitudinal incision is made down the labia majora through the fat pad until the bulbocavernosus muscle is located.

**5** The bulbocavernosus muscle is dissected out and transected above its insertion into the perineal body, leaving its blood supply from the branches of the pudendal artery intact. A tunnel approximately 3 cm wide is created from inside the vaginal canal with a Kelly clamp, and the bulbocavernosus muscle is drawn through this tunnel underneath the labia minora and hymenal ring.

**6** The bulbocavernosus muscle is sutured over the perirectal fascia with interrupted 3-0 Dexon sutures.

**7** The edges of the vaginal mucosa are then approximated with interrupted 2-0 Dexon sutures. The wound over the labia minora may be sutured by subcuticular 3-0 Dexon or interrupted 4-0 nylon sutures. Occasionally, there will be troublesome bleeding from the bed of the bulbocavernosus muscle. If this cannot be brought under adequate control by delicate clamping and suturing, it is often possible to pack this area with Avitene collagen hemostat. In this event, a small ¼-inch closed suction drain can be brought out from the inferior edge of the labial incision. To have the entire wound completely dry and avoid hemostatic agents or drains is preferred, however.

Care must be taken to ensure that the stool is completely soft and that there is no buildup of flatus above the sphincter. The latter can be accomplished by two techniques. One is to dilate the sphincter to 4–5 cm manually, thus temporarily paralyzing the rectal sphincter and leaving the patient fecally incontinent for approximately 1 week. The other is to incise the rectal sphincter at the 7 or 9 o'clockposition in one plane only. Multiple radial incisions in the rectal sphincter may produce permanent fecal incontinence. It is highly recommended that the patient use a stool softener for 3–6 months following fistula repair.

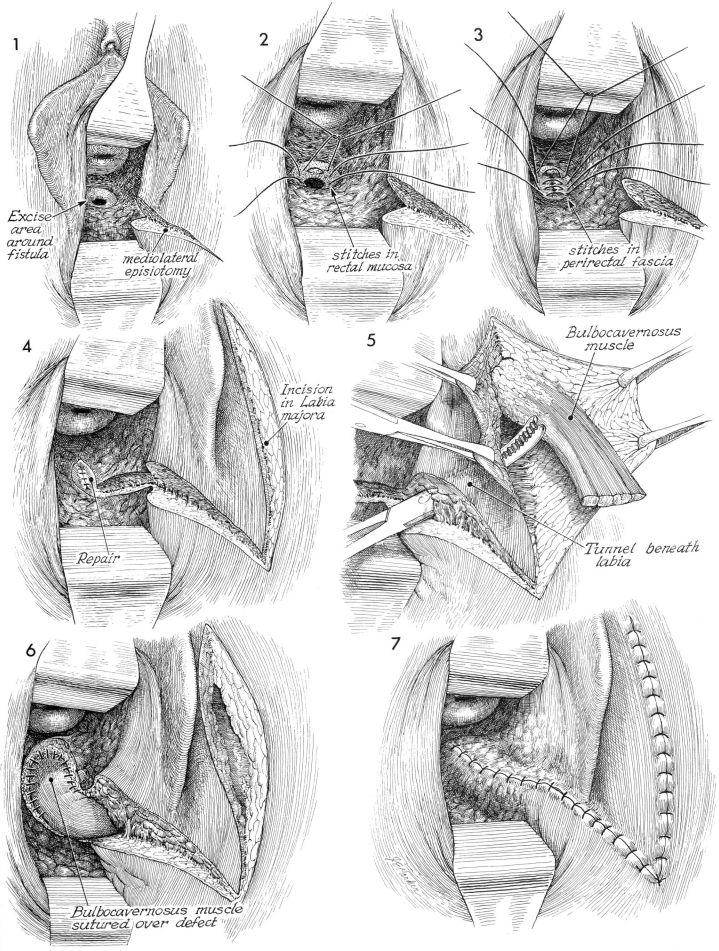

**1**

Excise area around fistula

mediolateral episiotomy

**2**

stitches in rectal mucosa

**3**

stitches in perirectal fascia

**4**

Incision in Labia majora

Repair

**5**

Bulbocavernosus muscle

Tunnel beneath labia

**6**

Bulbocavernosus muscle sutured over defect

**7**

# Reconstruction of the Urethra

Reconstruction of the urethra is indicated if a part of the urethra has been surgically removed or if there is a failure of fetal urogenital sinus development. Loss of a portion of the urethra may not be associated with total incontinence of urine. In cases of epispadias, however, there is total incontinence. In those patients who have lost the distal portion of the urethra and remain continent, considerable disability remains because the voided stream may be uncontrollable and, therefore, result in a significant esthetic problem.

When reconstruction of the urethra is required because of total epispadias, the patient may get a satisfactory anatomic result but remain incontinent unless the procedure is combined with a Goebell-Stoeckel fascia lata strap operation (see Section 2, page 116).

**Physiologic Changes.** An epithelial channel is constructed from the base of the bladder to the urethral meatus. Although this neourethra has no muscle, it acts as a conduit for the proximal urethra or bladder.

**Points of Caution.** The vaginal flap must be designed to ensure that the vascular supply to the base of the flap is sufficient to support the length of the flap needed.

If the tube flap technique (Figs. 7–11) is employed, adequate flaps of epithelium must be mobilized to meet in the midline without tension.

In both techniques, mobilization of the lateral labial epithelium is essential to cover and support the neourethra without tension.

# Reconstruction of the Urethra

## (Continued)

*Technique*

**1** A sagittal section of the pelvis without a urethra is shown. The patient is placed in the dorsal lithotomy position. The perineum is surgically prepared. Careful measurements should be made to design an adequate flap with 2 cm of width at the base for every 1 cm of length to ensure an adequate blood supply to the flap.

**2** The proposed flap should be marked off on the anterior vaginal wall. The mucosa is incised down to the pubovesical cervical fascia with a scalpel. A Foley catheter is inserted as indicated.

**3** The flap has been mobilized. Two parallel incisions are made approximately 2 cm apart to prepare the receptor bed for the edges of the flap. Plication sutures are placed in the pubovesical fascia from the apex of the vaginal incision to the neourethral vesical angle.

**4** The flap is sutured into position along the lateral grooves incised in the vestibule. This is performed with interrupted 4-0 synthetic absorbable suture. Lateral to the grooves, the labial tissue is mobilized by undermining it for a sufficient distance, usually 4 cm, to allow it to be brought to the midline without tension.

The vaginal wall defect should be closed with interrupted 2-0 synthetic absorbable sutures.

**5** The previously mobilized labial epithelium is sutured in the midline with 2-0 synthetic absorbable sutures to cover the flap and provide nutrition and support.

**6** The completed operation is shown.

**7** A second technique for reconstruction of the urethra involves rolling a tube flap, then covering it with a second layer of periurethral tissue. The flap is marked with brilliant green solution along the proposed new urethra. Care should be taken to ensure that sufficient tissue is mobilized to allow it to meet in the midline without tension. The margins of the flap are incised with a scalpel, and the tissue is mobilized medially.

**8** Tissue is then rolled toward the midline and sutured into place with interrupted 4-0 synthetic absorbable suture. The tissue lateral to the mobilized flap is undermined for a distance of about 4 cm.

**9** The lateral tissue is closed over the flap in two layers with interrupted 3-0 synthetic absorbable suture. A Foley catheter remains in the bladder.

**10** The epithelium is closed with interrupted 3-0 absorbable sutures.

**11** The completed operation is shown with the neourethra.

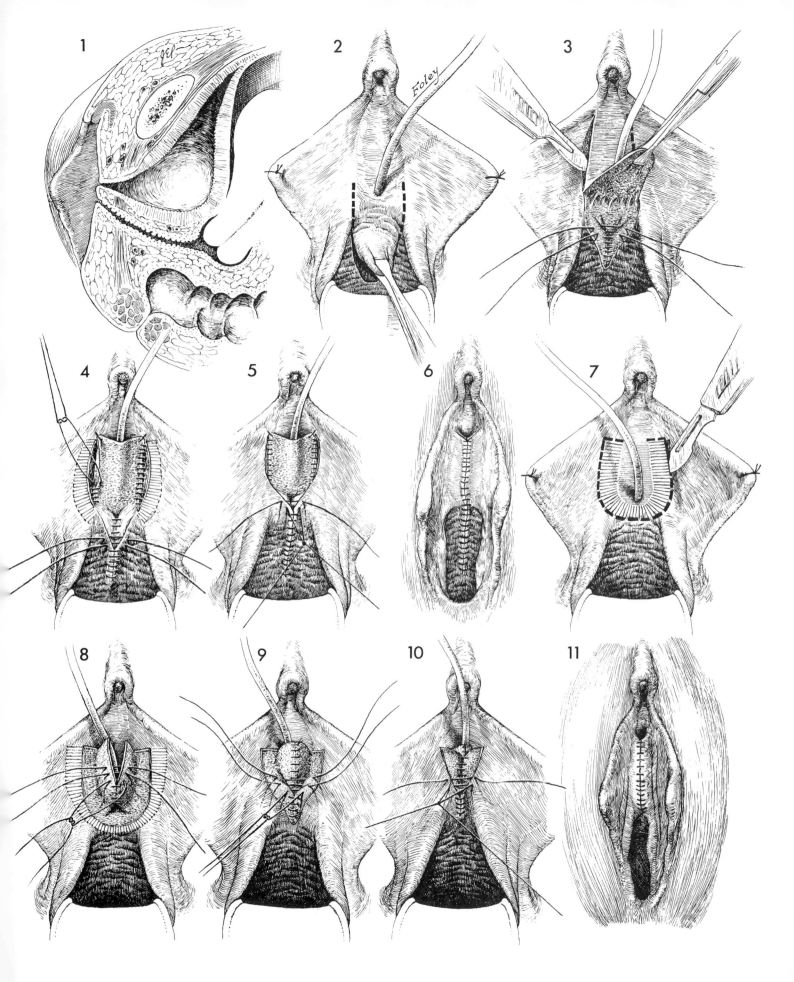

# Marsupialization of a Suburethral Diverticulum by the Spence Operation

Suburethral diverticulum in the distal one-third of the urethra can be treated by simple marsupialization of the diverticulum. In these cases, it is not necessary to perform all of the steps of a classic diverticular repair as described in Section 2, page 108. Although traditional operations for diverticula in the distal one-third of the urethra have produced problems with stenosis, marsupialization provides relief without complications.

**Physiologic Changes.** The suburethral diverticulum is marsupialized, and the source of chronic infection and urethritis is eliminated. Although the urethra is shortened by the marsupialization process, it is extremely rare for patients to experience urinary incontinence.

**Points of Caution.** The surgeon must be sure to marsupialize the entire suburethral diverticulum. When patients have multiple diverticula at the same site, each diverticulum must be opened during the operation and incorporated into the marsupialization.

## Technique

**1** Figure 1 is a sagittal view of a suburethral diverticulum. *B*, bladder.

**2** Figure 2 is a perineal view of the same diverticulum.

**3** With Metzenbaum scissors inserted into the urethra and the vagina, an incision is made through the posterior wall of the urethra down to the diverticulum and also through the anterior wall of the vagina down to and including the diverticulum.

**4** The diverticulum and urethra are now open. A 4-0 synthetic absorbable suture is used to marsupialize the epithelium of the vaginal mucosa to the urethral mucosa down to the sac of the diverticulum. The sac of the diverticulum is sutured to the anterior vaginal mucosa.

**5** The completed operation shows the posterior wall of the urethra and the entire sac of the suburethral diverticulum marsupialized to the anterior vaginal mucosa.

**6** Figure 6 is a sagittal view of the completed procedure. Note that although the urethra has been shortened, there has been no alteration in the pressure relationships between the lumen of the urethra and the bladder; therefore, urinary continence is not affected by the surgical procedure.

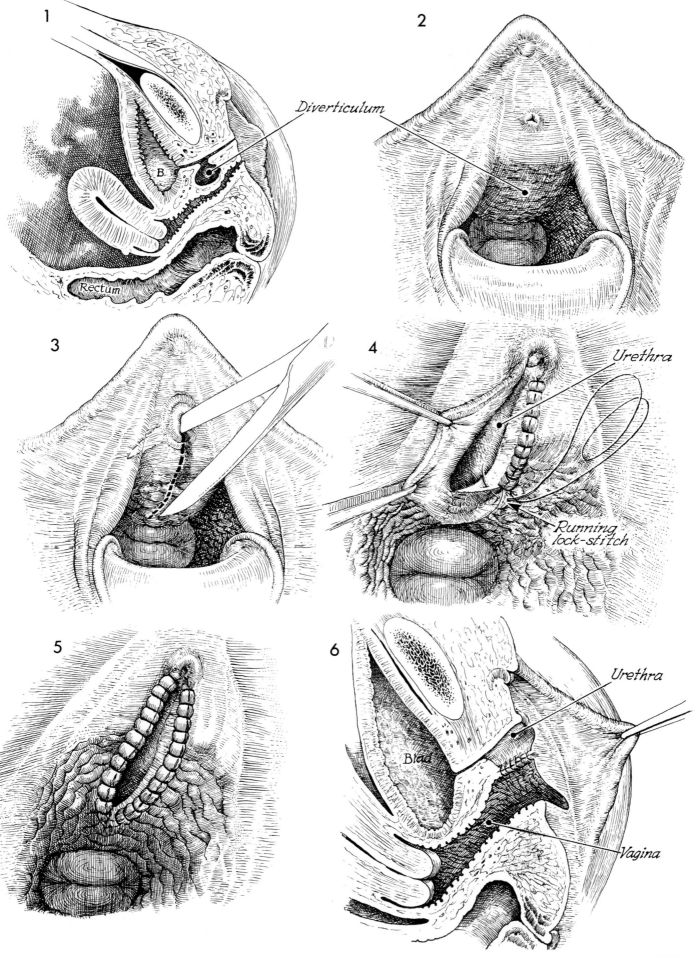

**1**

**2**

*Diverticulum*

*B*

*Rectum*

**3**

**4**

*Urethra*

*Running
lock-stitch*

**5**

**6**

*Urethra*

*Blad*

*Vagina*

107

# Suburethral Diverticulectomy
# via the Double-Breasted Closure Technique

Suburethral diverticula may be discovered in patients evaluated for recurrent or chronic urinary tract infection. The diverticula formation can be congenital or secondary to trauma of the female urethra.

The purpose of the operation is to remove the diverticulum and close the urethra without producing a stricture. This procedure should be utilized only for diverticula located in the middle and proximal thirds of the urethra. Suburethral diverticula in the distal one-third of the urethra are managed effectively by the Spence operation (Section 2, page 106).

**Physiologic Changes.** A source of chronic infection that is also a potential site of urethral stone formation is removed.

**Points of Caution.** After excision of the suburethral diverticulum, adequate mobilization of the surrounding tissues must be made to close the wound without tension and reduce the chance of urethral stricture. If the tissue is brought together under tension, necrosis can occur, and a fistula may develop.

## Technique

**1** Figure 1 is a sagittal section of the female bladder, urethra, and vagina, showing a suburethral diverticulum. Diverticula can be diagnosed either by urethroscopy or with the use of a Davis double-balloon catheter in which x-ray contrast media is injected under pressure.

This special catheter entraps x-ray contrast dye between the two inflated balloons, forcing dye into a diverticulum. A lateral x-ray film can demonstrate the diverticulum.

**2** The patient is placed in the dorsal lithotomy position, and the perineum is prepped and draped in the usual fashion. A uterine sound has passed through the urethra into the bladder. The vaginal mucosa is opened over the suspected diverticulum. Figure 2 shows the vaginal mucosa, pubovesical cervical fascia, and the urethral mucosa.

**3** The urethral mucosa is closed over the diverticulum with a running monofilament 4-0 synthetic absorbable suture. The sutures should be placed with the uterine sound in position to prevent stricture of the urethra. Notice that the pubovesical cervical (PVC) fascia has been developed into 2–3-cm-wide flaps of fascia. The vaginal mucosa has been dissected laterally and is held laterally with Allis clamps.

**4** The double-breasted closure technique is performed with monofilament delayed synthetic absorbable suture. The right pubovesical cervical fascia flap is sutured across to the base of the opposite pubovesical cervical fascia flap. It is best to place all these sutures prior to tying them. This will allow more accurate placement of the sutures.

Note that the vaginal mucosa is retracted laterally. On the patient's left, the opposite pubovesical cervical fascia is retracted out of the suture line.

**5** The left pubovesical cervical fascia flap is now sutured over the right pubovesical cervical fascia flap in a double-breasted fashion with monofilament delayed synthetic absorbable suture used.

**6** The vaginal mucosa is closed in the midline with 2-0 synthetic absorbable suture. Catheter drainage should be continuous for 1 week. This can be accomplished with a suprapubic Foley catheter or a transurethral Foley catheter.

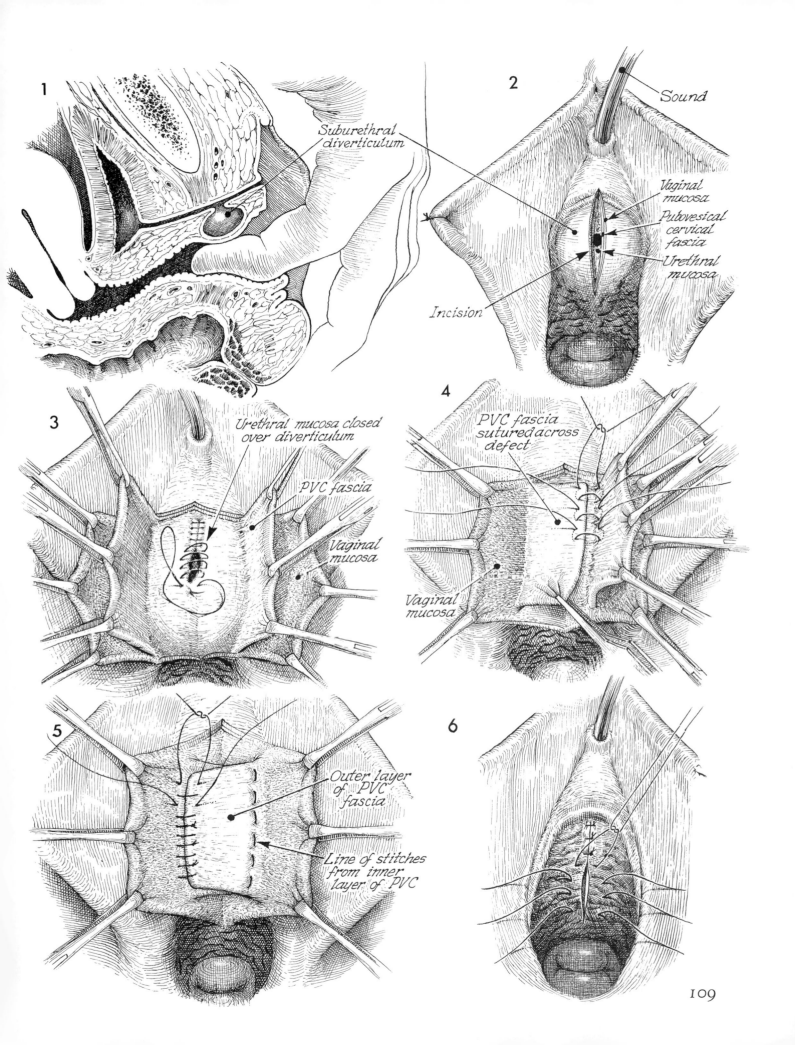

**1**

Suburethral diverticulum

**2**

Sound

Vaginal mucosa

Pubovesical cervical fascia

Urethral mucosa

Incision

**3**

Urethral mucosa closed over diverticulum

PVC fascia

Vaginal mucosa

**4**

PVC fascia sutured across defect

Vaginal mucosa

**5**

Outer layer of PVC fascia

Line of stitches from inner layer of PVC

**6**

109

# Urethrovaginal Fistula Repair
# via the Double-Breasted Closure Technique

Urethrovaginal fistulae are generally secondary to one of two conditions: (1) surgical trauma following anterior colporrhaphy or (2) obstetrical trauma.

In many instances, a urethrovaginal fistula exists, but the patient is still completely continent and has no problem voiding. Some patients with this condition, especially those with the fistula in the proximal one-third of the urethra, suffer a combination of incontinence and inability to control their urine stream when attempting to void. This technique is not applicable to fistulae in the distal one-third of the urethra. Those fistulae are adequately treated by the Spence operation from Section 2, page 106.

**Physiologic Changes.** In repairing a urethrovaginal fistula, the surgeon corrects the physiology of the urethra so that the patient may remain continent and the urinary stream may be emitted normally from the meatus. This procedure consists of three basic principles: (1) excise the scarred, devascularized tissue surrounding the fistula, (2) approximate healthy margins of tissue with multiple layers of closure, and (3) bring a source of blood supply and support to the base of the urethra to cover the fistula. This is particularly important in those cases where severe scarring and devascularization of tissue have occurred.

Preoperative evaluation of the patient should consist of a complete bladder-urethra workup including urodynamics, cystoscopy, urethroscopy, and urine culture.

**Points of Caution.** The margins of the fistula must be brought together without tension. The flaps of the pubovesical cervical fascia must be mobilized to allow the double-breasted closure technique. The size and caliber of the urethra must be adequate for voiding. The multiple-layer approach to fistula closure has stood the test of time and represents the best opportunity for permanent closure.

A vascular pedicle flap such as the bulbocavernosus muscle has reduced the incidence of recurrent fistula in high-risk patients.

# Urethrovaginal Fistula Repair via the Double-Breasted Closure Technique

## (Continued)

*Technique*

**1** With the patient in the dorsal lithotomy position, the fistula in the proximal third of the urethra is demonstrated. The vaginal mucosa is incised from the urethral meatus pass the fistula site.

**2** The pubovesical cervical fascia flaps are mobilized on each side. After complete mobilization of these flaps, the urethral mucosa of the fistula is closed with a running 4-0 monofilament synthetic absorbable suture. After closure of the urethral mucosa, the pubovesical cervical fascia flap on the patient's right is closed to the base of the pubovesical cervical fascia on the left with interrupted 3-0 monofilament delayed synthetic absorbable suture.

**3** The pubovesical cervical fascia flap from the patient's left is closed in double-breasted fashion over the flap of pubovesical cervical fascia from the right. This closure is completed with 3-0 monofilament delayed synthetic absorbable suture.

**4** If the fistula has been previously operated on or if there are factors such as radiation, a vascular flap should be brought over the suture line of the double-breasted pubovesical cervical fascia. The bulbocavernosus flap is initiated by an incision in the labia majora. The bulbocavernosus muscle with its associated fat pad is mobilized.

**5** The muscle is transected posteriorly; its blood supply comes from the vessels of the mons pubis. A Kelly clamp has been inserted on top of the pubovesical cervical fascia under the vaginal mucosal and enters the wound from the bed of the bulbocavernosus muscle.

**6** The bulbocavernosus flap is pulled through the defect created by tunneling under the vaginal mucosa, the labia minora, and the labia majora.

**7** The bulbocavernosus flap is sutured over the urethrovaginal fistula repaired with the double-breasted closure of the pubovesical cervical fascia.

**8** The skin over the labia majora is closed with interrupted monofilament synthetic absorbable suture. The vaginal mucosa is shown closed with interrupted synthetic absorbable suture. Ghosted under the closure of the vaginal mucosa is the bulbocavernosus flap.

A suprapubic Foley catheter should be inserted for 1 week to allow urethral mucosal healing before spontaneous voiding.

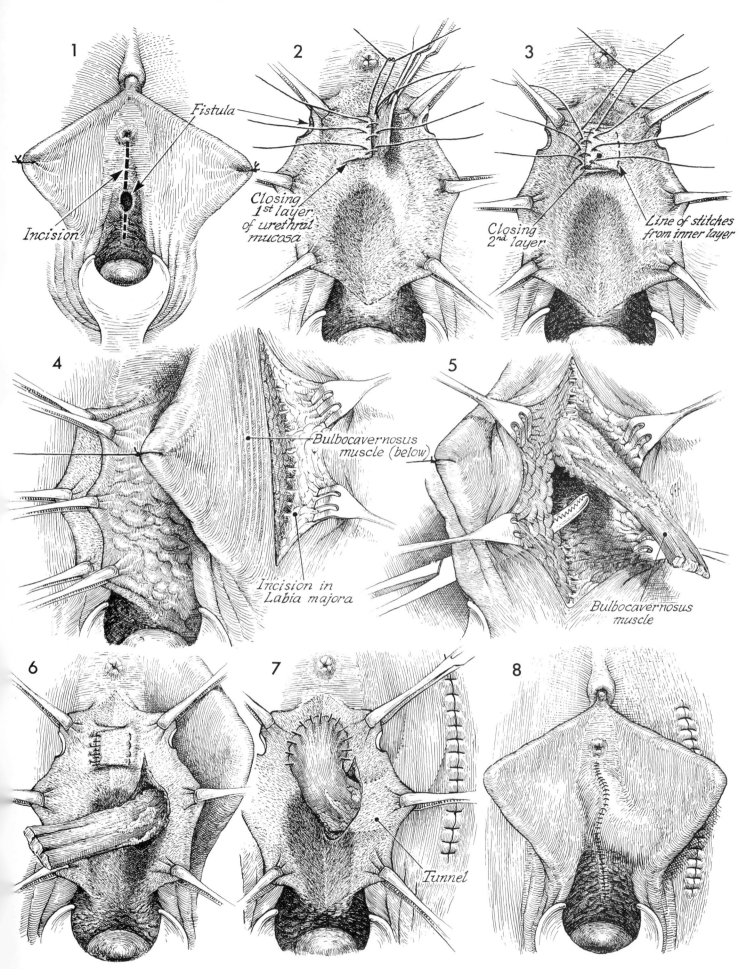

**1**

*Fistula*

*Incision*

**2**

*Closing
1st layer
of urethral
mucosa*

**3**

*Closing
2nd layer*

*Line of stitches
from inner layer*

**4**

*Bulbocavernosus
muscle (below)*

*Incision in
Labia majora*

**5**

*Bulbocavernosus
muscle (below)*

*Bulbocavernosus
muscle*

**6**

**7**

*Tunnel*

**8**

113

# Goebell-Stoeckel Fascia Lata Sling Operation for Urinary Incontinence

Surgery for stress incontinence of urine has a long history of numerous procedures designed to relieve patients of this disabling problem. There are procedures that reinforce the pubovesical fascia beneath the urethra, procedures that tack the urethra up to the rectopubic space, and procedures that elevate the urethrovesical angle by a suspension from the rectus fascia.

Long-term results reveal an interesting statistic. Most surgical procedures to correct all forms of urinary incontinence have a success rate of approximately 40–90%.

There are two ways to alter the anatomy and thus change the physiology to correct stress incontinence of urine. First, there are operations designed to increase the intraurethral pressure so that it exceeds the intravesical pressure in the resting and stress state. These include the Goebell-Stoeckel fascia lata sling, anterior repair with Kelly plication, Sexton perivaginal suspension, and the modified Marshall-Marchetti procedure in which the periurethral vaginal tissue is suspended from the conjoined tendon. Other procedures, such as the Marshall-Marchetti-Krantz operation, attempt to relieve urinary stress incontinence by making the vesical neck of the bladder an intra-abdominal organ.

The procedure demonstrating the best long-term result in our clinic is the Goebell-Stoeckel fascia lata sling.

We have used the Goebell-Stoeckel fascia lata sling in cases of primary stress incontinence of urine in elderly nulliparous patients, obese patients, and patients with congenital absence or traumatic loss of the urethra in conjunction with a primary reconstructive procedure to rebuild a urethra. In addition, we have used the Goebell-Stoeckel fascia lata sling for those cases of secondary stress incontinence of urine after an attempt to relieve the problem with one of the other surgical procedures has failed.

The operation is intended to relieve stress incontinence of urine.

**Physiologic Changes.** In this operation, the intraurethral pressure is elevated above the intravesical pressure by reducing the diameter of the urethral lumen. The increase in intraurethral pressure, however, should not be greater than the intravesical pressure at the moment of maximum detrusor contraction with normal voiding.

**Points of Caution.** There are several points of caution to observe in performing this operation. (1) The vaginal dissection at the urethrovesical angle should extend up behind the pubic bone to the level of the urogenital diaphragm so that the abdominal dissection down behind the symphysis pubis may be performed with blunt finger dissection only. In this way, the chance of inadvertently entering the bladder will be reduced. (2) The fascia strap should not be pulled too tightly. The strap should be loose enough to allow easy insertion of a Kelly clamp between the strap and the urethral vesical angle. When the strap is pulled too tightly, the patient will have postoperative urinary retention.

# Goebell-Stoeckel Fascia Lata Sling Operation for Urinary Incontinence

## (Continued)

## Technique

**1** The patient is placed in the dorsal lithotomy position and examined under anesthesia. The degree of cystourethrocele is assessed.

**2** The patient is changed to the right or left lateral decubitus position with flexion of both the hip and the knee at approximately 60°. A pillow should be placed between the knees in order to elevate the thigh to a level position. Two large pieces of tape are used to stabilize the patient and prevent her from moving to either side. The lateral thigh is prepped and draped. The *solid line* marks the site of the initial incision, and the *dotted line* marks the direction of the incision in the fascia lata.

**3** The Masson fascia stripper consists of two hollow metal tubes—one inside the other. The inner tube has a narrow opening near one end; the edge of the outer tube is sharpened to allow cutting of the fascia strip at the desired level.

**4** A longitudinal incision of 5 cm is made approximately 4 cm above the knee. This incision is carried down to the fascia lata. Small rake retractors are used to expose the fascia lata.

**5** The strap is started with the scalpel blade and should be approximately 3 cm wide. It is dissected off the muscle and the subcutaneous fat for a distance of at least 10–12 cm with the handle of the knife and index finger.

**6** The hand-carved portion of the strap is fed through the eye of the inner tube of the Masson fascia stripper. A 2-0 suture is placed through the fascia at the level of the eye to be used as a retriever in case the strap is inadvertently cut up inside the thigh. Two straight Kocher clamps are applied to the end of the strap for countertraction. The outer tube of the Masson fascia stripper is inserted over the inner tube, and they are locked together with a bolt action.

**7** With countertraction on the two Kocher clamps placed across the end of the strap, the Masson fascia stripper is advanced up the fascia lata until the desired length of fascia is obtained. At that point, the outer tube of the Masson fascia stripper is disengaged from the inner tube, and with a sudden shearing motion the inner tube is withdrawn from the outer tube, cutting the proximal end of the fascia strap.

**8** On occasion, the fascia strap will be too short, particularly in obese patients. Therefore, one end of the strap may be folded on itself, and several interrupted 2-0 Prolene sutures will need to be placed to anchor it. From the opposite end, an incision can be made down the length of the strap, thereby doubling the overall length.

**9** The incision in the thigh is closed with two layers—the inner layer with interrupted 3-0 synthetic absorbable suture and the outer layer with fine monofilament suture such as nylon or Prolene.

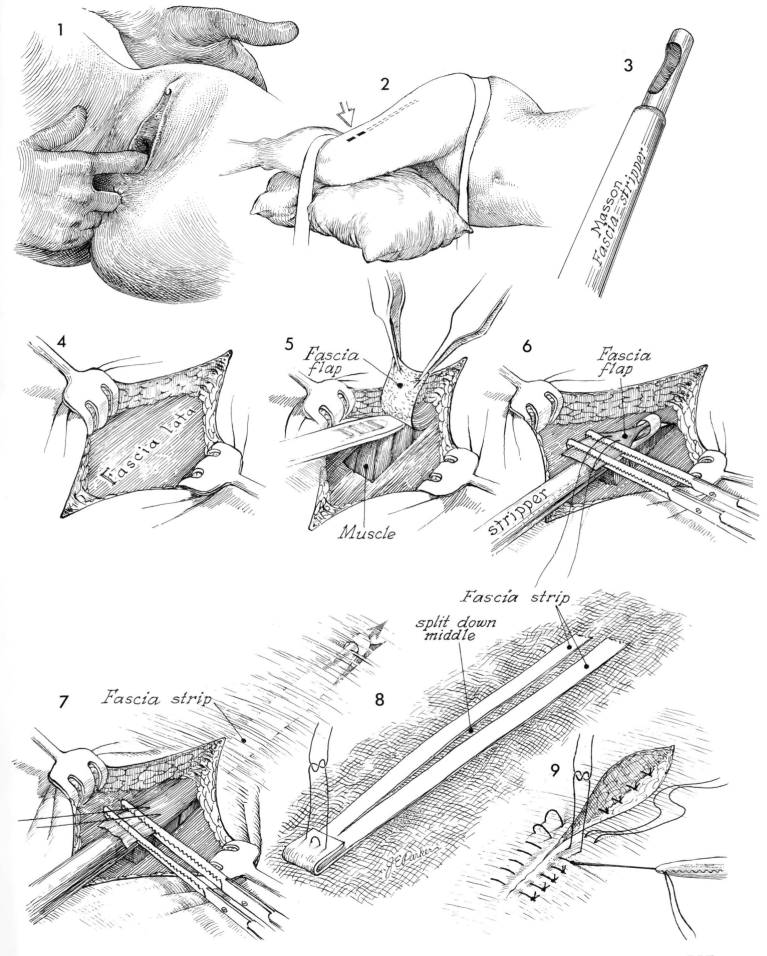

1

2

3

Masson Fascia stripper

4

Fascia lata

5

Fascia flap

Muscle

6

Fascia flap

stripper

7

Fascia strip

8

Fascia strip

split down middle

9

117

# Goebell-Stoeckel Fascia Lata Sling Operation for Urinary Incontinence

## (Continued)

**10** The patient is now changed from the lateral decubitus position to the dorsal lithotomy position. The vulva, vagina, and lower abdomen are prepped and draped.

**11** With the labia minora tacked to the perineum with interrupted sutures, a Foley catheter is inserted into the bladder, and tension is applied to define the urethrovesical angle.

**12** Two Allis clamps are applied at the urethrovesical angle, and a linear incision is made in the vaginal mucosa. This is carried down to the pubovesical cervical fascia.

**13** After sharp dissection has separated the vaginal mucosa from the pubovesical cervical fascia, blunt dissection with the finger can usually be carried out without difficulty lateral to the urethra up to the urogenital diaphragm. The same dissection should be carried out on the opposite side.

**14** The surgeon should make an 8-cm transverse incision approximately 8 cm above the pubic bone.

**15** This incision should be carried down to the rectus fascia, and two small oblique incisions large enough to admit a finger should be made in the rectus fascia.

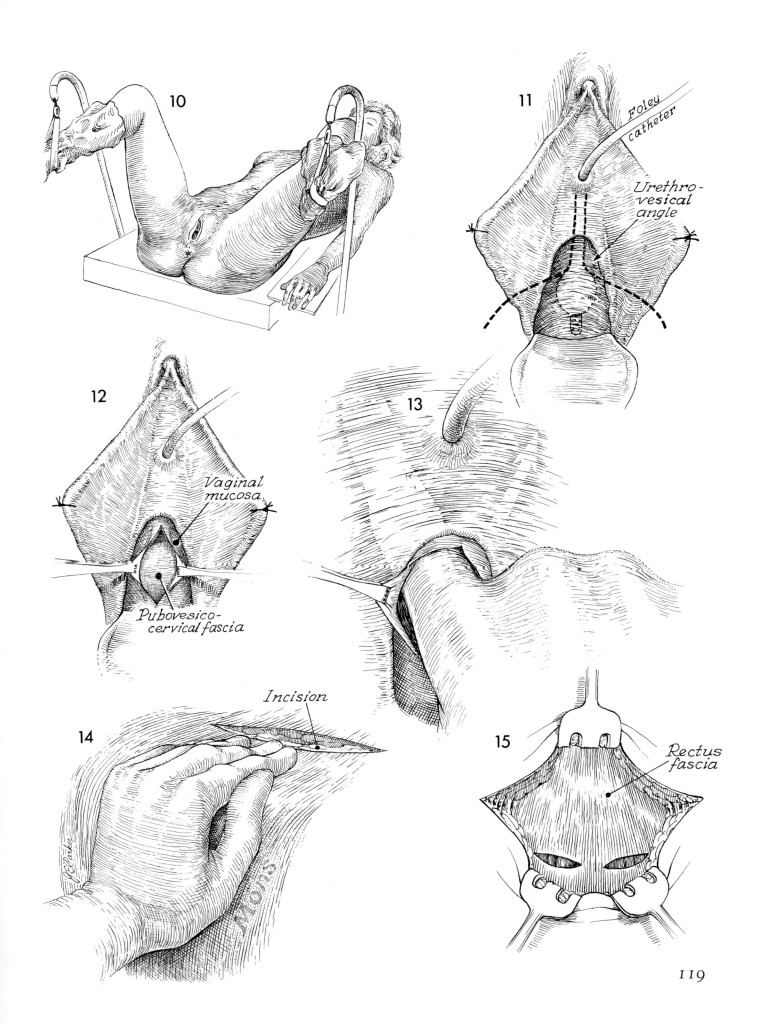

**10**

**11**
Foley catheter

Urethro-vesical angle

**12**
Vaginal mucosa

Pubovesico-cervical fascia

**13**

**14**
Incision

mons

**15**
Rectus fascia

119

# Goebell-Stoeckel Fascia Lata Sling Operation for Urinary Incontinence

## (Continued)

---

**16** Blunt dissection with a finger is used to create a space behind the pubic bone down to the urogenital diaphragm lateral to the urethra.

**17** A finger is inserted through the vaginal mucosa lateral to the urethra and up to the urogenital diaphragm. At the same time, a large Kelly clamp can be inserted through the rectus incision down to the point where it touches the finger.

**18** The Kelly clamp is then pushed through the urogenital diaphragm and out into the vagina. The clamp is used to grasp one end of the fascia strap.

**19** The strap is pulled up to the rectus abdominis incision and held with a small hemostat. A similar technique of dissection and strap pull-through is performed on the opposite side. A strap now is through both incisions in the rectus fascia and is around the urethrovesical angle.

Tension on the strap is adjusted so that there is enough space between the urethrovesical angle and the strap to easily insert a Kelly clamp.

**20** At this point, two 3-0 synthetic absorbable sutures are placed between the strap and the pubovesical cervical fascia at the urethrovesical angle. In addition, sutures are placed in the strap and rectus fascia.

**21** A suprapubic Foley catheter is inserted in the bladder as shown in Section 3, page 136. The abdominal incision is closed in layers; the vaginal mucosa is closed with interrupted 0 synthetic absorbable suture. The Foley catheter is left in place for at least 5 days, after which clamping of the catheter is started and the patient is encouraged to void.

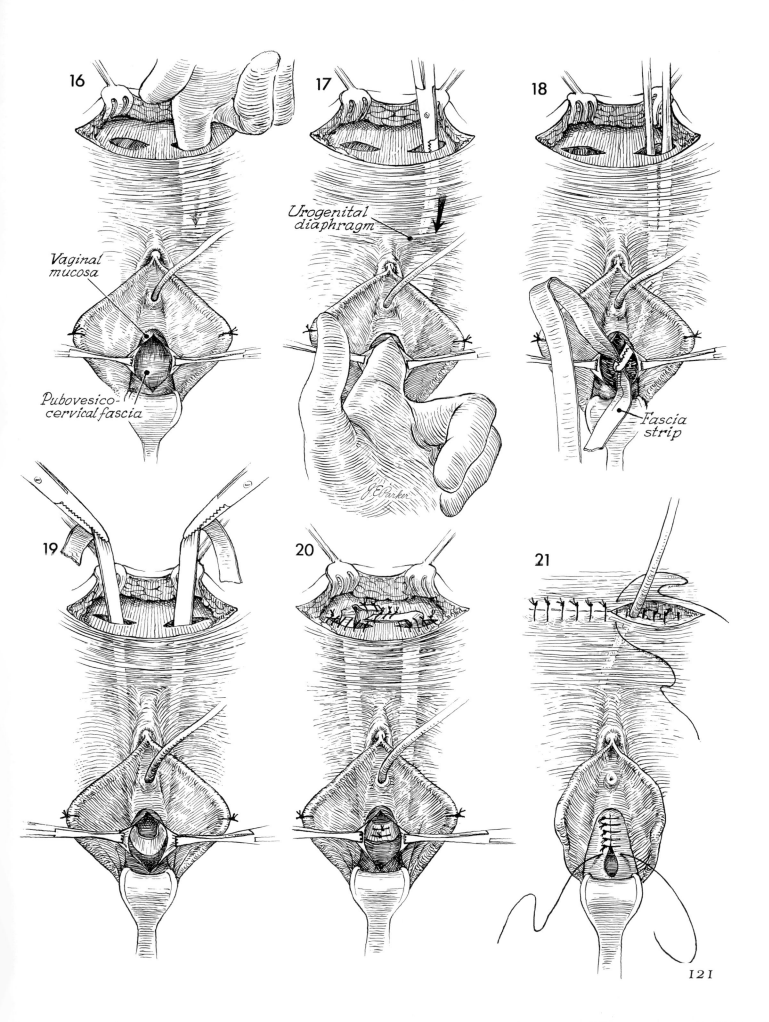

16

Vaginal
mucosa

Pubovesico-
cervical fascia

17

Urogenital
diaphragm

J.E.Parker

18

Fascia
strip

19

20

21

121

# Goebell-Stoeckel Fascia Lata Sling Operation for Urinary Incontinence

## (Continued)

**22** Figure 22 shows the physiologic changes in the anatomy that allow the Goebell-Stoeckel fascia lata sling procedure to correct urinary incontinence.

The central alteration in the anatomy is a reduction in size in the proximal and middle third of the urethral lumen, as noted in the *insert* to Figure 22 of the bladder and urethra. Continence is achieved by elevating the pressure inside this area above the pressure inside the bladder (*B*). *S* identifies the symphysis pubis.

It is important to note that unlike the retropubic "pin-up operations" (Marshall-Marchetti-Krantz, Burch, and Tenagho), the Goebell-Stoeckel fascia lata sling procedure does not make the bladder into an intra-abdominal organ. Instead, it increases the intra-urethral pressure (*pIU*) so that it becomes higher than the intravesical pressure (*pIV*) except when, on command, there is massive contraction of the detrusor.

Figure 22 illustrates a key point in this procedure. If the fascia strap is pulled too tightly, the chance of post-operative urinary retention will be greater than 30%. This is not a procedure to correct pelvic prolapse. The strap should not be used to bring the bladder back to an intra-abdominal organ like the Marshall-Marchetti-Krantz, Burch, and Tenagho procedures. Failure to recognize this point results in an unacceptable level of postoperative urinary retention.

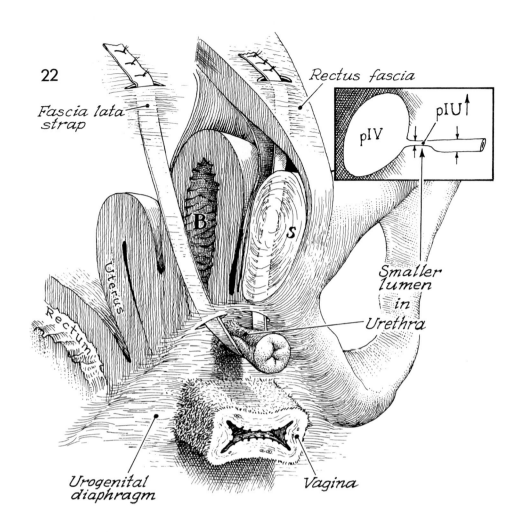

22

Fascia lata
strap

Rectus fascia

pIV

pIU↑

B

S

Uterus

Rectum

Smaller
lumen
in
Urethra

Urogenital
diaphragm

Vagina

# Transection of Goebell-Stoeckel Fascia Strap

The most serious drawback of the Goebell-Stoeckel fascia lata strap operation for restoration of urinary continence is the complication of postoperative urinary retention. In most cases, this results from the surgeon pulling the strap too tightly or from excessive contraction during healing, allowing the strap to pull itself too tightly. In general, the surgeon should allow 3 months before resorting to transection of the strap, since most cases of urinary retention are resolved with conservative therapy.

The purpose of the operation is to transect the strap without entering the urethrovesical bladder mucosa. When the strap alone has been transected, it separates approximately 1–2 cm and is densely adherent to the lateral periurethral tissue.

**Physiologic Changes.** With separation of the strap in the midline, the urethra is allowed to enlarge slightly. The intraurethral pressure is thereby reduced to a level that will allow the normal intravesical pressure on voiding to overcome the resistance in the urethra. The patient can then void and empty the bladder normally. Fortunately, in the majority of cases the dense adhesions of the strap to the lateral periurethral tissue continue to provide sufficient increase in the intraurethral pressure to avoid recurrent incontinence.

**Points of Caution.** The strap should be carefully identified (1) prior to making the vaginal incision, so that only the vaginal mucosa is separated, and (2) prior to cutting into the pubovesical cervical fascia.

---

## Technique

**1** The patient is placed in the dorsal lithotomy position with the vulva and vagina prepped and draped. A Foley catheter is placed in the bladder. The exact location of the fascia lata strap is located by palpation, and a 3–4-cm vaginal mucosal incision is made.

**2** The vaginal mucosa is separated with Allis forceps. The strap is located and picked up with thumb forceps and is transected with a small knife. G-S identifies the Goebell-Stoeckel strap.

**3** The edges of the vaginal mucosa are approximated in the midline with 3-0 synthetic absorbable suture. If necessary, a Foley catheter can be inserted transurethrally or suprapubically.

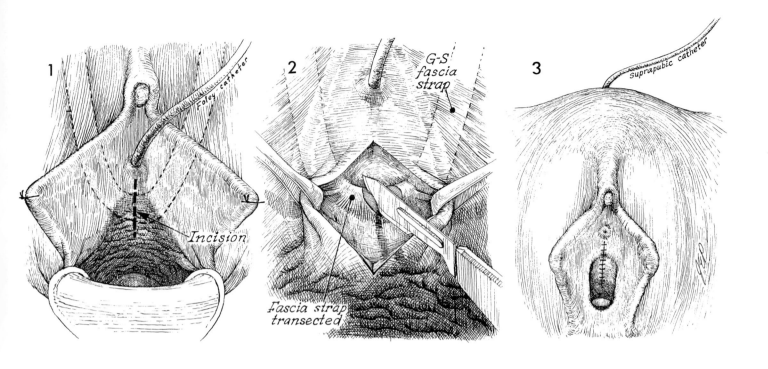

1    Foley catheter    Incision

2    G-S fascia strap    Fascia strap transected

3    suprapubic catheter

# Rectovaginal Fistula Repair via Musset-Poitout-Noble Perineotomy

Rectovaginal fistula in developed countries is predominately secondary to (1) gynecologic surgical procedures and (2) failed episiotomy repairs. In less developed countries, a rectovaginal fistula is generally the sequela from pressure necrosis of prolonged and obstructed labor.

Fistulae secondary to cancer therapy (surgical or radiation induced) require special techniques not required of rectovaginal fistulae associated with benign gynecologic surgery, failed episiotomies, and obstetrical delivery.

Modern surgical suture has a significant influence on the successful closure of these fistulae. Woven suture products, synthetic or nonsynthetic, are associated with microabscesses in the fistula repair. Bacteria become entwined in the woven suture product, and thus the suture product acts as a wick carrying bacteria to the wound. With the use of monofilament synthetic absorbable suture, we no longer return patients to the operating room on the eighth postoperative day for removal of permanent sutures such as woven Mersilene and silk. There is debate as to whether it is preferable to use monofilament delayed synthetic absorbable suture or a synthetic rapidly absorbable suture. Currently, we use the monofilament delayed synthetic absorbable suture on all layers of the fistula repair. Suture abscesses have been reduced. Therefore, until we have further data, we will continue to use the monofilament delayed synthetic absorbable suture polydioxanone rather than the monofilament synthetic absorbable suture poliglecaprone.

**Physiologic Changes.** The main physiologic change after repair of a rectovaginal fistula is to eliminate stool flowing from the rectum through the vagina. Concern may exist for the competence and continuity of the transected and reconstructed anal sphincter muscle. Transection of an otherwise competent anal sphincter and careful and proper reconstruction with suturing the fascia of the muscle should not be associated with incompetence of the sphincter and fecal incontinence secondary to that incompetent sphincter.

**Points of Caution.** Rectovaginal fistulae may present as multiple fistulae in a so-called honeycomb appearance or as one single fistula. It is important to excise the entire fistula tract of all fistulae.

# Rectovaginal Fistula Repair
## via Musset-Poitout-Noble Perineotomy
### (Continued)

---

## Technique

**1** Figure 1 shows several rectovaginal fistulae with a honeycomb appearance. An incision that encompasses the entire fistulae should be made in the posterior vaginal wall mucosa.

**2** The fistula tract has been removed down to the rectal mucosa. The margins of the vagina that remain are elevated and mobilized with sharp dissection. A perineotomy incision is made through the vagina, the superficial transverse peritonea (*STP*), the anal sphincter, and anal mucosa.

**3** Figure 3 illustrates the surgical removal of the fistulae, the perineotomy with the transected anal sphincter, the transected superficial transverse peritonea, and the rectovaginal space that has been developed surgically between the vaginal mucosa and the rectum (*R*).

**4** The rectum is repaired with a far-near–near-far Connell inverting suture that inverts the mucosa into the lumen of the rectum. Care is taken that the knot is tied in the rectum to prevent the knot from becoming a wick for bacteria in this area.

**5** The rectum is repaired down to the anal mucosa; the sutures are then cut. *1–5*.

**6** Figure 6 shows the anterior rectal wall with far-near–near-far sutures in place. The excess suture outside the knot can be cut. This differs from the traditional technique where woven suture products were used, since the sutures had to be left long so they could be removed from the wound on the seventh postoperative day. After the rectal mucosa has been sutured, a decision must be made to bring in an exterior source of blood supply, such as the bulbocavernosus muscles with their vestibular fat pad. If that is to be performed, it should be performed at this point, and the bulbocavernosus muscle with its fat pad should be sutured over the rectal suture line before beginning the posterior repair with plication of the levator muscle in the midline.

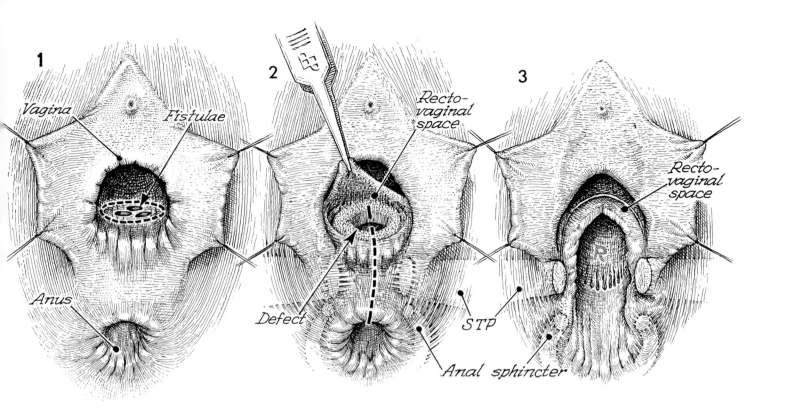

**1**

*Vagina*

*Fistulae*

*Anus*

**2**

*Recto-vaginal space*

*Defect*

*STP*

*Anal sphincter*

**3**

*Recto-vaginal space*

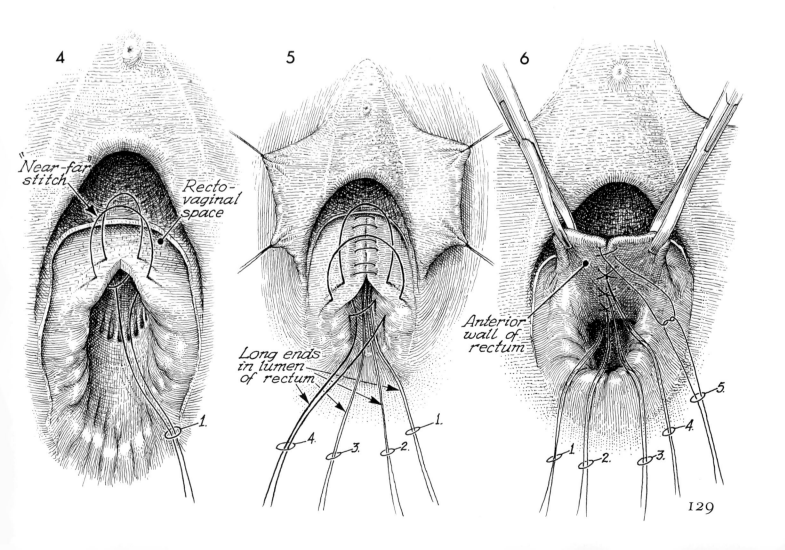

**4**

*"Near-far" stitch*

*Recto-vaginal space*

*1.*

**5**

*Long ends in lumen of rectum*

*4.* *3.* *2.* *1.*

**6**

*Anterior wall of rectum*

*1.* *2.* *3.* *4.* *5.*

# Rectovaginal Fistula Repair
# via Musset-Poitout-Noble Perineotomy

## (Continued)

**7** After the rectal mucosa has been sutured closed, the finger of the left hand is placed on top of the rectal suture line. This invagination produces prominence of the levator ani muscles. Delayed synthetic absorbable suture is placed in the levator muscles to plicate them on top of the rectal suture line.

**8** The levator plication has taken place over the rectal suture line. The stumps of the superficial transverse peritonea muscle must be identified, especially with their fascia sheaths. The anal sphincter muscle should be identified, and care should be taken to identify its fascia sheath. Sutures are placed through the fascia sheath and muscle. Generally, four sutures are used in a points-of-the-compass pattern.

**9** Figure 9 shows the rectal mucosa sutured. The levator ani muscles have been plicated over the rectal mucosa, the anal sphincter is plicated in the midline, and now the stumps of the superficial transverse peritonea (STP) muscle are identified, and sutures are placed in the fascia of this muscle in a points-of-the-compass pattern.

**10** The vaginal mucosa is closed with a running synthetic absorbable suture. Note that the knot is tied at the top of the vagina, and one strand of the knot is left long, coming on top of the levator repair underneath the vaginal mucosa. This strand of suture, when tied, will further plicate the top of the vagina posteriorly on top of the rectum, creating the so-called hockey-stick pattern of the vaginal canal.

**11** The suture has been extended out over to the skin of the peritoneal body. Note that the long end is tied to the end of the running suture. When this is performed, the upper vagina is pulled posteriorly onto the rectum.

**12** A finger could be inserted in the vagina, and a finger should be inserted in the rectum. These fingers should make a 90° angle. Postoperatively, the patient is placed on running daily doses of mineral oil and a low-residue diet. We would prefer the patient have loose watery stools every day for 2 weeks. After each watery stool, she should be cleaned with a septic solution.

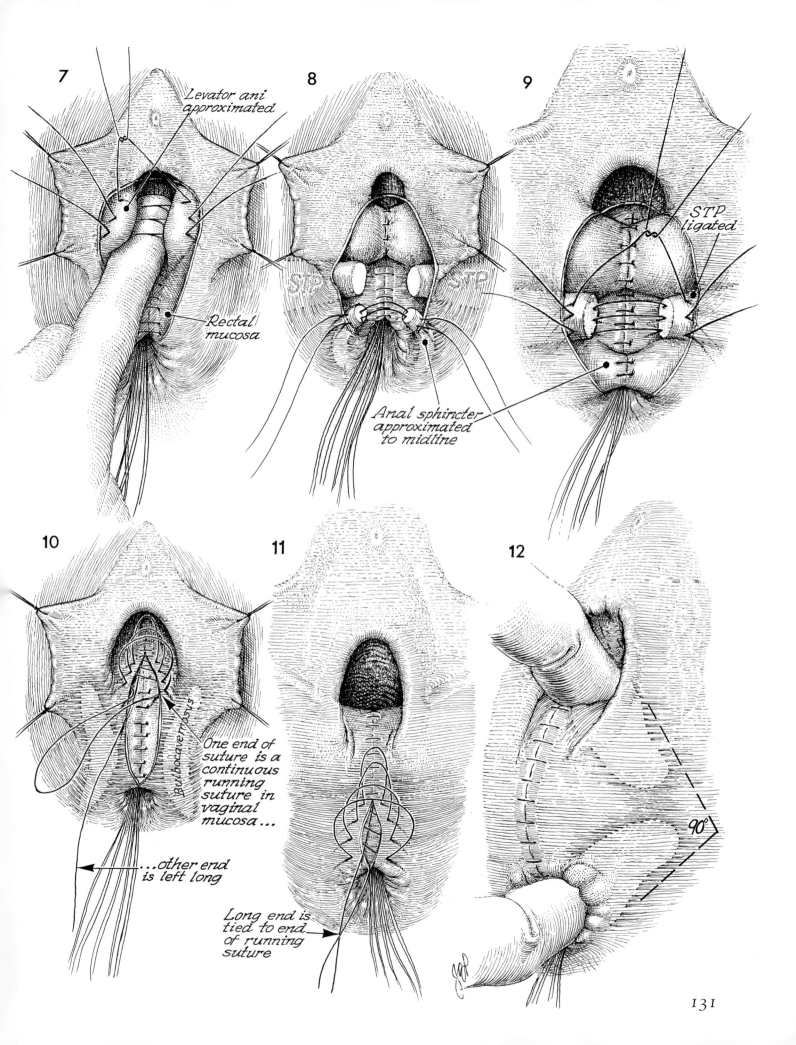

**7**

Levator ani
approximated

Rectal
mucosa

**8**

STP    STP

Anal sphincter
approximated
to midline

**9**

STP
ligated

**10**

Bulbocavernosus

One end of
suture is a
continuous
running
suture in
vaginal
mucosa...

...other end
is left long

**11**

Long end is
tied to end
of running
suture

**12**

90°

131

# Sigmoid Neovagina

The use of intestine for a neovagina adds an additional procedure to the formation of a neovagina. Traditional techniques for neovagina have included myocutaneous flaps, skin grafts, skin grafts applied to omental cylinders, and combinations thereof. The normal nonirradiated sigmoid colon may represent an ideal structure to become a neovagina. Unlike the small intestine, which has excessive necrotizing secretions, the mucosa of the sigmoid colon has secretions that are less necrotizing and less copious. The advantages of the sigmoid neovagina over skin grafts of various kinds are (1) it has its own inherent blood supply through the superior hemorrhoidal artery and sigmoid branches of that artery; and (2) it has distensibility through compliance unavailable in skin grafts. Although blood supply can be a positive aspect of sigmoid neovagina, the blood supply is critical. If for some reason the inferior mesenteric artery or the superior hemorrhoidal branch of the inferior mesenteric artery is compromised, the blood supply to the neovagina will be lost. A negative feature of sigmoid neovagina is that it requires an intestinal anastomosis between the descending left colon and the remaining rectum.

**Points of Caution.** Adequate mobilization of the descending colon must be achieved to prevent tension on the anastomosis. Adequate visualization of the superior hemorrhoidal artery and its sigmoid branches must be obtained.

The use of the vaginal form is controversial. There are those who believe that packing or a vaginal form is not necessary. Other surgeons routinely use foam rubber covered with a condom as a vaginal form to maintain dilation of the colon and/or neovagina.

---

## Technique

**1** Figure 1 shows a view of the pelvis in which a total supralevator exenteration has been performed. The stump of the urethral meatus, the stump of the vagina at the level of the introitus, and the stump of the rectum at the level of the peritoneum are noted.

**2** Sigmoid neovagina is begun by mobilizing the left colon including the splenic flexure of the transverse colon. The inferior mesenteric artery and its branches, the left colic artery and the superior hemorrhoidal artery, are carefully identified. A segment of sigmoid colon approximately 14 cm long is selected. The colon is transected, the marginal artery of the colon is divided, and the incision is extended along the *dotted line* into the mesentery. At this point, several branches of the superior hemorrhoidal artery that feed the sigmoid branches are identified. An incision is made in the mesentery to the sigmoid colon neovagina, leaving several branches of the superior hemorrhoidal artery intact to act as blood supply for the entire colonic segment neovagina via the margin artery of the colon. *IVC* indicates the inferior vena cava.

**3** The transection into the mesentery and parallel to the colon within the mesentery but beneath the network of marginal vessels to the colon is necessary for the segment to be rotated into the antiperistaltic position to reach the vaginal introitus. That is, the proximal end of the sigmoid neovagina is rotated 180°, and the distal end of the colon now becomes the proximal end of the neovagina. This 180° rotation prevents excessive tension on the superior hemorrhoidal artery, jeopardizing its integrity.

**4** The proximal end of the sigmoid colon is pulled through the vaginal introitus. A prolapse of colon protruding approximately 3 cm out of the introitus is created, and sutures are placed between the colonic wall and introitus. A 3–4-cm segment of prolapse is essential because in the immediate postoperative period there will be a tendency for retraction. If the surgeon transects the colon flush with the introitus, there will be postoperative retraction and stricture. Note here that the rectal stump is still in place for a very low end-to-end anastomosis between the left colon and the rectum with the EEA stapler, performed in the routine manner as seen in Section 7, page 335.

**5** The completed operation shows a soft foam rubber vaginal form in the sigmoid neovagina, which is protruding 3–4 cm outside the introitus and is sutured into place with interrupted sutures. This is left in place for a minimum of 2–3 weeks. Excess prolapsed colon can be trimmed with an electric cautery as an outpatient procedure. After the wounds have healed, we do not continue to use the neovaginal foam rubber form. Sexual intercourse is allowed as soon as the patient's wounds have healed and it becomes comfortable.

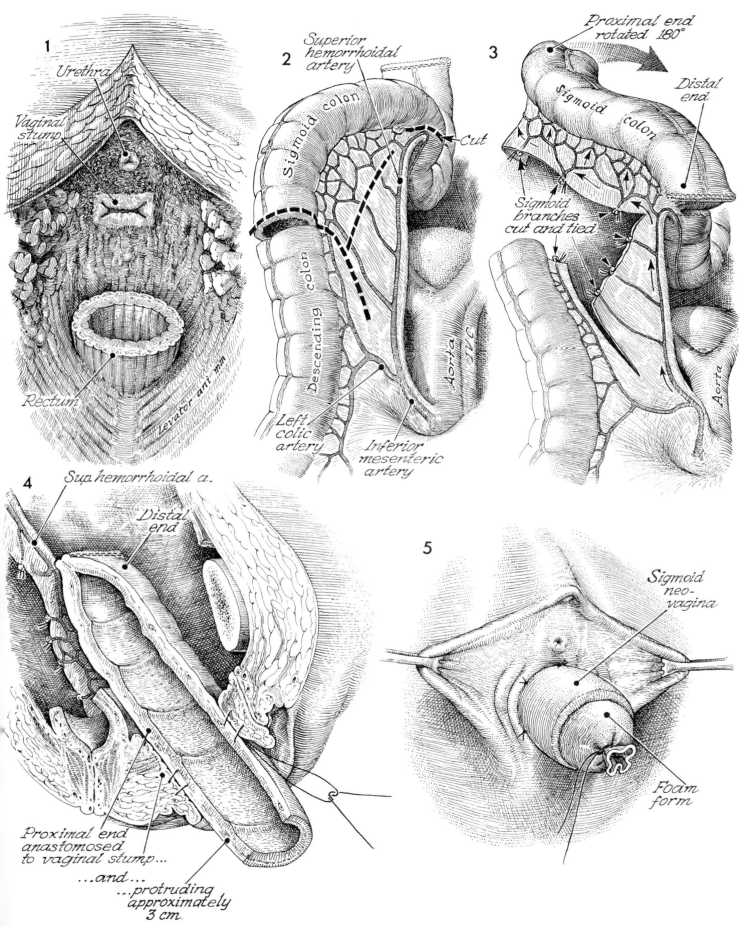

**1**

Urethra

Vaginal stump

Rectum

Levator ani mm.

**2**

Superior hemorrhoidal artery

Sigmoid colon

Descending colon

Cut

Aorta

I.V.C.

Left colic artery

Inferior mesenteric artery

**3**

Proximal end rotated 180°

Sigmoid colon

Distal end

Sigmoid branches cut and tied

Aorta

**4**

Sup. hemorrhoidal a.

Distal end

Proximal end anastomosed to vaginal stump...

...and...

...protruding approximately 3 cm.

**5**

Sigmoid neo-vagina

Foam form

# 3

## Bladder and Ureter

# Insertion of Suprapubic Catheter

Dissection at the base of the bladder to reach the anterior vaginal wall and uterine cervix creates edema, interrupts the small nerve pathways, and thereby sets up the physiologic changes that produce urinary bladder atony. Therefore, catheter drainage of the urinary bladder is an essential feature of many pelvic surgical procedures. Fortunately, in most cases, these conditions reverse themselves in 3–5 days, and catheter drainage is no longer needed.

Suprapubic bladder catheterization is superior to transurethral bladder catheterization because it is cleaner. It also leaves the urethra open for voiding when urinary function has returned. The use of an ordinary Foley catheter (No. 16 French with 5-mL bag) is preferable to the commercially available suprapubic catheter kits because a Foley catheter, when inserted as described in this section, is usually not dislodged from the bladder during sleep or activity. In addition, the Foley catheter is less costly and is available in all surgical clinics. The instrument used for insertion of the Foley catheter is an ordinary Randall stone forceps. The fulcrum of this instrument is toward the rear, which keeps the overall diameter of the axis virtually unchanged except at the jaws and gives it an advantage over a Kelly clamp.

The operation provides drainage of the urinary bladder through a clean surgical incision and ensures that the catheter does not slip out of the patient or become dislodged within the abdominal wall.

**Physiologic Changes.** The procedure reduces edema at the base of the bladder, allowing the return of normal vesical function.

**Points of Caution.** After grasping the catheter with the jaws of the Randall forceps (Fig. 4) and before inflating the Foley balloon, the catheter should be drawn through the bladder until the tip can be seen in the urethral meatus. This ensures that the catheter tip and balloon are in the bladder and not in the subcutaneous or subfascial space.

## Technique

**1** This procedure can be performed in the inpatient treatment rooms of a hospital, clinic, or doctor's office. Local anesthesia is adequate for most patients. The bladder does not have to be empty. The patient is placed in the dorsal lithotomy position. The periurethral area and suprapubic area are surgically prepped and draped. A routine pelvic examination is performed prior to placement of the suprapubic catheter. If local anesthesia is to be used, a 4 × 4-cm area around the insertion site is infiltrated with 1% lidocaine. Infiltration should include the fascia and, if at all possible, a small area of the bladder wall.

**2** A Randall stone forceps is inserted through the urethral meatus and used to elevate the dome of the bladder from the inside, pushing the suprapubic abdominal wall upward to the palpating finger.

**3** Upward pressure is maintained on the forceps, and a small incision is made in the suprapubic skin and fascia until the forceps can be felt with the blade of the knife.

**4** A sudden upward thrust of the forceps pierces the bladder wall and pushes the forceps through the incision. The jaws of the forceps are opened and used to grasp the tip of the Foley catheter.

**5** The Foley catheter is pulled through the bladder, and the forceps is withdrawn from the urethra until the tip of the Foley catheter can be seen in the urethral meatus.

**6** Traction is placed on the Foley catheter from above while the balloon is simultaneously inflated. This draws the catheter back into the body of the bladder.

**7** When 5 mL of sterile saline solution have completely filled the Foley balloon, the catheter is firmly retracted upward.

It is not necessary to suture the catheter to the abdominal skin. A sterile dressing is applied, and the Foley catheter is connected to straight drainage.

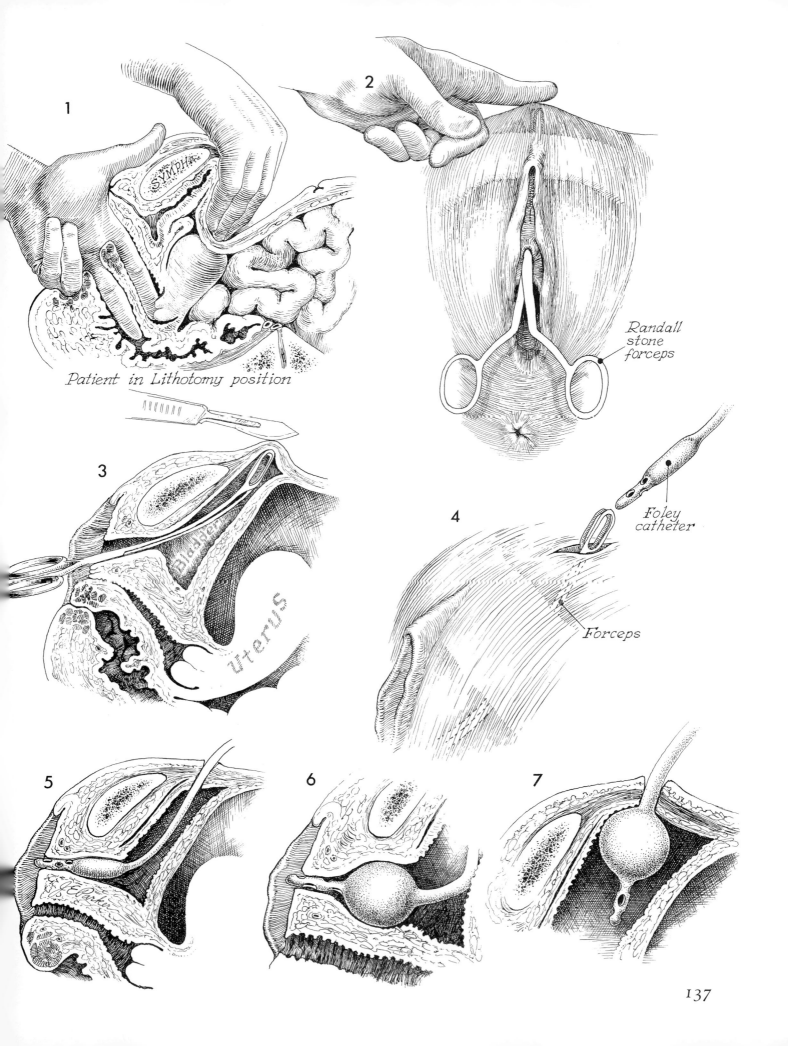

**1**

SYMPH

Patient in Lithotomy position

**2**

Randall
stone
forceps

**3**

Bladder

Uterus

**4**

Foley
catheter

Forceps

**5**

Bladder

**6**

**7**

# Retropubic Urethropexy: Marshall-Marchetti-Krantz and Burch Operations

The Marshall-Marchetti-Krantz (MMK) and Burch operations for stress incontinence of urine are two of the retropubic urethropexy "pin-up" operations that essentially return the urethrovesical angle to its role as an intra-abdominal organ and change the focal points of pressure applied through the abdomen during a Valsalva maneuver (coughing, sneezing, etc.).

Unlike other stress incontinence operations, the Marshall-Marchetti-Krantz and Burch operations do not, by themselves, produce significant changes in intraurethral or intravesical pressure to restore urinary continence.

The operations have evolved with several alterations since their original introduction by Marshall-Marchetti-Krantz and Burch. These procedures can be performed at the time of pelvic surgery for uterine or adnexal pathology.

The purpose of these operations is to eliminate stress incontinence of urine.

These operations do not correct a cystourethrocele. When this is present, it should be surgically corrected through the vagina.

**Physiologic Changes.** The Marshall-Marchetti-Krantz and Burch operations rarely change the relationship between intraurethral pressure and intravesical pressure. They make the proximal urethra and bladder neck an intra-abdominal organ and equalize intra-abdominal pressures on the bladder wall that are precipitated by a Valsalva maneuver.

**Points of Caution.** To ensure the integrity of the bladder and ureters, a cystotomy should be performed, and the bladder should be inspected under direct vision.

When operating in the space of Retzius, bleeding from the plexus of Santorini can be difficult to control. Total hemostasis is essential before these operations are completed.

# Retropubic Urethropexy: Marshall-Marchetti-Krantz and Burch Operations

## (Continued)

## Technique

**1** For the Marshall-Marchetti-Krantz and Burch operations, the patient is placed in the supine lithotomy position, i.e., the ski position. There are two acceptable incisions, the lower midline incision and the transverse incision. Each has its advocates. It is difficult to demonstrate superior results with either incision. The supine lithotomy position (ski) with a transverse incision is preferred unless the patient is undergoing surgery for a gynecologic oncologic problem.

The patient is prepped and draped, and a Foley catheter with a 30-mL bag is inserted.

**2** The incision is made in the rectus fascia. The fascia is excised.

**3** The space of Retzius is entered. The bladder and the urethrovaginal angle are identified with the aid of the Foley catheter.

**4** A finger is inserted in the vagina to identify the perivaginal and periurethral areas for placement of 0 Prolene suture. We prefer permanent monofilament suture. A small, curved Mayo needle is used, and the position of the suture is confirmed by palpating the bladder and inserting a finger in the vagina before making each suture. Notice blanching of the blood vessels in the plexus of Santorini. The blood vessels should be avoided in placing the sutures in the periurethral tissues.

**5** In **a,** showing the MMK operation, the suture that has been placed in the periurethral tissue is tied to the periosteum of the pubic symphysis. In **b,** showing the Burch operation, the suture that has been placed in the periurethral tissue has been brought through the conjoined tendon or Cooper's ligament.

In **a,** bleeding has been produced from the vessels in the plexus of Santorini.

**6** The bleeding produced from the plexus of Santorini can be easily stopped by elevating the finger in the vagina. This allows for fulgurating or grasping and tying each of the bleeders specifically. The blood vessels form the plexus of Santorini and are difficult to control if elevation of the vagina is not used to slow the bleeding process. The suture placed in the periurethral tissue is tied, respectively, to either the periosteum (MMK) **(a)** or Cooper's ligament (Burch) **(b).**

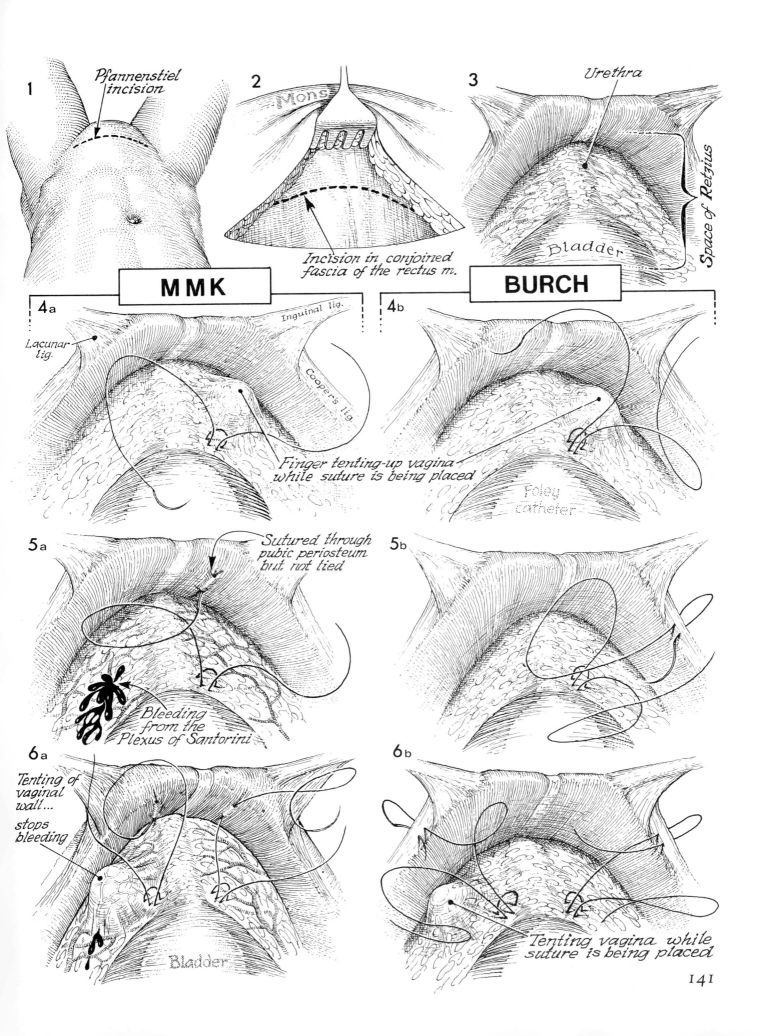

1.   Pfannenstiel incision

2.   Mons — Incision in conjoined fascia of the rectus m.

3.   Urethra — Bladder — Space of Retzius

**MMK**    **BURCH**

4a   Lacunar lig.    Inguinal lig.    Cooper's lig.    Finger tenting-up vagina while suture is being placed

4b   Foley catheter

5a   Sutured through pubic periosteum but not tied    Bleeding from the Plexus of Santorini

5b

6a   Tenting of vaginal wall... stops bleeding    Bladder

6b   Tenting vagina while suture is being placed

141

# Retropubic Urethropexy: Marshall-Marchetti-Krantz and Burch Operations

## (Continued)

**7** The sutures have been completely placed but not tied.

**8** In **a** (MMK), two vaginal fingers are used to tent up the anterior wall of the vagina while the sutures are being tied. The same is noted in **b** (Burch), as the sutures are tied to Cooper's ligament.

**9** In **a** (MMK), the sutures are completely tied to the periosteum of the symphysis pubis. An additional one or two sutures can be placed if desired.

In **b** (Burch), a finger is inserted between the conjoined tendon or Cooper's ligament and the suture in the periurethral tissue. A 2-cm space (1 fingerbreadth) is desirable to prevent total occlusion of the urethra and postoperative urinary retention.

**10** In **a** (MMK), the periurethral tissue with the adjacent pubovesical cervical (PVC) fascia sling is sutured to the periosteum of the symphysis pubis. The bladder (B) and proximal urethra have been brought back into the abdomen where intraurethral and intravesical pressures can be stabilized. In **b** (Burch), the urethra has been suspended by the pubovesical cervical fascia sling sutured to Cooper's ligament.

In reality, the pubovesical cervical fascia in both operations has been made into a sling to bring the proximal one-third of the urethra and the neck of the bladder back into the abdomen. This new position allows even disposition of external pressures on all surfaces of the bladder and proximal urethra. The rectum (R) and vagina (V) are shown in **a**.

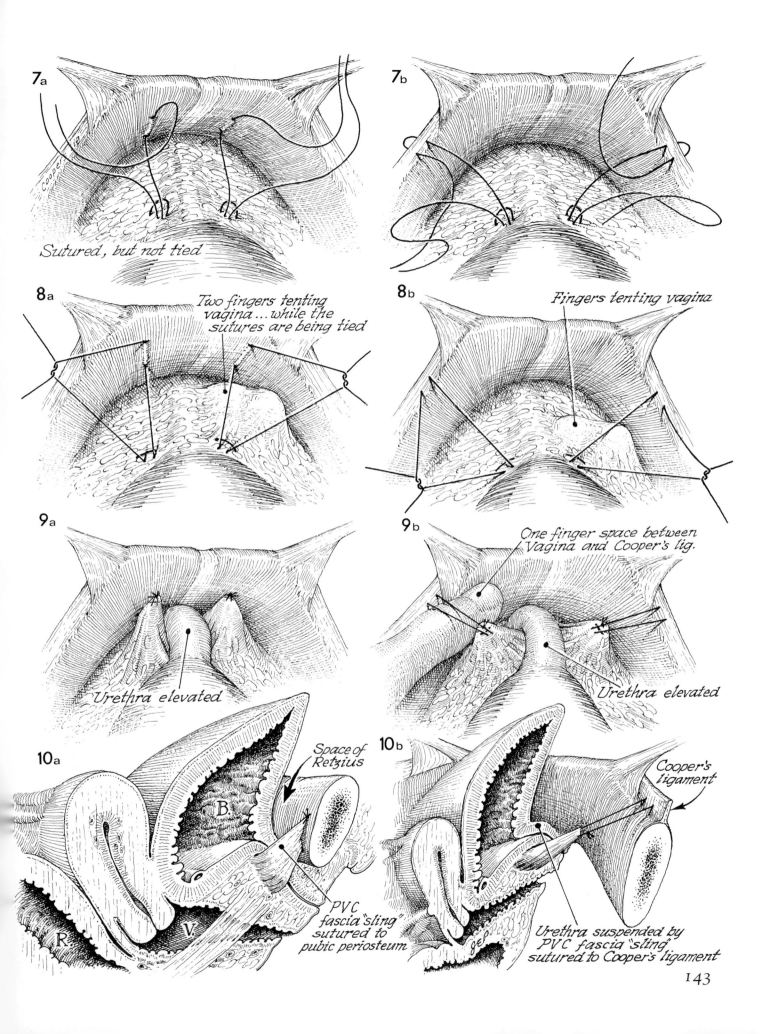

**7a**

*Sutured, but not tied*

**7b**

**8a**

*Two fingers tenting vagina...while the sutures are being tied*

**8b**

*Fingers tenting vagina*

**9a**

*Urethra elevated*

**9b**

*One finger space between Vagina and Cooper's lig.*

*Urethra elevated*

**10a**

*Space of Retzius*

B.

V.

R

*PVC fascia "sling" sutured to pubic periosteum*

**10b**

*Cooper's ligament*

*Urethra suspended by PVC fascia "sling" sutured to Cooper's ligament*

143

# Ureteroureterostomy

Injury to the ureter is occasionally high enough in the pelvis for a primary ureteroureterostomy to be performed without having to resort to a ureteroneocystostomy. In these cases, the ureter has been damaged at or near the pelvic brim while clamping, incising, and ligating the infundibulopelvic ligament or while excising an extensive ovarian carcinoma that has distorted the pelvic anatomy at or near the pelvic brim. Although less common than procedures for correcting lower injuries to the ureter, a ureteroureterostomy is preferable to a ureteroneocystostomy when it can be performed without tension on the anastomosis producing the stenosis.

The essential features of the procedure are the adequate mobilization of the cut ends of the ureter to prevent tension on the anastomosis, the use of a spatulated anastomosis, and the use of delicate suture, meticulous hemostasis, and drainage of the anastomosis site via a closed suction drain through the lower abdominal wall.

The purpose of the ureteroureterostomy is to anastomose the transected ureter.

**Physiologic Changes.** After a damaged or diseased portion of the ureter has been removed, the ureter is anastomosed. The sequelae of ureteral obstruction and/or laceration are relieved.

**Points of Caution.** Care should be taken to see that the ureter is anastomosed without tension.

A soft Silastic indwelling catheter should be placed through the anastomotic area and fed into the bladder caudad and the renal pelvis cephalad.

The drain should be placed in the area of the anastomosis and brought out through the right or the left lower quadrant and kept in place until all external drainage has ceased.

## Technique

**1** The patient is placed in the dorsal position, and the abdomen is opened through a lower midline incision.

**2** The pelvis is cleared of adhesions and intestinal contents. Exposure of the pelvic structures is essential at all times. The pathologic site in the ureter is identified, and the peritoneum overlying the ureter at its junction with the common iliac artery is incised. Dissection of the ureter is carried down to the site of damage and/or stenosis.

**3** An appropriate segment of ureter is dissected out of its bed and mobilized between soft Silastic drains. Care is taken not to damage the ureteral sheath or the delicate network of vessels beneath the sheath that are vital to the vascularity of the ureter. The pathologic portion of ureter is excised with scissors.

**4** A Silastic ureteral catheter is inserted up to the renal pelvis and down into the bladder. Interrupted 4-0 synthetic absorbable sutures are placed through the entire wall of the ureter.

**5** The anastomosis has been completed over a Silastic ureteral catheter. Vessel loops are shown elevating the ureter.

**6** A closed suction drain site in the lower quadrant of the abdomen is selected. A Kelly clamp is passed down retroperitoneally, and a soft closed suction drain is brought out through the lower quadrant and is left adjacent to the anastomosis. The drain is used to prevent the collection of urine in the area of the anastomosis and should be left in place until all urinary drainage through it has ceased.

**7** The peritoneum is closed with interrupted 3-0 synthetic absorbable sutures over the ureteroureterostomy so that the ureter remains retroperitoneal.

The Silastic ureteral catheter is removed at the time of water cystoscopy 10–12 days postoperatively. A urologic workup should be performed 6 weeks following the anastomosis and 3 months thereafter to ensure against stenosis and hydronephrosis.

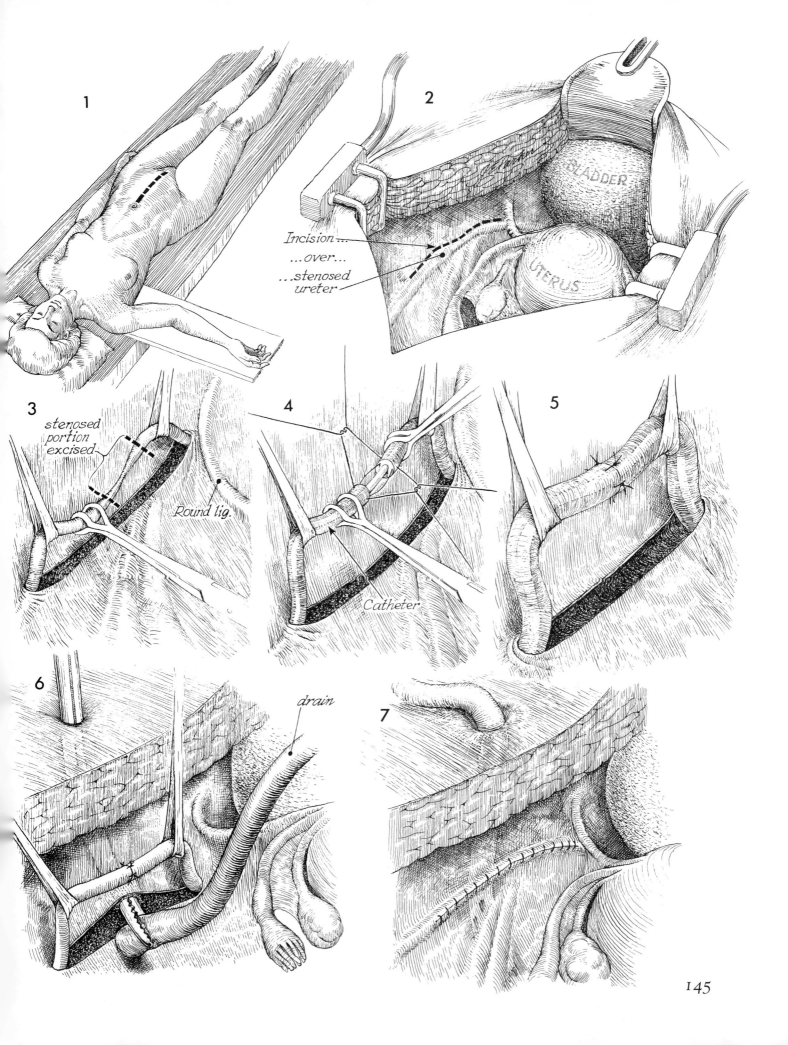

**1**

**2**

Incision...

...over...

...stenosed ureter

BLADDER

UTERUS

**3**

stenosed portion excised

Round lig.

**4**

Catheter

**5**

**6**

drain

**7**

145

# Ureteroneocystostomy and Ureteroneocystostomy With Bladder Flap

Reimplantation of the ureter into the bladder is necessary in cases of congenital anomaly or damage to the ureter secondary to pelvic surgery or irradiation. If there is total obstruction of the ureter, a percutaneous needle nephrostomy should be attempted, and surgical repair should be delayed until ideal conditions for repair are achieved. Every hour that the kidney remains totally obstructed, progressive damage to the kidney occurs.

Important points in the procedure are (1) full mobilization of the bladder to prevent tension on the anastomosis; (2) leaving a Silastic ureteral stent catheter in the ureter for at least 10–14 days; (3) adequate drainage of the implantation site to prevent urinary ascites; and (4) thorough postoperative cystoscopic evaluation with intravenous pyelogram.

**Physiologic Changes.** The ureter is reimplanted into the bladder, if possible, and if not possible, a flap of bladder can be developed into a tube that can be made and anastomosed to the ureter at or near the pelvic brim.

The issue of tunneling the ureter through the bladder wall to prevent reflux remains an open question. In some cases, reflux of urine and its associated urinary tract infection can produce pathologic changes of the upper urinary tracts. Reflux is unusual, however, in adults who do not have a congenital neuromuscular malformation within the walls of their ureter. This problem is generally confined to children or young adults with a neuromuscular malformation in the ureter.

**Points of Caution.** The surgeon must be confident that the ureter can be reimplanted without tension.

A mucosal-to-mucosal anastomosis should be performed. A Silastic catheter stent should be inserted through the anastomosis and coiled into the bladder, with the opposite end placed in the renal pelvis.

The bladder flap must have sufficient width to its base to provide an adequate blood supply at the tip of the flap.

---

## Technique

### URETERONEOCYSTOSTOMY

**1** A thorough bimanual and speculum examination of the pelvis should be performed prior to ureteroneocystostomy.

**2** Two mL of indigo carmine solution are injected intravenously prior to the procedure to provide a urinary marker for fast identification of the ureter in the distorted pelvic anatomy. If there is confusion as to whether a tubular structure is a ureter or a blood vessel, aspiration with a 21-gauge needle and a 5-mL syringe will yield the blue dye from the indigo carmine if the structure is the ureter.

**3** The patient is operated on in the supine position. A lower midline incision is made.

**4** The peritoneum is entered, and the omentum and intestinal contents are dissected out of the pelvic cavity.

**5** The peritoneum over the ureteral area is incised at the bifurcation of the common iliac artery, and the dissection is continued into the pelvis until the damaged portion of the ureter is exposed.

**6** The ureter is transected above the damage, and the distal end is tied with 0 synthetic absorbable suture. The proximal portion is dissected out of its bed with careful surgical technique to ensure the continuity of the ureteral sheath that is so important for adequate blood supply to the ureter.

**7** The bladder is mobilized by entering the space of Retzius behind the pubic symphysis and dissecting the bladder cephalad so that a portion of posterior bladder wall meets the proximal portion of ureter to be implanted. The dome of the bladder is picked up with Allis clamps, and a cystostomy is made by cautery.

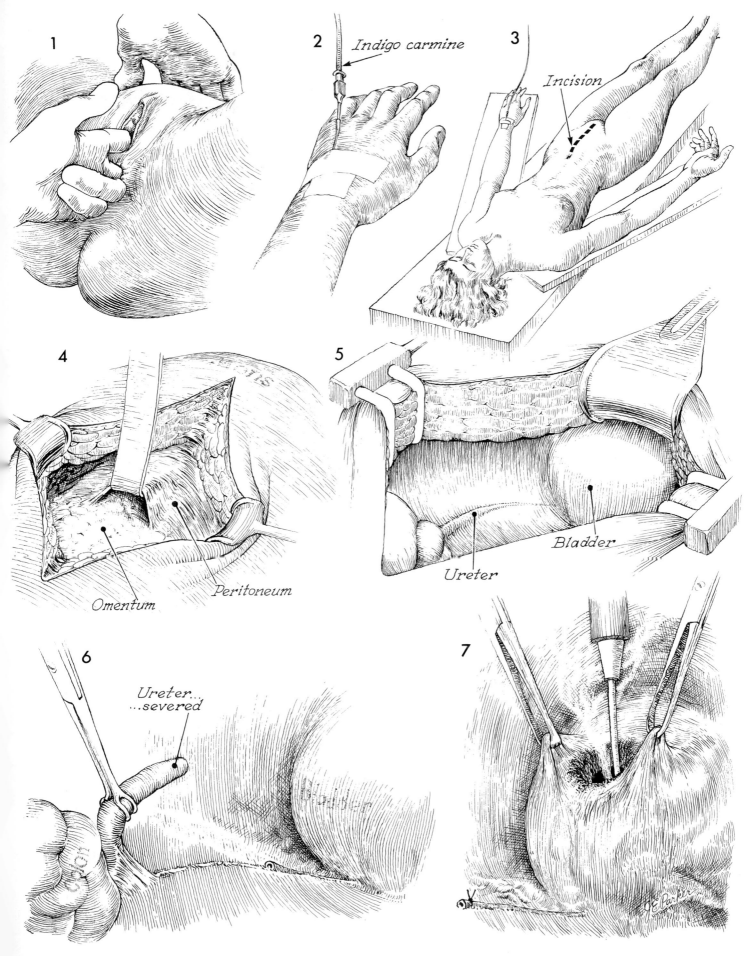

**1**

**2** *Indigo carmine*

**3** *Incision*

**4** *Omentum*    *Peritoneum*

**5** *Ureter*    *Bladder*

**6** *Ureter... ...severed*

**7**

# Ureteroneocystostomy and Ureteroneocystostomy With Bladder Flap

## (Continued)

**8** The defect is expanded by blunt dissection with the finger to reduce bleeding.

**9** The bladder is brought into position adjacent to the proximal portion of the ureter to ensure that there is adequate mobilization of the bladder and that the anastomosis will be free of tension.

**10** A Kelly clamp is inserted in the bladder through the cystostomy and pressed against the bladder wall at a point adjacent to the ureter to be implanted. The Kelly clamp is advanced through the bladder wall and opened sufficiently to allow at least a 2-cm defect. The tip of the ureter is sutured with a 3-0 suture and grasped with the Kelly clamp.

**11** The ureter is drawn into the bladder through the cystostomy.

**12** A No. 8 French Silastic double-J ureteral stent catheter is inserted into the ureter and advanced to the renal pelvis. A small fish-mouth incision is made at the 3 and 9 o'clock positions in the ureter with scissors or a scalpel to prevent iris contracture at the anastomosis.

**13** Under direct vision the ureter is anastomosed mucosa to mucosa to the bladder with interrupted 4-0 synthetic absorbable suture.

**14** A Finney "J" catheter stent is inserted up into the ureter. The J catheter stent is designed to prevent peristalsis from pushing the catheter out of the ureter and into the bladder. We prefer to leave the catheter in the bladder for a minimum of 12 days and, in irradiated patients, for approximately 3 weeks.

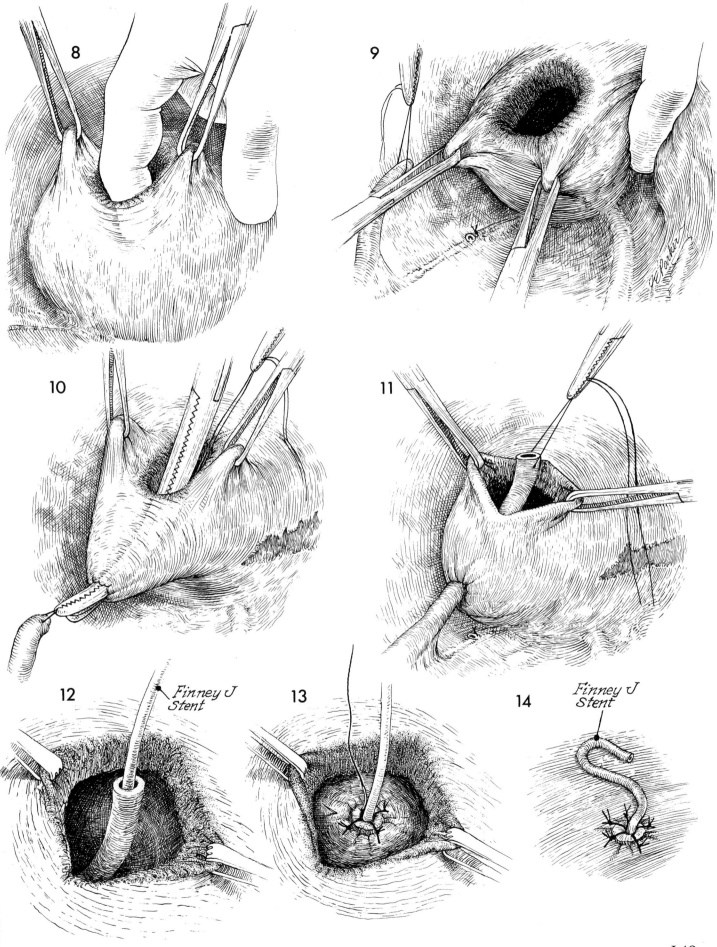

8

9

10

11

12    *Finney J*
      *Stent*

13

14    *Finney J*
      *Stent*

# Ureteroneocystostomy and Ureteroneocystostomy With Bladder Flap

## (Continued)

**15** To ensure that the anastomosis will be free of tension, a site on the psoas fascia is located, and the dome of the bladder is sutured to it with multiple interrupted 0 synthetic absorbable sutures. The bladder is mobilized by entering the space of Retzius.

**16** A soft closed suction drain is placed through the lower quadrant of the abdomen adjacent to the ureteroneocystostomy. The cystostomy in the dome of the bladder is closed with interrupted 3-0 synthetic absorbable sutures in two layers. Three of the first layer sutures are shown.

**17** A running 3-0 synthetic absorbable suture is used to close the bladder musculature and serosa.

**18** An additional closed suction drain is placed through the opposite lower quadrant and brought adjacent to the anastomosed area. These drains should remain in place until no urinary drainage is noted.

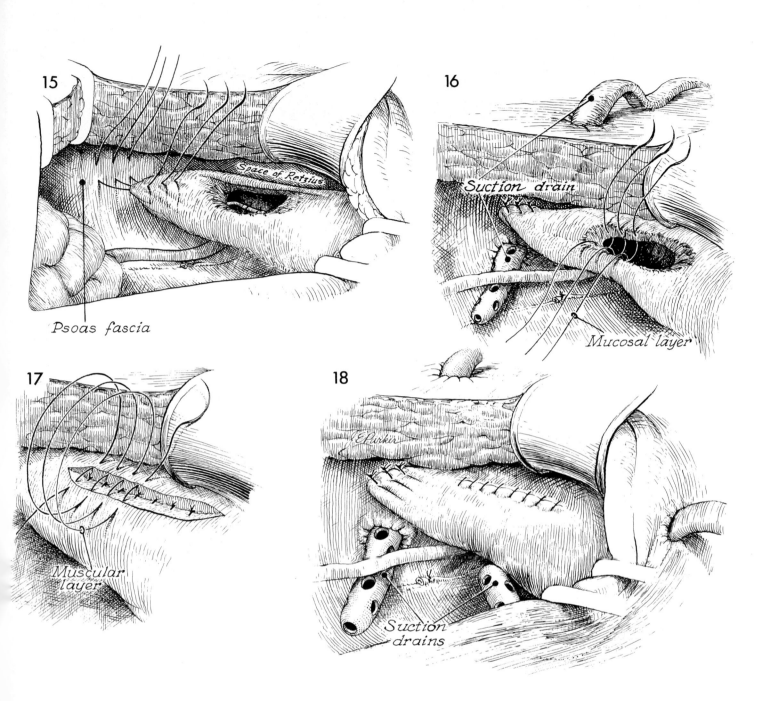

15

Space of Retzius

Psoas fascia

16

Suction drain

Mucosal layer

17

Muscular layer

18

E. Parker

Suction drains

# Ureteroneocystostomy and Ureteroneocystostomy With Bladder Flap

## (Continued)

BLADDER FLAP

**19** Occasionally, the excised portion of ureter is so great that anastomosis with the bladder cannot be made without tension. This is frequently the case in ureteral stricture resulting from irradiation. Rather than chance placing the ureteroneocystostomy under tension that will result in retraction of the ureter, stenosis, and eventually hydronephrosis, it is preferable to create a bladder flap from the dome of the bladder that can extend to the transected ureter. This is begun by measuring the distance between the bladder wall and the proximal portion of the ureter. This distance, usually 8–9 cm, is marked off on the posterior bladder wall with brilliant green in the area of insertion of the superior vesical artery. The flap is incised out of the bladder wall by use of scissors or scalpel. The base of the flap should be wider than the length. A No. 8 French Silastic ureteral catheter is inserted into the ureter to the renal pelvis.

**20** The flap is raised and brought into a position adjacent to the proximal portion of the ureter. Care must be taken at this point to ensure that there is no tension on the anastomosis. If an inadequate flap has been developed, the flap incisions may be extended at the base of the flap. The flap is rolled in a tubular fashion and closed with interrupted 4-0 synthetic absorbable suture over the catheter.

An end-to-end anastomosis between the proximal ureter and the tube flap is then made with interrupted 4-0 synthetic absorbable suture. A single layer of through-and-through 4-0 synthetic absorbable suture is used for closure of the tube flap, rather than the two-layer technique normally used on the bladder wall. This alteration in technique guards against stenosis in the bladder flap that could result from a two-layer closure.

**21** The bladder wall is closed by using the two-layer technique, the first layer on the bladder mucosa and the second layer on the muscle and serosa (as in Figs. 16 and 17). A closed suction drain is brought into the anastomosis site through the lower quadrant of the abdomen. The ureteral catheter is left in place for a minimum of 2 or 3 weeks. It is removed by water cystoscopy.

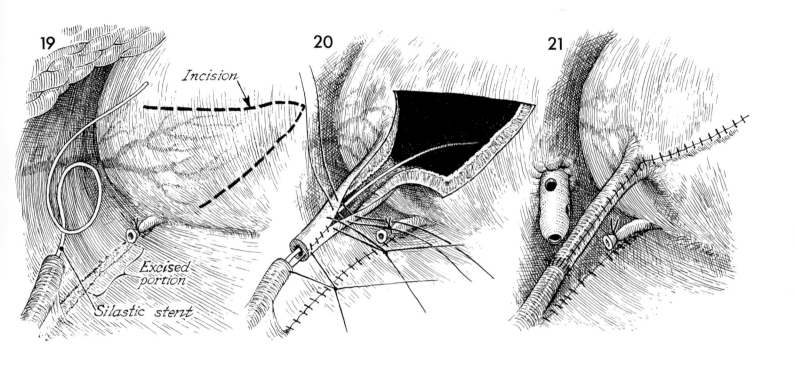

19    *Incision*

*Excised portion*

*Silastic stent*

20

21

# Transperitoneal Ureteroureterostomy (End-to-Side Anastomosis)

In some patients, resection of the terminal ureter is required for complete removal of a pelvic malignancy. In these cases, diversion of the urine must be achieved by either ureteroneocystostomy or transperitoneal ureteroureterostomy.

If the opposite ureter is normal and healthy and if there is any sizeable distance between the damaged ureter and the bladder, transperitoneal ureteroureterostomy is preferred. Postoperative stricture formation following ureteroneocystostomy is frequently produced by tension on the anastomotic suture line. Therefore, in these cases, end-to-side transperitoneal ureteroureterostomy may allow a tension-free anastomosis.

In those cases associated with pelvic irradiation, transperitoneal ureteroureterostomy allows diversion of the urine at a site outside the fields of irradiation without tension, thus avoiding the problem of stenosis in a surgical anastomosis within heavily irradiated tissue.

The basic concept of transperitoneal ureteroureterostomy is to bring the ureter from one side across the peritoneal cavity under the mesentery of the intestine to the healthy ureter on the opposite side and to anastomose it. We prefer to perform all of these anastomoses over a Silastic catheter stent that is left in place for approximately 2 weeks.

The purpose of the operation is to save the kidney, when its ureter has been injured or obstructed, by implanting that ureter in a healthy ureter on the opposite side to allow the free flow of urine from both kidneys through one ureter to the bladder.

**Physiologic Changes.** If stricture is avoided at the anastomotic site and if there is no obstruction to the terminal portion of the recipient ureter, few if any physiologic changes occur. A single ureter is capable of carrying the entire flow of urine from both kidneys. If the disease process has obstructed the ureter on one side, however, it may eventually obstruct the ureter on the opposite side, thus requiring a second diversion by ileal loop.

**Points of Caution.** Care should be taken to excise the damaged portion of the injured ureter. The affected ureter should be handled in a delicate manner to avoid damaging the network of vessels under the ureteral sheath that provides the blood supply to the ureter from the renal pelvis to the bladder. A 1 × ½-cm segment of the wall in the recipient ureter is removed for the anastomosis rather than making an incision into the ureter for the anastomosis. This, we feel, reduces the incidence of postoperative stricture formation. We prefer (1) to spatulate all ureteral anastomoses to prevent iris contracture and (2) to perform the anastomosis over a Silastic tube stent. The site of the anastomosis should be drained retroperitoneally through the lower quadrant by a closed suction drain.

# Transperitoneal Ureteroureterostomy (End-to-Side Anastomosis)

## (Continued)

*Technique*

**1** The patient is placed on the operating table in the dorsal supine lithotomy position. A Foley catheter has been placed in the bladder. The abdomen is opened through a lower midline incision.

**2** The peritoneum over the common iliac vessels of the affected side is elevated and opened with Metzenbaum scissors, exposing the entire path of the diseased or damaged ureter. The diseased portion of the ureter is identified. The distal segment of ureter going to the bladder is cross-clamped and tied with a 0 synthetic absorbable suture. The proximal segment of the ureter for implantation is carefully mobilized, preserving the blood supply by preventing damage to the ureteral sheath and the underlying network of vessels. All damaged portions of the ureter should be removed, and in cases of pelvic irradiation, the entire irradiated portion of the ureter should be removed. The peritoneum covering the mesentery of the large bowel is opened, and a tunnel is created under the mesentery. Care is taken to prevent damage to the vessels in the mesentery of the large bowel.

**3** The damaged ureter is brought through the tunnel in the mesentery of the large bowel. The peritoneum overlying the common iliac artery on the opposite side is elevated and opened. The healthy ureter is identified and dissected for an appropriate distance.

**4** The recipient ureter is elevated with a vein retractor. The ureter to be implanted is brought adjacent to the recipient ureter at a convenient site. Extreme care should be taken at this point to ensure that there is proper mobility and that there will be no tension on the suture line. The damaged ureter should be brought to the normal ureter. The normal ureter should be mobilized only enough to perform the anastomosis.

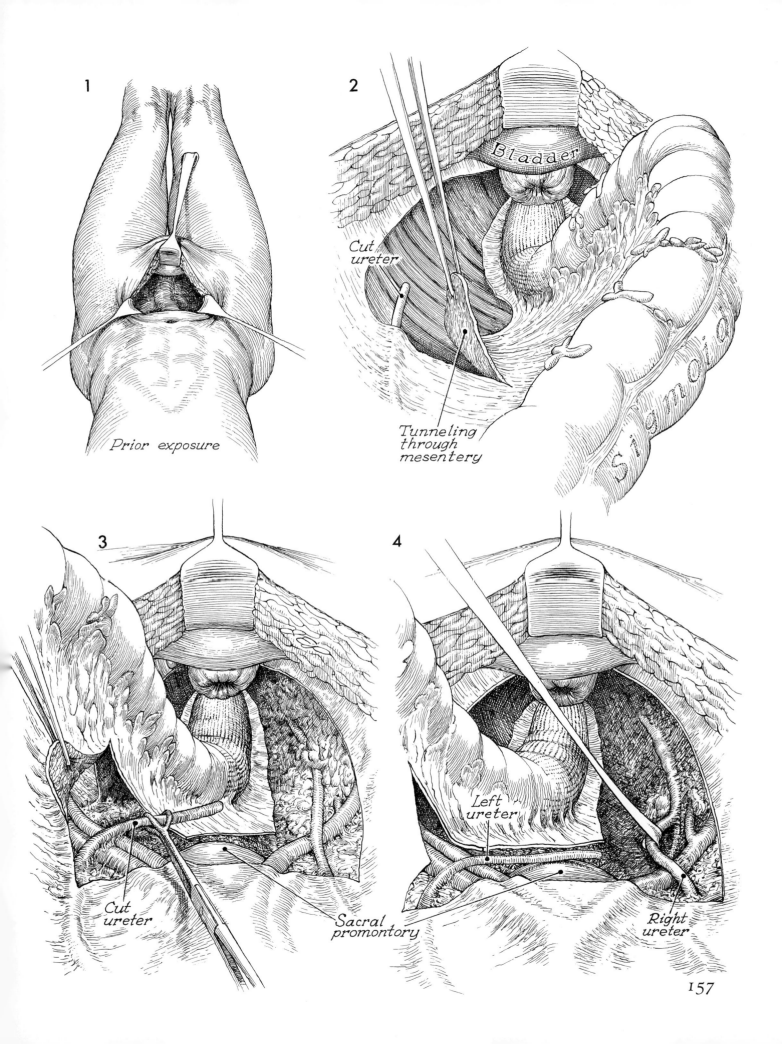

**1**

Prior exposure

**2**

Bladder

Cut
ureter

Tunneling
through
mesentery

Sigmoid

**3**

Cut
ureter

Sacral
promontory

**4**

Left
ureter

Right
ureter

157

# Transperitoneal Ureteroureterostomy (End-to-Side Anastomosis)

## (Continued)

**5** We prefer to perform all ureteral anastomoses over a Silastic tube stent. It is difficult to insert a flexible Silastic tube stent down the recipient ureter into the bladder. Therefore, we have evolved the following technique to bring a flexible Silastic tube into the bladder. A cystotomy is performed, and a No. 5 French whistle-tip ureteral catheter is inserted through the ureteral orifice up the recipient ureter to the area of ureterotomy. The No. 5 French whistle-tip ureteral catheter is passed through the defect in the recipient ureter and sutured to the Silastic T-tube with a 4-0 Prolene suture.

**6** The Silastic tube stent is then pulled through the distal ureter with the ureteral catheter into the bladder. The arms of the T-tube are passed into the recipient and the implanted ureters.

**7** The Silastic T-tube is coiled in the bladder. The cystotomy in the bladder is closed in two layers with 3-0 synthetic absorbable suture. The second arm of the T-tube is fed into the ureter to be implanted.

**8** The ureteroureterostomy end-to-side anastomosis is performed with interrupted 4-0 synthetic absorbable sutures in a through-and-through technique, creating a mucosa-to-mucosa anastomosis. A spatulated ureteral anastomosis is less likely to develop an iris contracture.

**9** The peritoneum is closed over the ureteral anastomosis. A closed suction drain is placed through the lower quadrant of the abdomen and brought retroperitoneally up to the site of the ureteroureterostomy. It is left in place until drainage ceases. A water cystoscopy is performed 2–3 weeks postoperatively, and the Silastic T-tube stent is removed. An intravenous pyelogram (IVP) is performed at that time and repeated every 2 months until the surgeon is satisfied with the results of the anastomosis.

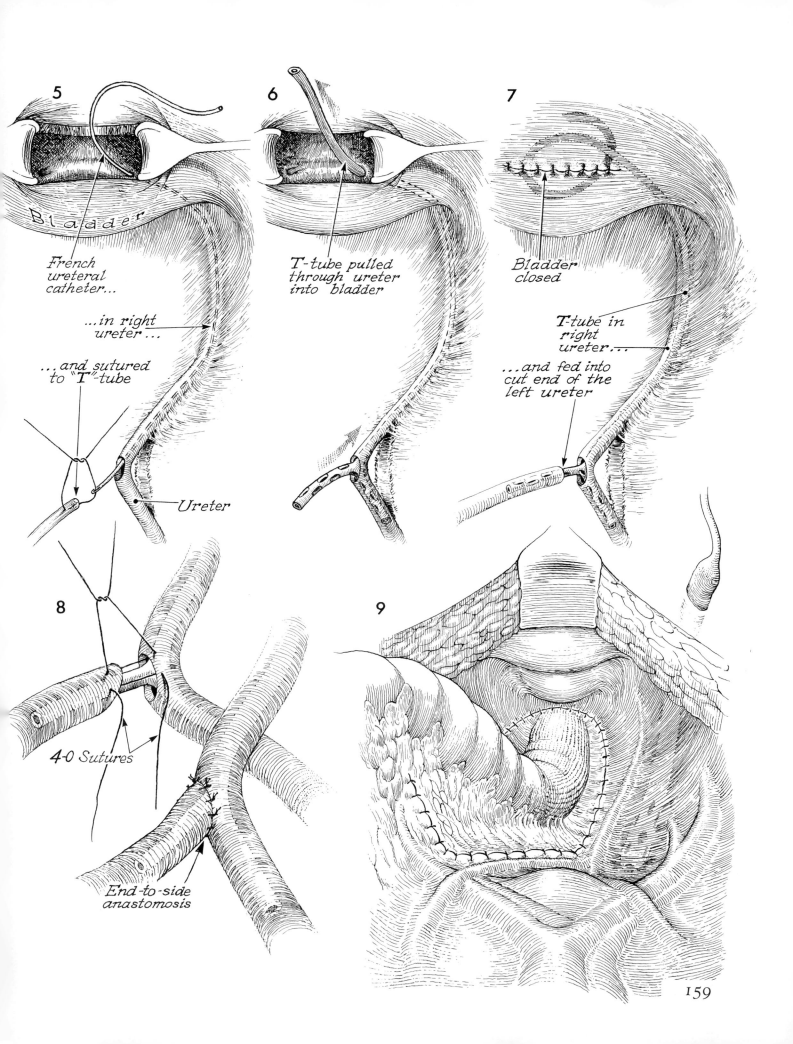

**5**

Bladder

French
ureteral
catheter...

...in right
ureter...

...and sutured
to "T"-tube

Ureter

**6**

T-tube pulled
through ureter
into bladder

**7**

Bladder
closed

T-tube in
right
ureter...

...and fed into
cut end of the
left ureter

**8**

4-0 Sutures

End-to-side
anastomosis

**9**

159

# Intestinal Loop Urinary Diversion

There are several ways in which the urinary system can be diverted: nephrostomy, cutaneous ureterostomy, ureterosigmoidostomy, intestinal loop urinary diversion, and continent urostomy. Intestinal loop is a good procedure for diverting the urine in elderly patients or in patients without sufficient bowel to perform one of the continent urostomies. This procedure began as an ileal loop urinary diversion. The colon loop urinary diversion eliminates the need for a bowel resection in the terminal ileum. This is particularly important when the patient has had total pelvic irradiation. Hyperchloremic acidosis associated with implantation of the ureters into the intact sigmoid colon does not occur with colon loop urinary diversion because the average length of the colon loop, 8–10 cm, is too short for significant absorption of urine from the colonic mucosa.

The purpose of the intestinal loop urinary diversion is to divert the urine following removal of the bladder at the time of anterior or total exenteration or if the bladder and lower ureters have lost their neurologic function and a continent urostomy is contraindicated.

**Physiologic Changes.** The most significant physiologic change of an intestinal loop urinary diversion is the rapid runoff of urine from the isolated intestinal loop.

Because of this, the incidence of urinary tract infection is less than that encountered when the ureter is implanted into a functional segment of the rectosigmoid colon.

A negative change in intestinal loop diversion is the problem of contaminated reflux from the loop of the renal pelvis. This produces loss of upper renal units in 65% of patients.

**Points of Caution.** The ureters should be transected as low in the pelvis as possible. Excess ureter can be trimmed away if necessary. Silastic catheters should always be inserted up the ureter and through the intestinal loop to splint the anastomosis for 10–12 days. This alone has significantly reduced the incidence of ureteral stricture and separation from the intestinal anastomotic site.

Another point of caution concerns the design of the loop. In general, it should be selected from bowel that has had the least irradiation. The length should be long enough to reach the abdominal wall, usually 8–12 cm. Care should be taken to close mesenteric defects in the reanastomosed intestine and those between the loop and the abdominal side wall to prevent internal hernia.

# Intestinal Loop Urinary Diversion

## (Continued)

*Technique*

**1** The patient is placed in the supine position, and the abdomen is opened through a lower midline incision. Occasionally, extension of the incision around the umbilicus is required. The pelvis is thoroughly explored, and both ureters are identified and traced as deep in the pelvis as is technically possible.

**2** The loop of bowel to be used, colon or ileum, is selected. Figure 2 shows the terminal ileum and the colon. The appropriate length of bowel is measured, selected, and marked. The mesentery of the bowel is carefully illuminated with a bright light to delineate the vascular arcades. This confirms that the loop is adequately nourished by a generous blood supply from the vascular branches of the arcade. The mesentery of the loop is opened for approximately 4–5 cm, and the small vessels are clamped and tied. The loop can be transected in the classic way between Kocher clamps. Today, however, the automatic surgical stapler with TA-55 premium absorbable staples for the proximal end of the loop is often used. If wire or permanent suture is used in the proximal end of the loop, stone formation may occur.

As shown here, a GIA (gastrointestinal anastomosis) stapling and division device can be applied to the distal portion of the loop. A standard TA-55 wire staple can be applied to the proximal portion of the bowel, but a TA-55 premium absorbable staple is preferable for the proximal portion of the loop. If staples are not available, the proximal loop can be closed with synthetic absorbable suture.

After all of these staples are fired, the loop can be transected between the TA-55 wire staples and the TA-55 absorbable staples. A standard bowel anastomosis can be made between the proximal and distal ileum or proximal and distal colon as outlined in the technique in Figures 7–10.

**3** The ureter is identified deep in the pelvis and mobilized, preserving the delicate ureteral sheath that surrounds the ureter from the renal pelvis to the bladder. After transecting the ureter, the distal stump is tied with 0 synthetic absorbable suture. The proximal ureter is catheterized with a Silastic "J" ureteral anastomosis catheter that contains either a suture sleeve or a suture rib.

If the ileal segment of bowel has been selected, the mesentery of the rectosigmoid colon must be opened to allow the left ureter to be transported through the

mesentery to bring it into position for anastomosis to the ileum. If the sigmoid colon has been selected for the loop, this is not necessary, since the mesentery will already be open.

**4** The intestinal segment has been cross-clamped with the GIA stapler, so that both proximal and distal ends of the segment are stapled closed. A small opening must be made in the distal segment of the loop to admit a narrow arterial forceps that is advanced down the segment of bowel to within 3 cm of the distal end. At that point, the arterial forceps is slightly elevated, and an incision is made over the tip of the arterial forceps until the intestine is entered. A small button of bowel wall measuring approximately 1 × 1 cm in diameter may be removed. The forceps is advanced through this opening and grasps the Silastic catheter that is in the ureter. A 4-0 synthetic absorbable suture on two small needles has been previously placed through the Silastic suture sleeve or suture rib on the Silastic catheter.

If an ileal segment of bowel is to be used as seen in **b**, a defect has to be created in the mesentery of the sigmoid colon to allow the left ureter to be brought through that defect and into position for an anastomosis to the ileum. In **b**, the right ureter is seen in the approximate position for anastomosis.

**5** This sagittal section of the intestinal segment illustrates the technique of suturing the Silastic catheter sleeve with a fine 4-0 synthetic absorbable suture to the wall of the intestine to hold the Silastic catheter in place and prevent peristalsis of the ureter from pushing the catheter into the loop and thus out of the ureter. This step is unnecessary if the stent has a "J" or "pigtail" configuration that prevents expulsion. The Silastic catheter should stay in the ureter, stenting the anastomosis, for at least 10–12 days. The sutures for the ureteral intestinal anastomosis are placed full thickness through the bowel wall and the ureter so that, when tied, a mucosa-to-mucosa anastomosis is performed.

**6** The ureter is anastomosed to the intestinal wall with interrupted 4-0 synthetic absorbable sutures. Generally, 4–5 sutures are needed to complete the anastomosis. In addition, some periureteral peritoneum is anchored across the anastomosis to take tension off the suture line. The opposite ureter is sutured to the intestine in a similar manner.

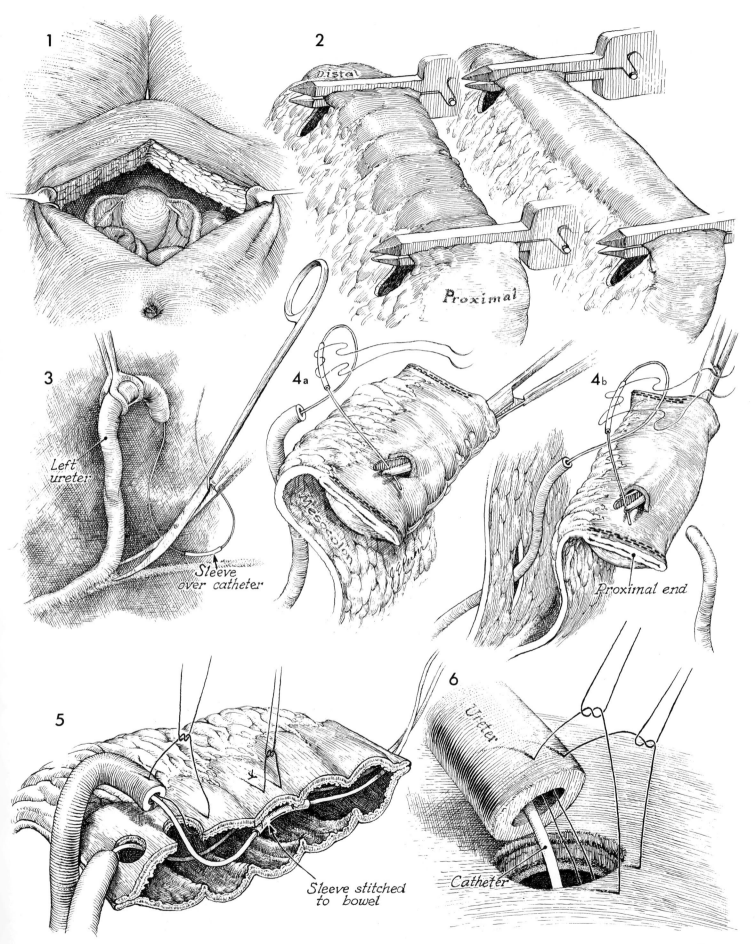

1

2

Distal

Proximal

3

*Left
ureter*

*Sleeve
over catheter*

4a

Mesocolon

4b

*Proximal end*

5

*Sleeve stitched
to bowel*

6

*Ureter*

*Catheter*

163

# Intestinal Loop Urinary Diversion

## (Continued)

**7** The intestinal segments are lifted superior to the constructed loop, allowing an end-to-end functional anastomosis to be completed between the segments of bowel. If a segment of rectosigmoid colon is used, the intestinal loop is moved medially to allow an end-to-end colocolostomy.

Figure 7 shows the anastomosis being performed on the descending colon, but the technique of the stapler anastomosis is the same for both large and small bowel.

**8** Both blades of the GIA stapler are passed into the colon along the antimesenteric border. The stapler is activated, and a V-shaped ostium is created along the antimesenteric border for a distance of approximately 5 cm with a double row of staples on each side and an incision down the middle.

**9** The edges of the remaining defect are picked up with Babcock clamps and brought through the activated TA-55 stapler. Any excess bowel is trimmed away with curved Mayo scissors.

**10** The functional end-to-end anastomosis is completed. The mesentery is sutured with interrupted 3-0 synthetic absorbable sutures.

**11** The distal portion of the intestinal urinary loop, with the ureters anastomosed in place, is pulled through the abdominal wall defect, which should be at least 2 fingersbreadth or 4 cm in diameter. The excess Silastic catheter is trimmed away.

**12** The stoma is sutured to the skin of the abdominal wall with a rosebud stitch, as shown in the operation for end sigmoid colostomy (see Section 7, page 325), which raises the stoma approximately 1 cm above the level of the skin and allows urine to drip off the stoma into its bag without contact with the skin. The mesentery of the intestinal segment must be carefully closed to the lateral pelvic wall to prevent internal hernia.

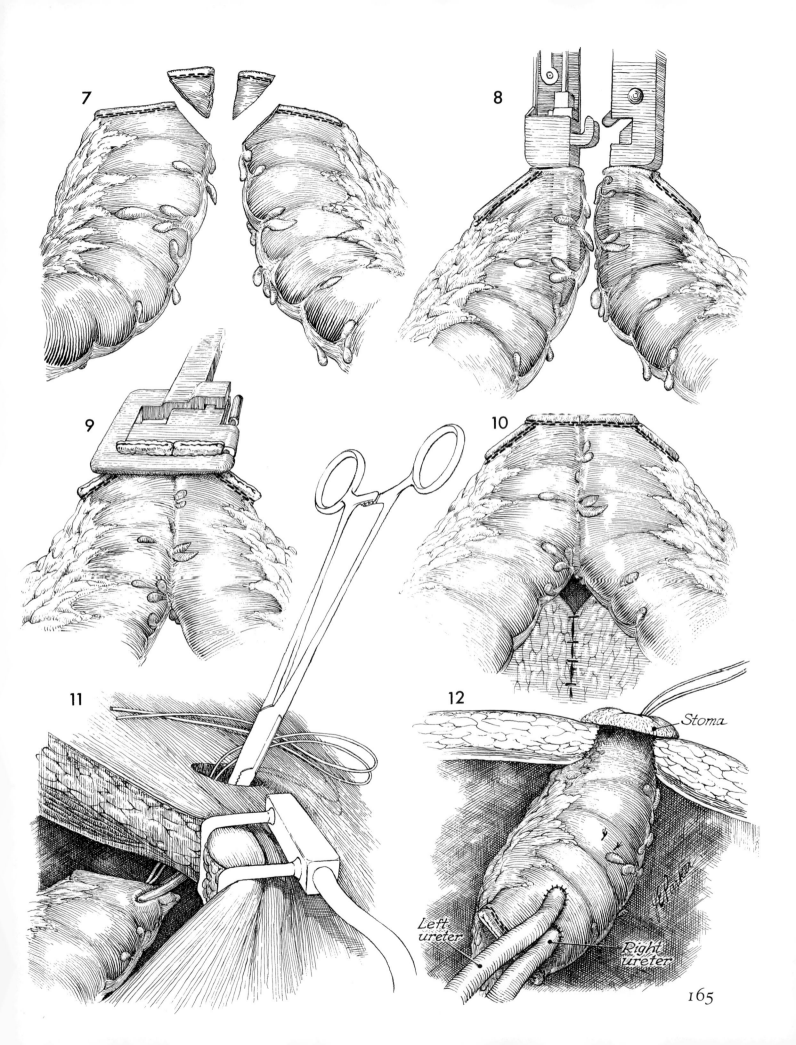

7

8

9

10

11

12

*Stoma*

*Left ureter*

*Right ureter*

165

# Percutaneous Nephropyelostomy

A suture ligature, excessive radiation, scarring from radical surgery, or clamping the ureter all lead to hydroureter and eventual hydronephrosis and loss of the kidney. If the ureter is transected, urinary ascites will result and eventually lead to infection and abscess.

The incidence of injury to the ureter associated with pelvic disease and/or surgery ranges from 0.3% to 5%.

Injury to the ureter is a medical emergency. Time is of importance, since for every hour that the kidney is obstructed, there is further damage to the renal collecting system.

A straightforward and simple procedure has been developed that avoids major surgery and relieves the sequelae of ureteral injury and obstruction in most cases—percutaneous needle nephropyelostomy.

**Physiologic Changes.** Percutaneous nephropyelostomy relieves the obstruction and prevents death of the renal nephron unit while corrective surgery can be planned.

**Points of Caution.** Fluoroscopy and ultrasound are used to guide the needle through the cortex of the kidney into the renal pelvis. Once the needle is in the renal pelvis, the guidewire should be advanced down into the urinary tract as far as the bladder if possible.

An attempt should be made to totally implant the J or pigtail stent. Not having a catheter through the renal parenchyma will reduce repeated episodes of gross hematuria. In some cases, however, this cannot be done, and the stent must be brought out through the renal cortex, flank wall, and skin and connected to a drainage bag.

## Technique

**1** The patient is placed in the prone position and rolled into the modified lateral decubitus position with the hip and the knee flexed. The side representing the normal kidney should be down, with the hip and the knee on that side extended. Dye for an intravenous pyelogram has been injected. The hydronephrosis is seen in the right kidney.

**2** Under fluoroscopic control, the 16-gauge Tuohy-type needle should be advanced through the abdominal wall in the costovertebral angle area. The renal cortex should be perforated, and the needle should be advanced into the renal pelvis. Injection of a small amount of x-ray dye will confirm that the needle is in the renal pelvis. At this point, a flexible guidewire is threaded through the needle, down the ureter, under fluoroscopic control. The area of damaged ureter is approached, and if possible, the guidewire is manipulated through this area of damage into the bladder. If this is not possible, the guidewire should be threaded as close as possible to the area of damage.

**3** The needle is withdrawn, and a double-J or pigtail catheter is inserted over the guidewire through the flank wall, through the renal cortex, into the renal pelvis, and down the ureter. Ideally, the double-J catheter should be inserted through the area of ureteral damage into the bladder. Injection of small amounts of contrast medium can confirm its position.

**4** By using a tubular pusher over the guidewire, the surgeon can advance the proximal end of the J catheter through the flank wall and the renal cortex into the renal pelvis. This leaves the proximal end of the catheter stent in the renal pelvis and the other end in the bladder.

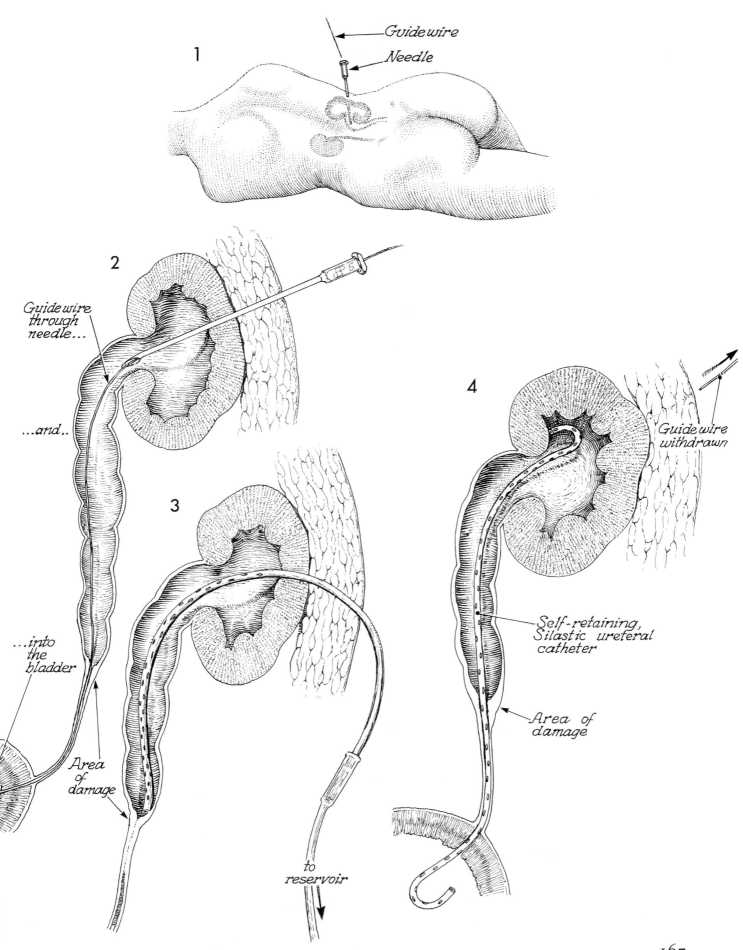

**1**

Guidewire

Needle

**2**

Guidewire
through
needle...

...and..

...into
the
bladder

Area
of
damage

**3**

to
reservoir

**4**

Guidewire
withdrawn

Self-retaining,
Silastic ureteral
catheter

Area of
damage

# Ureteroileoneocystostomy

When a large segment of the ureter must be excised as a result of radiation stenosis and/or chronic ureteritis, it is unwise to try to anastomose the remaining stenosed, radiated, and inflamed ureter to the bladder. Therefore, if the patient's kidney is reasonably healthy, the surgeon may choose among three procedures: (1) a cutaneous nephrostomy, (2) a transureteroureterostomy, and (3) a ureteroileoneocystostomy. This last procedure has the advantage of using nonirradiated materials in the entire system.

**Physiologic Changes.** The most important physiologic changes are that (1) obstruction is taken away from the ureter and (2) the kidney is allowed to survive. The loss of a 10–15-cm segment of terminal ileum has few long-term sequelae. If a longer portion of the ileum is removed, however, vitamin $B_{12}$ should be administered systemically.

**Points of Caution.** All diseased ureter should be removed. The anastomosis of ileum into the renal tract can be made from the renal pelvis, along the ureter, down to the bladder. Frequently, this is unnecessary, as the proximal portion of the ureter coming off the renal pelvis may be nonirradiated and noninflamed. As in all cases of ureteral surgery, the ureter should be stented with medical grade Silastic double-J catheters.

---

## Technique

**1** A segment of terminal ileum is selected. The vascular branches in the mesentery of the ileum are observed by transillumination prior to transection of the terminal ileum. An incision is made into the avascular plane of Treitz medial to the ileocolic artery. The terminal ileum does not have to be selected; proximal ileum or even terminal jejunum can also be used.

**2** An ileoileostomy is performed either with sutures or with staples.

**3** All diseased ureter has been removed. In this particular figure, a stump of ureter is shown coming off the renal pelvis and out of the bladder. The surgeon should not hesitate, however, to make a cystostomy in the bladder and to excise any diseased ureter noted.

**4** The proximal stump of ureter is opened longitudinally to prevent iris contracture at the anastomotic site. A Silastic-grade double-J catheter has been inserted up into the renal pelvis.

**5** The segment of ileum is moved into place. The medical grade Silastic double-J catheter has been brought through the lumen of the ileum. Anastomosis of the ileum to the ureter is made with interrupted synthetic absorbable suture.

**6** The Silastic double-J catheter is inserted down the distal portion of the ileum into the bladder.

**7** The ileum is shown anastomosed to the distal ureter. The Silastic double-J stent is in place. A Jackson-Pratt suction drain is placed adjacent to the anastomosis. Both the Jackson-Pratt suction drain and the stent can be removed in 2–3 weeks.

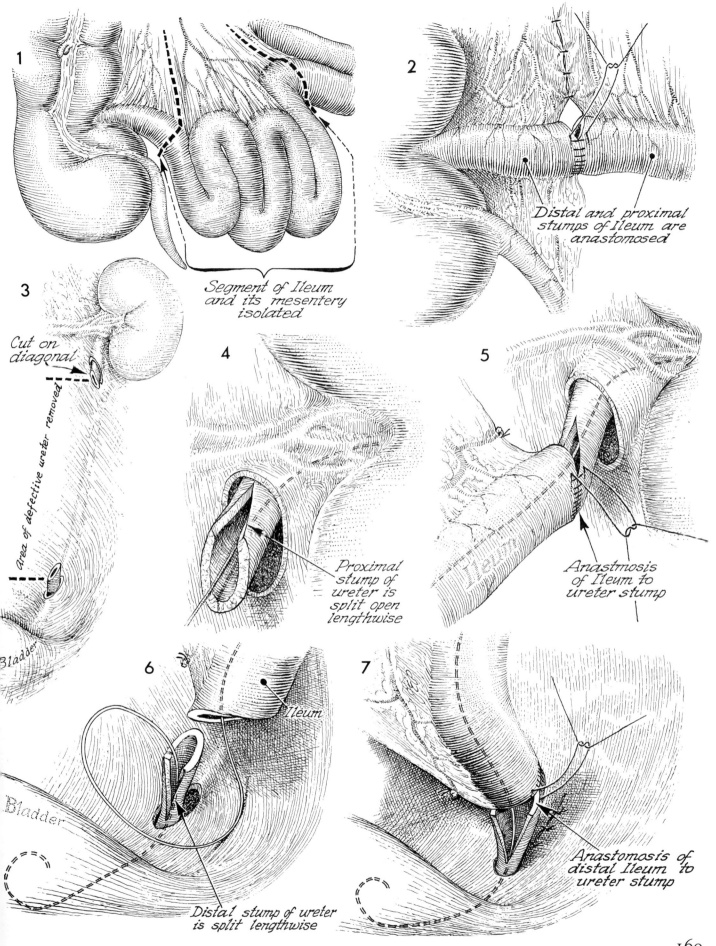

**1**

Segment of Ileum
and its mesentery
isolated

**2**

Distal and proximal
stumps of Ileum are
anastomosed

**3**

Cut on
diagonal

Area of defective ureter removed

Bladder

**4**

Proximal
stump of
ureter is
split open
lengthwise

**5**

Ileum

Anastmosis
of Ileum to
ureter stump

**6**

Ileum

Bladder

Distal stump of ureter
is split lengthwise

**7**

Anastomosis of
distal Ileum to
ureter stump

# "Clam" Gastrocystoplasty

Pelvic radiation is frequently necessary for the treatment of gynecologic cancer. Normally, the bladder tolerates irradiation therapy up to 7000 cGy without significant sequela. In some patients, however, radiation fibrosis develops, creating a small stiff bladder with low capacity and high pressure resulting in total incontinence of urine. Frequently, these patients have a low urethral pressure but an extremely high vesical pressure. The usual urogynecologic pin-up surgical procedures, e.g., the Marshall-Marchetti-Krantz or Burch operations, will not alter the physiologic changes that created the problem, i.e., radiation fibrosis of the bladder.

A source of nonirradiated highly vascular tissue placed in the wall of the bladder for augmentation can relieve this disabling and incapacitating situation.

There are cases in which the patient has received no radiation but has a severe detrusor instability of the bladder with total incontinence. Transecting the bladder in the longitudinal plane produces some denervation of the bladder and reduction of detrusor instability. The augmentation of stomach to the transected bladder is referred to as a "clam" procedure and can relieve the incontinence.

**Physiologic Changes.** The physiologic sequela of removing a small gastric flap from the greater curvature of the stomach has few if any consequences. The augmentation of an opened bladder with this gastric flap has significant physiologic changes. The bladder capacity increases significantly. The usual bladder capacity of a radiation-fibrosed bladder is less than 100 mL. The gastric flap increases the bladder capacity from 300 to 500 mL.

The gastric flap secretes acid. This gives the patient an acid urine that creates an unfavorable environment for bacterial growth.

The gastric flap is quite distensible. Because of this distensibility the bladder, when full of urine, will have a low pressure, usually in the range of 30–40 cm of water. If the urethral pressure has a natural pressure of 70–80 cm of water, continence will be restored. If the urethral pressure is low, continence will be improved if a Goebell-Stoeckel fascia lata sling operation in addition to the clam gastrocystoplasty is performed (see Section 2, page 115, for discussion of the Goebell-Stoeckel fascia lata sling).

# "Clam" Gastrocystoplasty

## (Continued)

### Technique

**1** Figure 1 shows the esophagus, stomach, spleen, and omentum. The left gastroepiploic artery for this flap is shown, although the right gastroepiploic artery works equally well. The defects in the mesentery between the short gastric arteries are made, and each short gastric artery is cut and tied. The right gastroepiploic artery is transected at the junction of the duodenum, and each of the branches of the right gastroepiploic artery are transected and tied. The GIA (gastrointestinal anastomosis) stapler is placed across the stomach for approximately 6 cm. The base of this triangular flap will be approximately 6 cm.

**2** The right gastroepiploic artery has been transected (*bottom*). The right side of the wedge of stomach has been cut and stapled. The left portion of the wedge flap is shown with the GIA stapler dividing both the anterior and the posterior gastric wall.

**3** The defect in the stomach is shown, and small incisions are made for a gastrotomy in the proximal and the distal stomach.

**4** A GIA stapler is placed in the small gastrotomy incisions on the greater curvature. The GIA stapler reapproximates the stomach and then cuts between the edges to reestablish continuity.

**5** The remaining defects created by the small stab wound gastrotomies are picked up with Babcock clamps and cross-clamped and stapled with a TA-55 4.8 stapler. The TA-55 stapler closes the two gastrotomy defects. Excessive tissue is cut away.

**6** A feeding tube gastrostomy is placed in the stomach for decompression and possible total enteral nutrition if needed. The procedure is initiated by placing the automatic pursestring suture device across the stomach wall 8–10 cm proximal to the resected and reconstituted gastric flap.

**7** A small gastrotomy is made in the center of the pursestring suture. A stab wound is made in the left upper quadrant of the abdomen, and a No. 22 French Malecot catheter is brought through the abdominal wall to be inserted into the lumen of the stomach.

**8** Figure 8 shows the stomach lumen, the abdominal wall, and the feeding tube gastrostomy catheter (Malecot) in place. The visceral peritoneum of the stomach is sutured to the parietal peritoneum to prevent leakage of gastric juice until mesothelialization has sealed the wound.

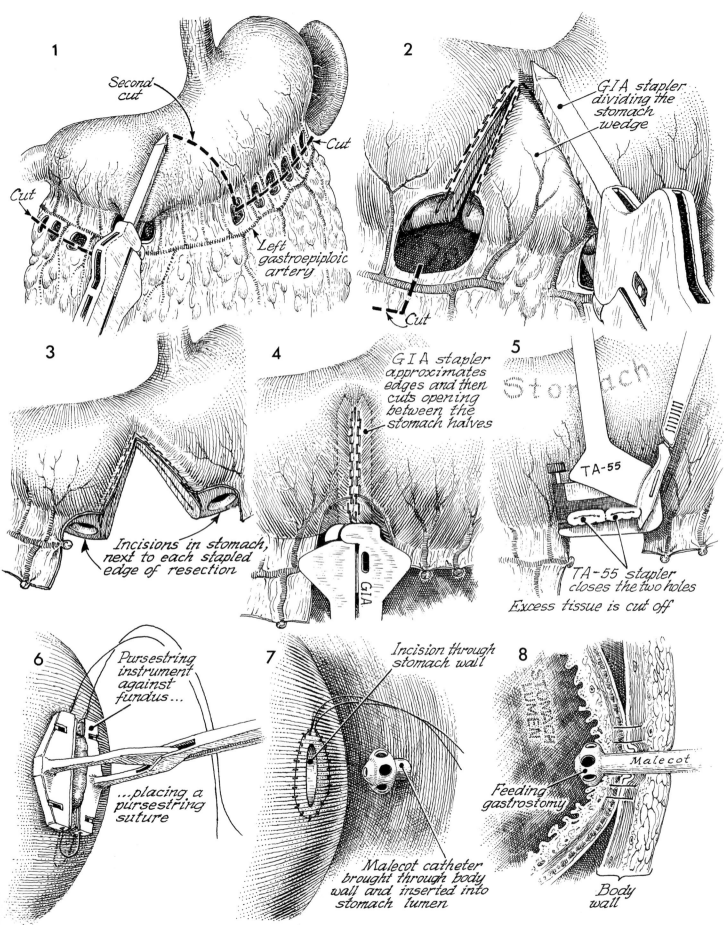

**1**

Second cut

Cut

Cut

Left gastroepiploic artery

**2**

GIA stapler dividing the stomach wedge

Cut

**3**

Incisions in stomach, next to each stapled edge of resection

**4**

GIA stapler approximates edges and then cuts opening between the stomach halves

GIA

**5**

Stomach

TA-55

TA-55 stapler closes the two holes

Excess tissue is cut off

**6**

Pursestring instrument against fundus...

...placing a pursestring suture

**7**

Incision through stomach wall

Malecot catheter brought through body wall and inserted into stomach lumen

**8**

STOMACH LUMEN

Malecot

Feeding gastrostomy

Body wall

# "Clam" Gastrocystoplasty

## (Continued)

**9** The right gastroepiploic artery on the greater curvature of the stomach, a branch of the celiac artery, is shown transected and tied. The remaining short gastric branches of the left gastroepiploic artery are seen transected and tied. The omentum with its attached gastric flap is shown lateral to the left colon. It is placed in the left descending colonic gutter along the line of Toldt. The wedge of stomach with omentum attached is brought down into the lower pelvis. In the bottom portion of this figure, the incision line into the bladder is shown, thus creating an opening shaped like a sea clam. This linear incision (*broken line*) in the bladder offers a wide defect. The defect partially deinnervates the bladder. Those patients with severe detrusor instability have reduced, uncontrolled contractions of their bladder.

**10** Figure 10 shows the left gastroepiploic artery with its short gastric branches feeding the wedge of the gastric flap. All staples must be completely removed. The presence of staples will create stones in the bladder. The triangle gastric flap is open and now forms the shape of a diamond.

**11** The longitudinally opened bladder is shown—thus its description as a clam. The gastric diamond-shaped flap is sutured into the bladder defect. The suture material should be synthetic absorbable.

**12** At the bottom, the diamond-shaped wedge of stomach is seen sutured in place to the clam gastrocystoplasty-opened bladder, while the reconstituted stomach with its staple line is shown at the top.

We frequently place two Foley catheters in the reconstructed bladder. A transurethral No. 16 French Foley catheter with a 5-mL bag is placed through the urethra into the reconstructed bladder. We frequently perform a small cystotomy 3 cm away from the gastric wedge suture line to insert a second Foley catheter as a suprapubic cystotomy. This double drainage guards against the possibility of mucus produced by the gastric artery plugging up one of the Foley catheters, thus allowing the possibility of a disrupted suture line through elevated hydraulic pressure. A Jackson-Pratt suction drain is brought through the anterior abdominal wall and placed near the bladder suture line. The Foley catheter is left in the bladder for approximately 2 weeks. When drainage has ceased, the Jackson-Pratt suction drain is removed. The patient initiates timed voiding by bearing down. The patient should void every 4–6 hours. Patients are discouraged from getting up at night to void; they are encouraged to void immediately upon arising.

All feedings are initiated when there are excellent bowel sounds and a bowel movement. At this time it will be safe to remove the tube gastrostomy.

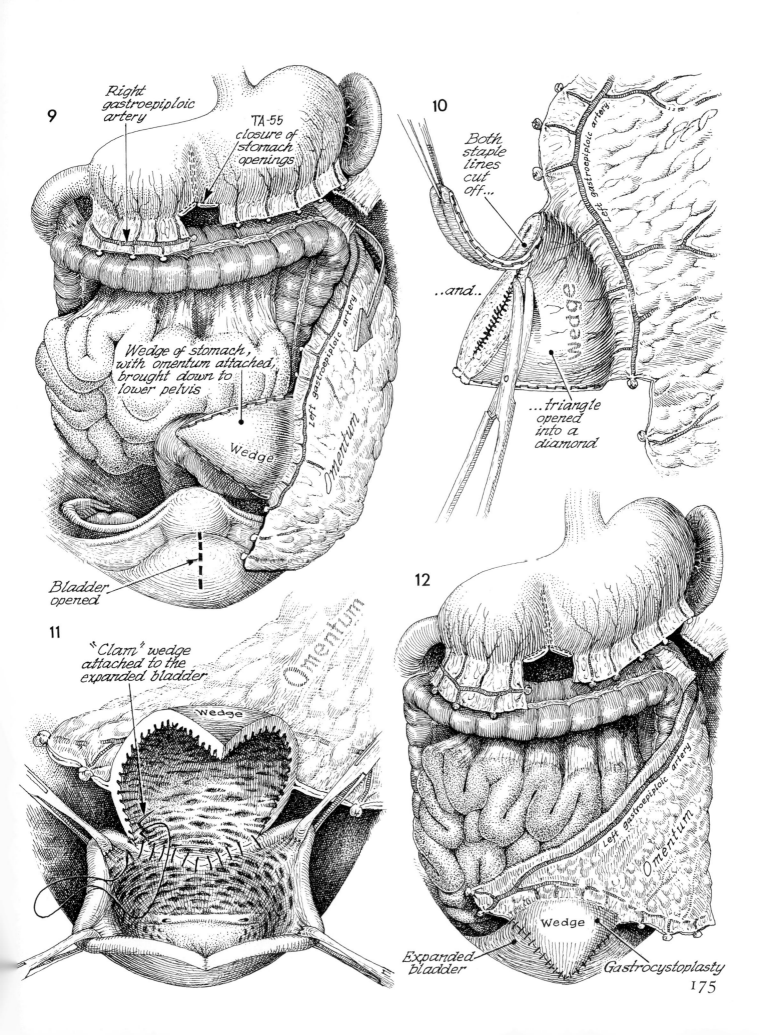

**9**

Right gastroepiploic artery

TA-55 closure of stomach openings

Wedge of stomach, with omentum attached, brought down to lower pelvis

Wedge

left gastroepiploic artery

Omentum

Bladder opened

**10**

Both staple lines cut off...

...and...

left gastroepiploic artery

Wedge

...triangle opened into a diamond

**11**

"Clam" wedge attached to the expanded bladder

Omentum

Wedge

**12**

left gastroepiploic artery

Omentum

Wedge

Expanded bladder

Gastrocystoplasty

# 4

## Cervix

# Biopsy of the Cervix

Randomized biopsy of the cervix is indicated whenever a gross lesion of the cervix is seen. All too often, gross lesions are diagnosed on sight as cervical "erosions or eversions" without histologic confirmation. The Papanicolaou smear alone is not sufficient for diagnosing gross lesions of the cervix.

The purpose of the operation is to obtain a histologic specimen of the squamocolumnar junction of the cervix.

**Physiologic Changes.** None.

**Points of Caution.** Cervical carcinoma begins at the squamocolumnar junction. Therefore, it is essential that this junction be taken in any biopsy of the cervix.

This operation has been illustrated in conjunction with Section 5, page 202 (Dilatation and Curettage).

## Technique

**1** The cervix is exposed and immersed in Schiller's iodine solution. The iodine solution will rapidly stain cells storing glycogen. Those cells with rapid nuclei division are generally glycogen depleted and therefore will not stain with the iodine solution. These areas are known as "Schiller white areas."

A sharp alligator-mouth biopsy forceps is placed at the junction of the Schiller dark and Schiller white areas; a liberal biopsy is obtained. This process is repeated in at least four other quadrants. Rarely is cauterization or suture of the biopsy site needed. A vaginal tampon is applied to the cervix to absorb the cervical bleeding. If hemostasis is required, a 4-0 synthetic absorbable suture or Avitene collagen hemostat can be applied to the cervix.

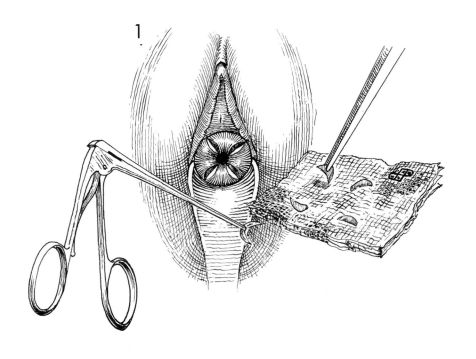

# Directed Biopsy of the Cervix at Colposcopy

Colposcopy as an adjunctive diagnostic tool in the assessment of cervical intraepithelial neoplasia is a significant aid to the pelvic surgeon in selecting the appropriate method of therapy in certain cases. Its use is indicated in all patients having abnormal Papanicolaou cytologic smears or gross lesions.

To obtain accurate cytologic specimens for study, the surgeon must be trained not only in performing a colposcopy but also in selecting the proper instruments for the examination.

The purpose of the operation is to visualize the cervix under high magnification and delineate abnormal zones of cervical epithelium. In addition, it is designed to allow precise, accurate biopsies to be obtained from these abnormal zones of epithelium.

**Physiologic Changes.** None.

**Points of Caution.** A direct Papanicolaou smear should be taken prior to any manipulation of the cervix.

A detailed survey of the cervix should be performed prior to any surgical manipulation.

Directed biopsies, oriented to prevent tangential cutting, should be placed on small pieces of wet paper towel and sent to the pathologist.

## Technique

**1** The patient is placed on an ordinary gynecologic examining table, and a nonlubricated speculum is placed in the vagina. The colposcope is moved into appropriate position and focused. A routine cytologic smear as well as a wet mounted smear for *Trichomonas* and *Monilia* are taken. The cervical mucus is then cleared by applying 4% acetic acid to the cervix and removing the solution with either a small suction cannula or a cotton-tip applicator. The cervix is studied carefully with the green filter lens in place to enhance the appearance of the cervical blood vessels.

**2** Appropriate biopsy instruments, designed for taking crisp, sharp, directed biopsies from zones of abnormal tissue located by the colposcope, are selected.

**3** An endocervical speculum is inserted to appropriately inspect the endocervical canal.

**4–6** Because there are significant patterns important to the diagnosis of cervical intraepithelial neoplasia, the surgeon searches specific zones for signs of abnormal epithelium.

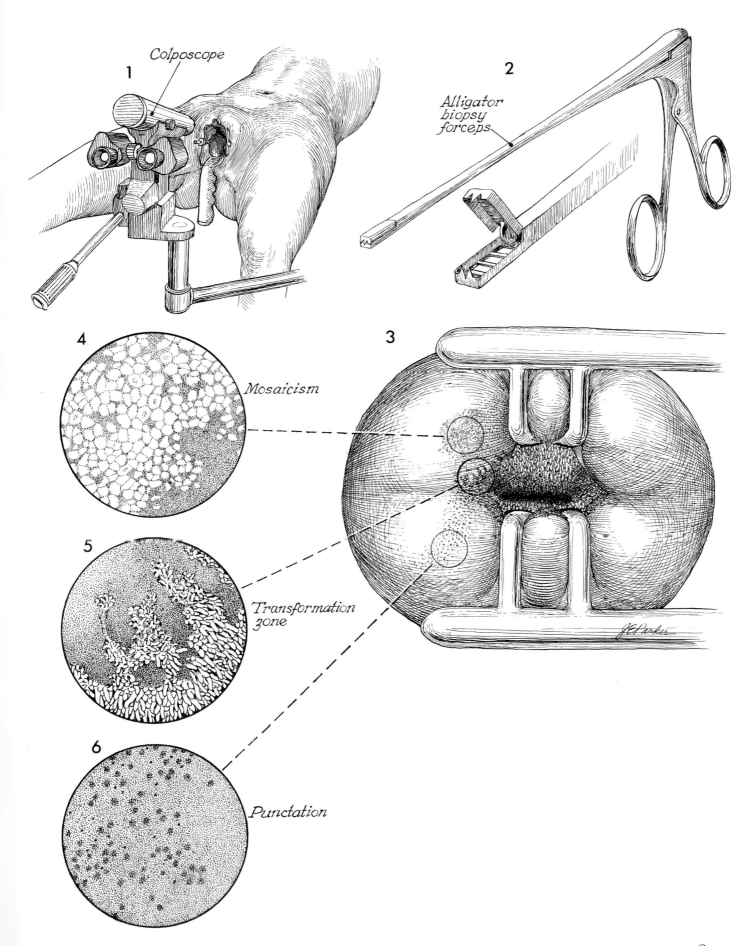

1

Colposcope

2

Alligator
biopsy
forceps

4

Mosaicism

5

Transformation
zone

6

Punctation

3

J.E.Parker

# Endocervical Curettage at Colposcopy

Colposcopy as an adjunctive diagnostic tool in the assessment of cervical intraepithelial neoplasia is a significant aid to the pelvic surgeon in selecting the appropriate method of therapy in certain cases. Its use is indicated in all patients having abnormal Papanicolaou cytologic smears or gross lesions.

To obtain accurate cytologic specimens for study, the surgeon must be trained not only in performing a colposcopy but also in selecting the proper instruments for the examination.

The purpose of the operation is to visualize the cervix under high magnification and delineate abnormal zones of cervical epithelium.

Endocervical curettage enables the surgeon to take specimens from the endocervical canal that may not be visible even with the colposcope.

**Physiologic Changes.** None.

**Points of Caution.** A direct Papanicolaou smear should be taken prior to any manipulation of the cervix.

A detailed survey of the cervix should be performed prior to any surgical manipulation.

The endocervical curettings should be sent as a second specimen.

## Technique

**1** The patient is placed on an ordinary gynecologic examining table, and a nonlubricated speculum is placed in the vagina. The colposcope is moved into appropriate position and focused. A routine cytologic smear as well as a wet mounted smear for *Trichomonas* and *Monilia* are taken. The cervical mucus is then cleared by applying 4% acetic acid to the cervix and removing the solution with either a small suction cannula or a cotton-tip applicator. The cervix is studied carefully with the green filter lens in place to enhance the appearance of the cervical blood vessels.

**2** A sagittal section of the uterus and upper vagina shows the area of the endocervix to be curetted. The cervix should not be dilated, since dilation would increase the possibility of the curet entering the endometrial cavity.

**3** The endocervical curet is placed in the cervix up to the internal os. The curet is moved back and forth in the cervical canal, collecting tissue within the rectangular box. The tissue is then sent to the pathologist. This movement is repeated in a 360° circle until the entire cervical canal has been curetted.

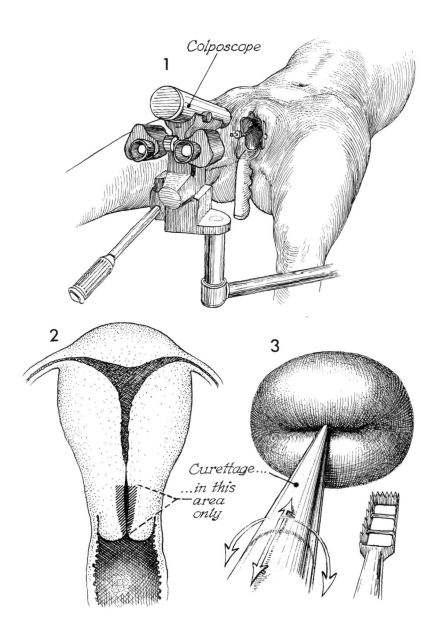

1

Colposcope

2

Curettage...

...in this
area
only

3

# Conization of the Cervix by the Loop Electrical Excision Procedure (LEEP)

The indications for conization of the cervix are (1) the limits of the lesion in the cervix cannot be completely defined by colposcopy and directed biopsy, or the lesion is noted to extend up into the cervical canal and, therefore, is inaccessible to histologic examination by directed biopsy; (2) there is severe cervical intraepithelial neoplasia (CIN) or carcinoma in situ in a young patient for whom a hysterectomy is contraindicated because of age and desire for fertility; and (3) there is a failure of agreement between cytology, colposcopy, and histology. The purpose of conization of the cervix by the LEEP is to remove a cone-shaped piece of cervical tissue that will encompass the squamocolumnar junction. The procedure can be diagnostic as well as therapeutic.

**Physiologic Change.** This operation removes the endocervical glands and in some patients has been associated with infertility because it reduces the production of cervical mucus. In addition, it may weaken the internal os of the cervix and, therefore, can be associated with second-trimester abortion.

**Points of Caution.** The surgical specimen should be adequate to provide an accurate diagnosis and remove the entire lesion. Hemostasis after conization is essential. These patients should be informed that there may be a small incidence of persistent cervical intraepithelial neoplasia following conization by the LEEP. Therefore, follow-up cytology and colposcopy are essential to this form of therapy.

# Conization of the Cervix by the Loop Electrical Excision Procedure (LEEP)

## (Continued)

### Technique

**1** The patient may be anesthetized with general or local anesthesia. Local anesthesia consists of paracervical injections of 1% lidocaine at the 3, 5, 7, and 9 o'clock positions around the cervix. The cervix is stained with an iodine solution such as Schiller's solution to demarcate zones of glycogen depletion and thus neoplasia. If the patient is under general anesthesia, a solution of Pitressin diluted with 10 IU to 30 mL of normal saline is injected around the entire surface of the cervix. If the patient is under local anesthesia, the Pitressin can be mixed with the lidocaine. Vascular constricture and blanching of the cervix will be noted. The injection of Pitressin solution is contraindicated in patients with cardiovascular disease and/or hypertension. A pursestring vascular cerclage to control bleeding is rarely indicated.

**2** With the lesion adequately stained with Schiller's solution, the loop device with suction attached to the rod removes the smoke or flume. The loop is placed outside the lesion in the area of normal cervix. The electrocoagulator is adjusted to a blend between the cutting and the electrocoagulation current. The loop device is inserted through the cervical tissue to the depth of the available loop and is slowly moved from one side of the portio of the cervix to the other side. By inserting the loop to the full depth of the cervix, the cone should contain the entire lesion. When the surgeon has reached the opposite limits of the lesion as noted by Schiller's white area, the loop is lifted forward, and the specimen is removed.

**3** Electrocoagulation of any bleeding surfaces with the ball cautery is performed.

**4** The lesion is larger than (extends outside the limits of) the available steel loops and must be removed in sections (see also Figs. 5–8). The electric wire of the loop is inserted and swept across the cervix in a routine fashion as shown in Figures 1–3.

**5** Excessive lesion remains outside that removed by the LEEP.

**6** The cone is removed, but excessive lesion can still be seen outside the excised area.

**7** The remaining lesion can be removed by repeating the standard procedure, moving the electrical loop from one side to the other. The lesion that was outside the original cone has been removed.

**8** The lesion on the anterior lip of the cervix is removed in a similar manner.

**9** The three cone specimens of the cervix removed by the LEEP are (1) the original cone, (2) the posterior portion, and (3) the anterior portion.

**10** When the original lesion extends high into the endocervical canal, the cone specimen of the cervix is removed as shown here. Conization by the LEEP is moved from the patient's right to her left in the same technique as previously shown.

**11** Most of the lesion has been removed by the LEEP.

**12** The exterior lesion on the portio is completely removed, but neoplasia remains in the cervical canal.

**13** A smaller loop is placed up the canal. The remaining portion of the endocervical canal is removed by the LEEP.

**14** The two pathologic specimens, the cylinder and the cone, are shown here. Hemostasis can be achieved as shown in Figure 3 by the ball cautery. The specimens are sent to pathology clearly marked as upper cervical canal and lower squamous columnar junction of the cervix.

We have found it advantageous to dip a tampon in a ferrous sulfate solution such as Monsel's. The tampon with the tip soaked in Monsel's solution is placed in the cervical cone for additional hemostasis.

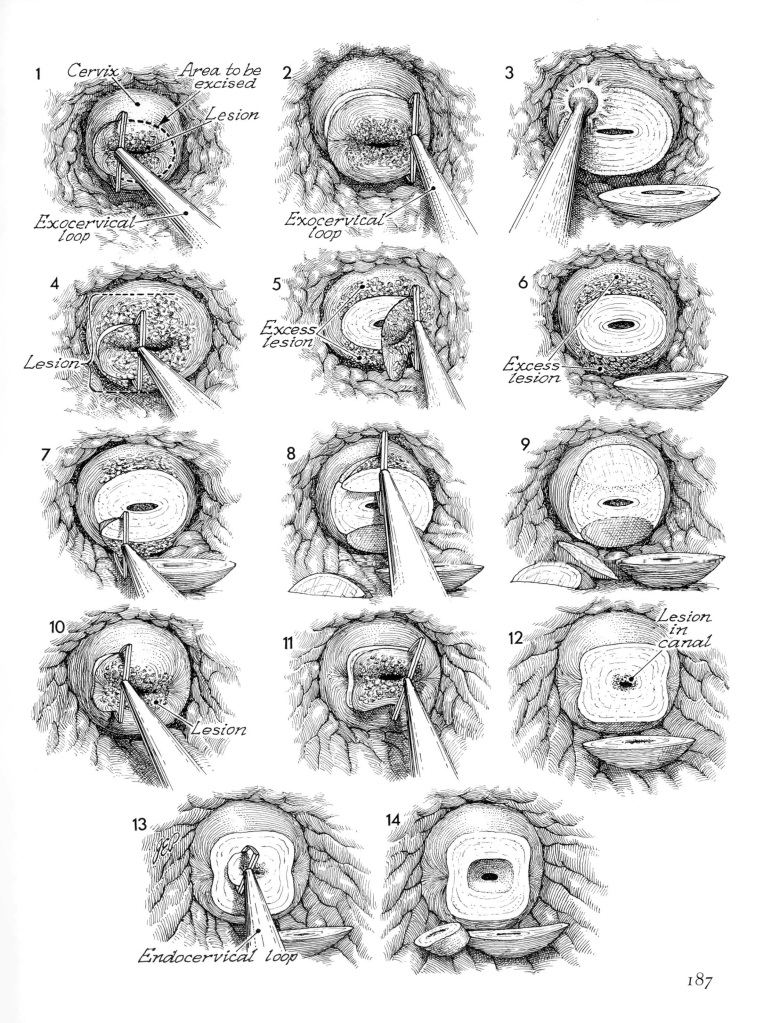

1 Cervix    Area to be excised    Lesion

Exocervical loop

2 Exocervical loop

3

4 Lesion

5 Excess lesion

6 Excess lesion

7

8

9

10 Lesion

11

12 Lesion in canal

13 Endocervical loop

14

187

# Abdominal Excision of the Cervical Stump

Fortunately, subtotal abdominal hysterectomy is a relatively rare procedure today. The pelvic surgeon may, however, encounter a patient who underwent this operation in the past and has developed neoplasia or myoma in the cervical stump. In such cases, surgery is indicated.

Care should be exercised in removal of the stump. The bladder and/or the rectum may have been used to reestablish the peritoneal lining of the pelvis after the subtotal abdominal hysterectomy. Therefore, these organs may be injured during the resection.

The transverse incision is useful in those conditions where overall abdominal exploration and exposure are not needed. The vaginal cuff is left open for drainage to reduce the incidence of postoperative pelvic infection and abscess.

The purpose of this operation is to remove the cervical stump via the abdominal route.

**Physiologic Changes.** The diseased cervix is removed.

**Points of Caution.** Because of previous surgery, the ureters may be densely adherent to the cervical stump. Care must be taken to properly identify these and to free them both laterally and vertically during the dissection of the bladder from the cervix.

# Abdominal Excision of the Cervical Stump

## (Continued)

*Technique*

**1** The patient is examined under anesthesia. At this time, the vagina and abdomen should be surgically prepped, and a Foley catheter should be inserted into the bladder and connected to straight drainage.

**2** The patient is placed in the supine position, and a transverse incision 12–14 cm in length is made following the skin lines above the mons pubis. By keeping the incision slightly above the mons pubis, the surgeon can avoid the vascular plexus within the mons and aid hemostasis.

**3** The incision is carried down to the rectus fascia, which is incised transversely, exposing the rectus abdominal muscles.

**4** The rectus abdominal muscles can be separated in the midline, and greater exposure can be achieved by undermining the rectus abdominal muscles lateral to the inferior epigastric artery. If greater mobility is required or if the rectus muscle needs transection, the inferior epigastric artery and vein should be ligated prior to extensive mobilization and/or muscle transection. The peritoneum is elevated and can be opened in the transverse or longitudinal plane.

**5** A self-retaining retractor is placed in the incision. The pelvis and abdomen are explored. The patient is placed in the moderate Trendelenburg position, and the bowel is packed off with wet, warm gauze packs. Frequently, the bladder peritoneum has been closed over the cervical stump, and the only recognizable structures are (1) the round ligaments as they enter the pelvic wall and (2) the tubes and ovaries. The round ligaments should be identified first, elevated with an Ochsner clamp and suture ligated. By elevating the transected round ligament, a plane of dissection can be achieved that in most cases will allow the surgeon to free the bladder from the cervix. The round ligaments in these cases have generally been sutured back to the cervical stump and, therefore, appear to be originating from the upper lateral area of the cervical stump. The tube and suspensory ligament of the ovary are frequently involved in the attachment to the cervical stump; and to avoid hemorrhage, these structures should not be cut.

**6** With adequate elevation of the cervical stump via the round ligaments, the anterior leaf of the broad ligaments can be identified. Sharp dissection is used to incise the bladder peritoneum as well as the posterior leaf of the broad ligament and the peritoneum overlying the cul-de-sac and the rectum.

**7** By elevating the bladder and vesical peritoneum with the bladder blade of the retractor, the filmy attachments of the bladder to the cervix can be identified and taken down with blunt or sharp dissection. This is facilitated by placing cephalad retraction on the cervical stump.

**8** If the tubes and ovaries remain, it may be advisable to remove them by identifying the infundibulopelvic ligament and undermining the ligament with the ovarian artery and vein below the brim of the pelvis. Care at this point should be taken to identify the ureter, since, as a result of previous scarring, it may have been diverted into the general field of the infundibulopelvic ligament and, therefore, be accessible to damage.

**9** The infundibulopelvic ligament should be doubly clamped with Ochsner clamps and transected.

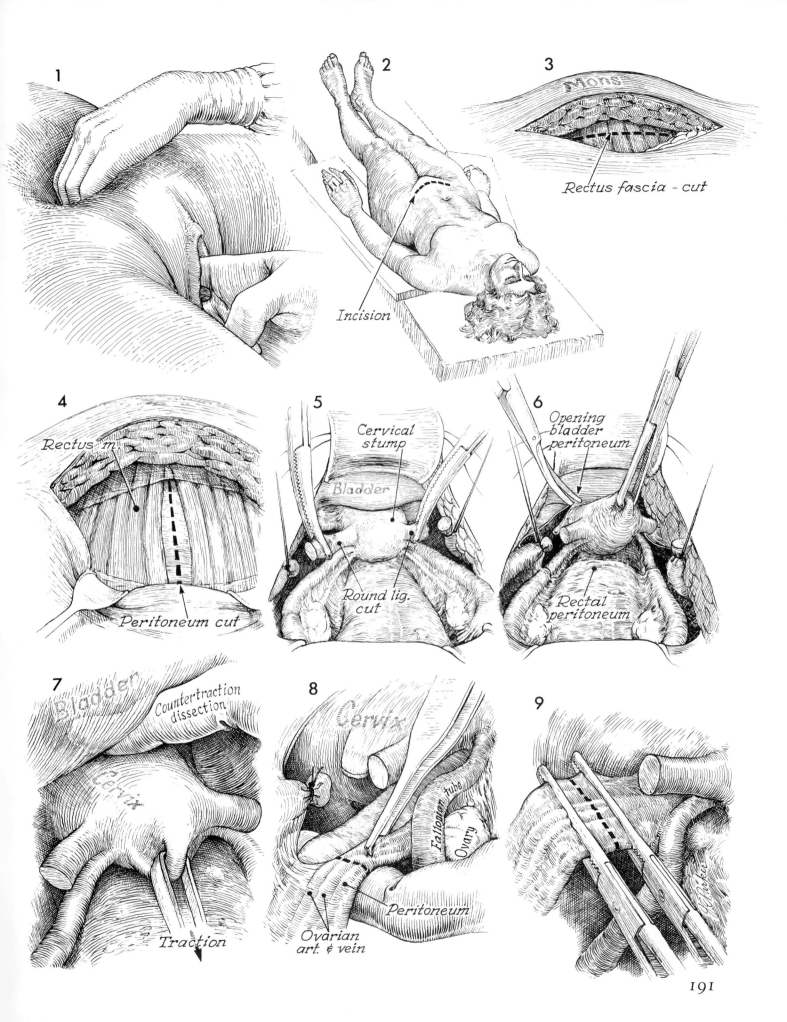

**1**

**2**

Incision

**3**

Mons

*Rectus fascia - cut*

**4**

Rectus m

Peritoneum cut

**5**

Cervical stump

Bladder

Round lig. cut

**6**

Opening bladder peritoneum

Rectal peritoneum

**7**

Bladder

Countertraction dissection

Cervix

Traction

**8**

Cervix

Fallopian tube

Ovary

Ovarian art. & vein

Peritoneum

**9**

# Abdominal Excision of the Cervical Stump

## (Continued)

**10** Two ligatures are customarily applied to the stump of the infundibulopelvic ligament: a tie of 2-0 synthetic absorbable suture and a suture placed through the midportion of the stump and tied on both sides.

**11** The cervical stump has now been freed from the round ligament and infundibulopelvic ligament. The peritoneum has been opened with a 360° arch around the cervical stump. The upper portions of the cardinal ligaments have been clamped and tied. The remaining cardinal ligaments and uterosacral ligaments remain to be cut and tied.

**12** Cephalad retraction is placed on the dome of the cervical stump. Straight Ochsner clamps are applied to the lateral edge of the cervix and allowed to slide off into a "groove" immediately lateral to the cervix, clamping any remaining portions of the uterine vessels and the cardinal ligament. The cardinal ligament is then transected with a scalpel, leaving an adequate stump protruding from the Ochsner clamp to prevent retraction of the stump of the cardinal ligament through the clamp.

**13** A second or, possibly, a third application of the Ochsner clamp is needed to completely clamp and transect the cardinal ligament. The last application of the Ochsner clamp encompasses in one bite the remaining portion of the cardinal ligament and the uterosacral ligament. By uniting the cardinal and uterosacral ligaments in one pedicle, the first step in resuspension of the vaginal cuff is created. This is incorporated into the angle of the vagina in later steps to facilitate suspension and to prevent enterocele.

**14** With cephalad retraction on the cervical stump, the anterior wall of the vagina is picked up by an Ochsner clamp, and the vagina is entered with curved Mayo scissors or by a stab wound with a scalpel. The curved Mayo scissors is then used to transect the remaining vaginal canal, and the cervical stump, the tubes, and the ovaries are removed.

**15** The space between the rectum and the vagina is closed with 0 synthetic absorbable suture.

**16** The 0 synthetic absorbable suture is continued in a running lock fashion around the edge of the vagina. Care is taken to place several sutures into the stump of the uterosacral and cardinal ligaments to firmly attach them to the angle of the vagina.

**17** The peritoneum of the pelvis is reestablished with a running 3-0 synthetic absorbable suture approximating the anterior peritoneum to the posterior peritoneum.

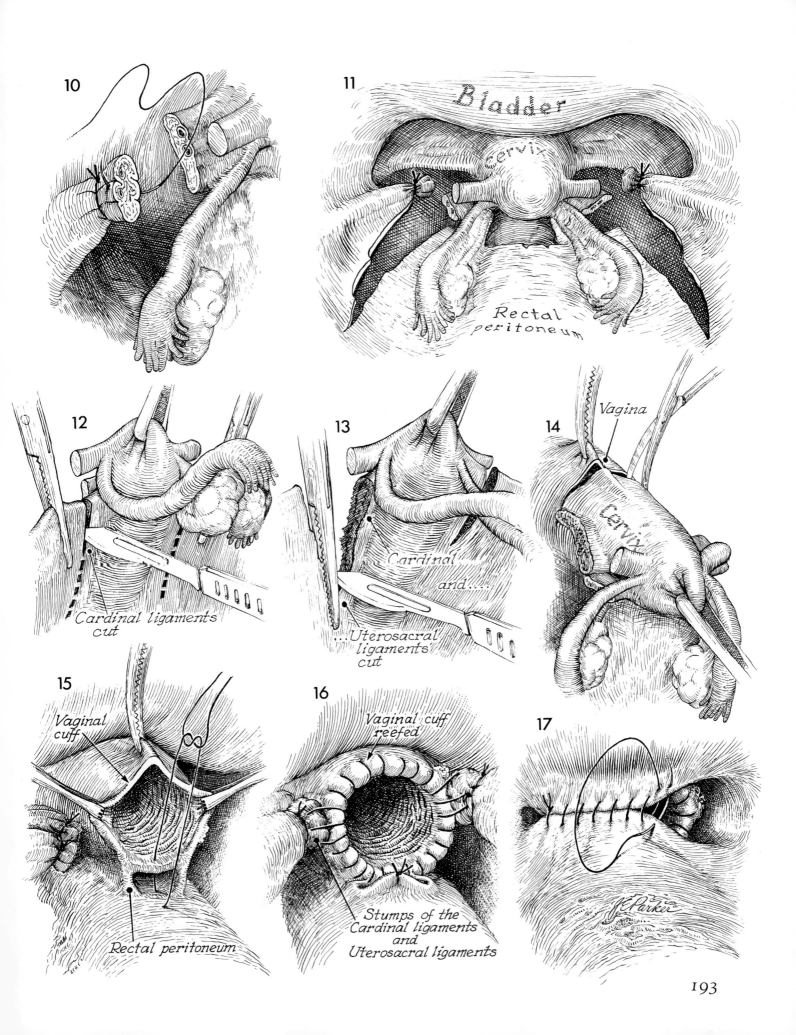

10

11

Bladder

cervix

Rectal
peritoneum

12

Cardinal ligaments
cut

13

Cardinal
and...

...Uterosacral
ligaments
cut

14

Vagina

cervix

15

Vaginal
cuff

Rectal peritoneum

16

Vaginal cuff
reefed

Stumps of the
Cardinal ligaments
and
Uterosacral ligaments

17

JCParker

193

# Correction of an Incompetent Cervix by the Shirodkar Technique

Patients who have habitually experienced second-trimester abortions may have an incompetent cervical os. Of the several surgical alternatives available to correct this problem, the Shirodkar technique, with fascia lata used, is an excellent choice for patients in the nonpregnant state.

The purpose of the operation is to restore competence to the cervix and thereby prevent the cervix from dilation during the second-trimester pregnancy.

**Physiologic Changes.** The restoration of appropriate strength to the internal cervical os prevents sudden dilation as the pregnancy progresses.

**Points of Caution.** Patients having this operation should be delivered at term by cesarean section.

Care must be taken to adequately mobilize the bladder to prevent injury from application of the fascia strap.

If the tunnel made on the lateral side of the cervix is made too high, the uterine vessels may be perforated, and copious hemorrhage may result.

## Technique

1 The patient is placed in the dorsal lithotomy position. The vulva and vagina are prepped with a surgical soap solution. A weighted posterior retractor is placed in the vagina, and the cervix is grasped with a wide-mouthed tenaculum on the anterior lip. A transverse incision approximately 2–3 cm wide is made at the junction of the vaginal mucosa and the portio of the cervix. The incised edge of the vagina is picked up with an Allis clamp or thumb forceps.

2 Allis clamps are applied to the lateral edge of the transverse incision, and a gloved finger is used to dissect the bladder off the cervix. The bladder should be dissected up to the vesicouterine peritoneal fold, thus avoiding injury when the strap is placed.

3 The posterior vaginal epithelium overlying the cul-de-sac is exposed. A transverse incision is made approximately 2–3 cm at the junction of the posterior vaginal mucosa and the cervical portio. With Metzenbaum scissors, the peritoneum of the cul-de-sac is dissected from the posterior cervix.

4 A piece of fascia lata that has been previously taken from the lateral thigh (see Section 2, page 115, for the Goebell-Stoeckel fascia lata sling procedure including the technique for obtaining the strip of fascia lata) is used for the Shirodkar strap. An aneurysm needle is maneuvered under the vaginal mucosa from the anterior incision into the posterior incision. A suture of 2-0 Prolene is placed in the end of the fascia lata strap and tied to the aneurysm needle.

5 The fascia strap is pulled from the posterior transverse incision into the anterior transverse incision. In a similar manner, the other aneurysm needle is used to dissect under the left side of the remaining vaginal mucosa and likewise is attached to the opposite end of the fascia strip with 2-0 Prolene.

6 The fascia lata strap is fixed to the posterior surface of the cervix with a single interrupted 2-0 synthetic absorbable suture.

7 A right-angle retractor lifts the bladder up and away from the anterior cervix; the fascia lata strap is trimmed to fit snugly around the cervix at the level of the internal os. The fascia strap is anchored to the anterior cervical tissue with several interrupted 2-0 Prolene sutures.

8 The anterior vaginal mucosa is returned to position and resutured with interrupted 3-0 synthetic absorbable suture.

9 This illustrates the results of the operation in the midplane. The internal os is closed enough to admit only a uterine sound or a 4-mm Hegar dilator. Thus, it becomes obvious that cesarean section will have to be performed to accommodate delivery.

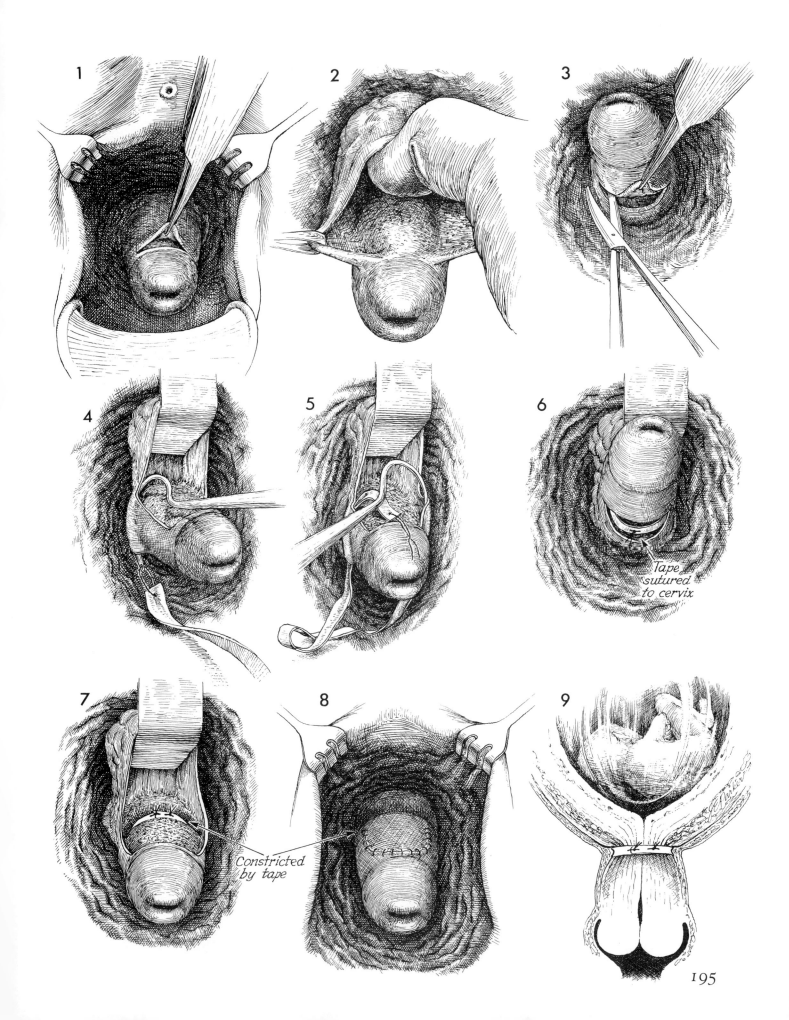

1

2

3

4

5

6

*Tape
sutured
to cervix*

7

*Constricted
by tape*

8

9

# Correction of an Incompetent Cervix by the McDonald Operation

The McDonald operation is used in a pregnant patient with an incompetent cervix. It may be performed under local anesthesia with minimal irritation to the uterus. It should be performed as early in the pregnancy as possible and must be done prior to effacement and complete dilation of the cervix.

Rupture of the membranes, leading to the loss of the pregnancy, may be associated with the procedure. The suture must be cut prior to labor to prevent severe laceration of the cervix.

In the McDonald operation, a suture is strategically placed to give additional strength to the cervix and thereby prevent second-trimester abortion.

**Physiologic Changes.** By suturing the cervix, the products of gestation are held in the uterine cavity until the fetus is viable.

**Points of Caution.** Care must be taken not to lacerate the soft pregnant cervix with the instruments.

The suture must be placed near the internal cervical os, but care must be exercised not to enter the bladder with the suture anteriorly.

---

## Technique

**1** The patient, who may be given light sedation with Demerol and Valium, is placed in the dorsal lithotomy position. The vulva and vagina are prepped with a surgical soap solution, and the weighted posterior retractor is placed in the vagina to expose the cervix. An effort is made to place a minimum of retraction instruments upon the cervix; if a retraction instrument is needed, however, a wide-mouthed toothless instrument such as a sponge forceps is preferable to a single-toothed cervical tenaculum. A large, monofilament nonabsorbable suture such as Prolene or nylon is selected. The first bite of the McDonald stitch is placed at the 12 o'clock position on the cervix at the junction of the vaginal mucosa and portio of the cervix at the level of the internal os.

**2** Repeated pursestring sutures are placed in 4 or 6 bites around the cervix at the level of the internal os.

**3** The pursestring suture is tied.

**4** A cross section of the cervix reveals the way the McDonald suture closes the internal os. The suture must be cut prior to labor and delivery of the fetus.

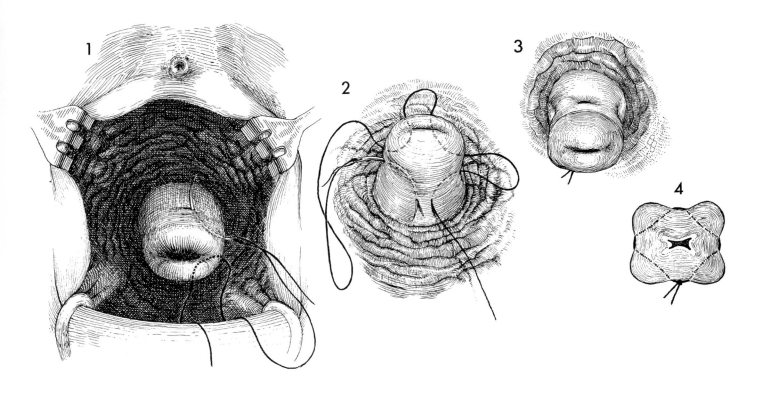

# Correction of an Incompetent Cervix by the Lash Operation

Patients with habitual second-trimester abortions occasionally show a defect in the wall of the cervix. This is usually at the 12 o'clock position at the internal cervical os and may be related to failure of fusion of the Müllerian duct. In any case, it results in a weakened internal cervical os. Repair is best performed in the nonpregnant state.

The purpose of the Lash operation is to correct the defect in the cervical wall and restore competence to the cervix, thereby allowing gestation to proceed to term.

**Physiologic Changes.** The cervix regains the strength to hold the developing fetus in utero until term, thus preventing second-trimester abortion.

**Points of Caution.** Patients undergoing the Lash operation should be delivered at term by cesarean section. Dilation and effacement of the cervix following this procedure are unpredictable.

Care must be taken to ensure that the bladder is properly retracted in order to prevent the placement of sutures through the bladder in the closing of the cervical defect.

## Technique

**1** The patient is placed in the dorsal lithotomy position under general anesthesia, and the vulva and vagina are prepped in a surgical manner. A weighted posterior retractor is placed in the vagina. The cervix is exposed and is placed on traction with a wide-mouthed tenaculum such as a Jacobs tenaculum. A uterine sound is placed in the cervical os, and the defect is demonstrated in the cervical wall. A transverse vaginal incision is made for approximately 2–3 cm at the junction of the vaginal mucosa and the portio of the cervix. This may require extending the mucosal incision laterally in a "block U."

**2** The bladder is dissected off the cervix with blunt dissection.

**3** The defect is exposed, and the unhealthy cervical tissue is excised with a knife. The opening is closed in two layers with interrupted 2-0 Dexon suture.

**4** The bladder is elevated by a right-angle retractor to separate it from the suturing procedure. Interrupted 2-0 delayed absorbable Lembert inverting sutures are placed in a second row.

**5** The sutures are tied, inverting the defect into the cervical canal. A uterine sound is passed through the cervical canal to ensure that the canal has not been obliterated.

**6** The vaginal mucosa is reapproximated with interrupted 3-0 synthetic absorbable sutures. The patient should be protected from pregnancy for a minimum of 3 months to allow maximum healing of the cervical incision.

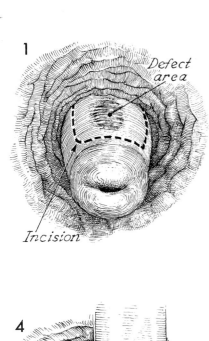

1

Defect area

Incision

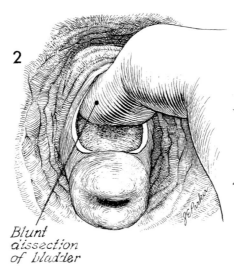

2

Blunt
dissection
of bladder

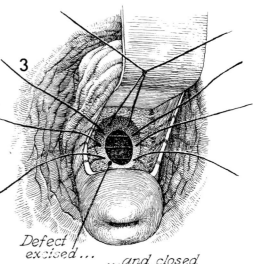

3

Defect
excised...

...and closed
in 2 layers

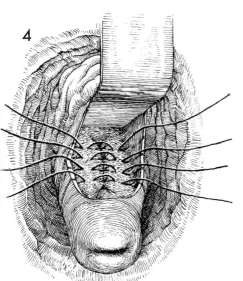

4

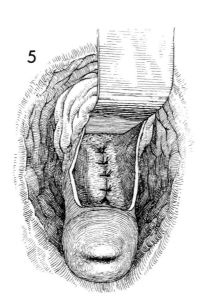

5

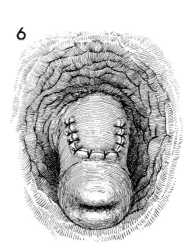

6

# 5

## Uterus

# Dilatation and Curettage

Dilatation and curettage unrelated to pregnancy is best performed with the patient under general anesthesia to allow the gynecologist to perform a more thorough pelvic examination.

The purpose of the operation is to remove as much hyperplastic, proliferative, and necrotic endometrium as possible to allow an accurate pathologic diagnosis to be made and to arrest dysfunctional uterine bleeding.

Excessive bleeding will usually discontinue for at least several months.

**Physiologic Changes.** Removal of the endometrium back to the stratum basale will not change the physiology of the hypothalamic-pituitary-ovarian axis in regard to ovulation.

**Points of Caution.** Care must be taken in dilating the cervix to avoid perforation of the uterus.

---

## Technique

**1** The patient is placed in the dorsal lithotomy position with the legs in appropriate gynecologic stirrups.

**2** A thorough bimanual examination, including a rectovaginal examination, should be performed prior to the procedure.
The perineum and vagina should be washed with surgical soap. Shaving the perineal hair, however, is not necessary for this procedure.

**3** Adequate exposure to the cervix can be achieved by the use of a Sims posterior retractor. Some gynecologists prefer a weighted posterior retractor, but in most cases this is unnecessary. The procedure is begun by grasping the anterior lip of the cervix with a wide-mouthed Jacobs tenaculum. The endometrial cavity is sounded for both depth and direction.

**4** The cervical canal is progressively dilated with Pratt dilators until a diameter of approximately 8 mm is reached.

**5** A ureteral stone forceps is helpful in exploring the uterine cavity and searching for polyps. Polyps can frequently be missed by the sharp curet itself. If polyps are found, they should be removed by twisting them from their stalks. They should be sent to the pathology laboratory in a separate specimen.

**6** A sharp curet is advanced through the dilated cervical canal to the fundus. The endometrial cavity is curetted with a systematic back-and-forth movement of the curet so that all possible endometrium is sampled.

**7** The cervix should be stained with Lugol's solution, and four random quadrant biopsies should be taken from the squamocolumnar junction.

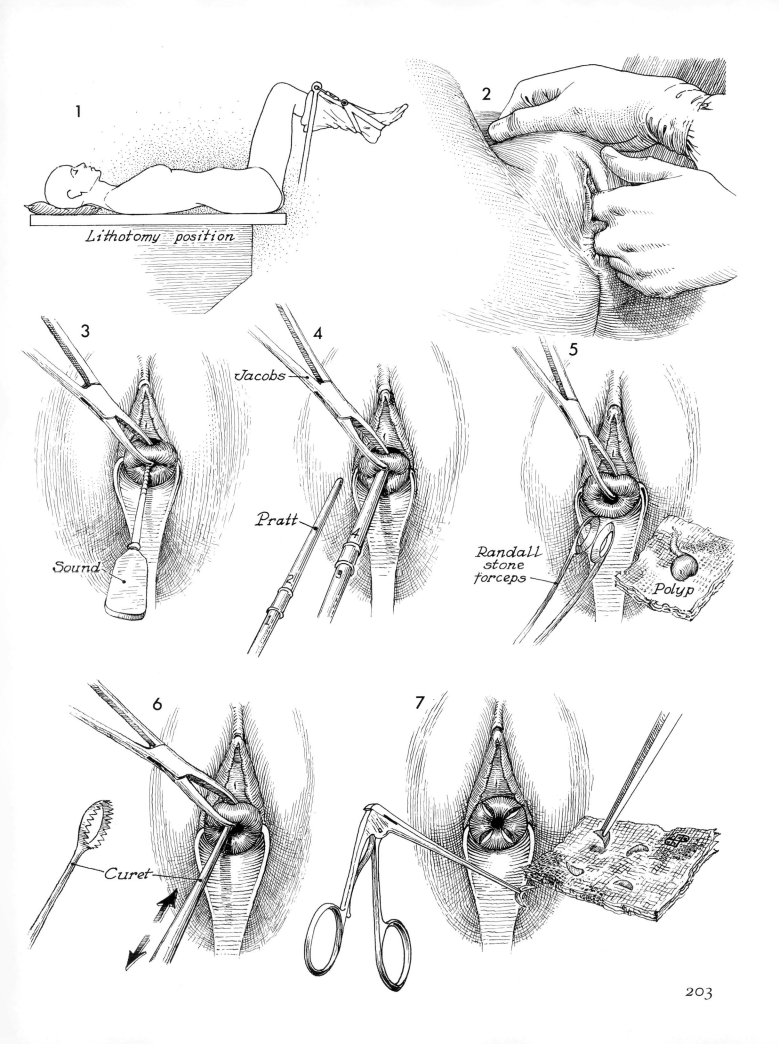

1

*Lithotomy position*

2

3

*Sound*

4

*Jacobs*

*Pratt*

5

*Randall stone forceps*

*Polyp*

6

*Curet*

7

203

# Suction Curettage for Abortion

Suction curettage has proven to be the most efficacious technique for evacuation of the uterus in the first trimester of pregnancy. It has advantages over sharp curettage in that it has a lower incidence of uterine perforation and less blood loss.

The purpose of the operation is to evacuate the gravid uterus in the first trimester.

**Physiologic Changes.** The use of a strong vacuum through a suction catheter placed through the dilated cervix into the uterine cavity rapidly shears away the first-trimester placenta from the uterine wall.

When a vacuum pump producing 70 mm Hg and 100 mL of airflow per minute is used, the products of conception are rapidly separated from the uterine wall, allowing their removal from the endometrial cavity and inducing uterine contraction, thereby reducing blood loss.

**Points of Caution.** Care must be taken to determine the length of gestation of the pregnancy. This should be done by history and by physical examination of the pelvis. In addition, the uterine cavity should be accurately measured with a sound prior to initiating the procedure. In this way, pregnancies exceeding 13 weeks should be diagnosed, and suction abortion performed, in those circumstances where the potential benefits outweigh the risks of performing a second-trimester abortion with the suction technique.

The surgeon should be sure that adequate airflow through the suction pump is maintained at all times. An airflow in the system of approximately 100 mL/minute is preferred. For most standard suction curettage machines, this means turning the pump to the maximum setting. Reduced or low airflow through the system allows retained products of conception and therefore increases the risk of hemorrhage and postpartum infection.

If perforation of the uterus is suspected, the vacuum should be turned off, and the curet should be removed with caution to prevent injury to the intestine.

# Suction Curettage for Abortion

## (Continued)

*Technique*

**1** The patient is placed in the dorsal lithotomy position after appropriate anesthesia (general, regional, or local) has been administered.

**2** A careful pelvic examination is performed to accurately ascertain the gestational size of the uterus.

**3** A Sims posterior retractor is used to obtain adequate exposure to the upper vagina and cervix. Lateral retractors or self-retaining retractors are rarely needed for this procedure.

The anterior lip of the cervix is grasped with a wide-mouthed Jacobs tenaculum. Single-toothed tenacula should be avoided, as they tend to tear the pregnant cervix. A uterine sound is passed through the undilated cervix until the fundus is reached. The length of the uterine cavity is recorded.

**4** Tapered cervical dilators, such as Pratt dilators, are used to progressively dilate the cervix, usually to 10 mm in diameter. Nontapered dilators, such as Hegar dilators, should be avoided because they are difficult to pass through the cervix, particularly in nulliparous patients, and produce a greater amount of cervical trauma.

**5** After appropriate dilatation, a suction cannula is introduced through the cervix. We prefer large-diameter straight suction cannulae, such as 10-mm straight cannulae, rather than the curved or angulated variety. This is because 360° arcs of the cannulae must be made to adequately remove all gestational tissue. When 360° arcs are made with angulated cannulae, the diameter of the arc created in the intrauterine cavity by the angulated suction cannulae is excessive.

The suction curet should be introduced all the way to the fundus.

**6** The suction is applied to the curet. The curet is rotated in a 360° arc and is slowly withdrawn in 1-cm increments.

The suction curet should be introduced 2–3 times to ensure that all products of conception have been adequately removed.

It is efficacious at this point to administer 50 IU of Pitocin in an intravenous drip and 0.2 mg of Methergine given intravenously. This has significantly reduced blood loss by inducing uterine contraction.

**7** An ovum or sponge forceps is introduced into the endometrial cavity and are opened, closed, and withdrawn several times to ensure that all gestation tissue has been removed.

The patient is observed for 2 hours for hemorrhage prior to discharge.

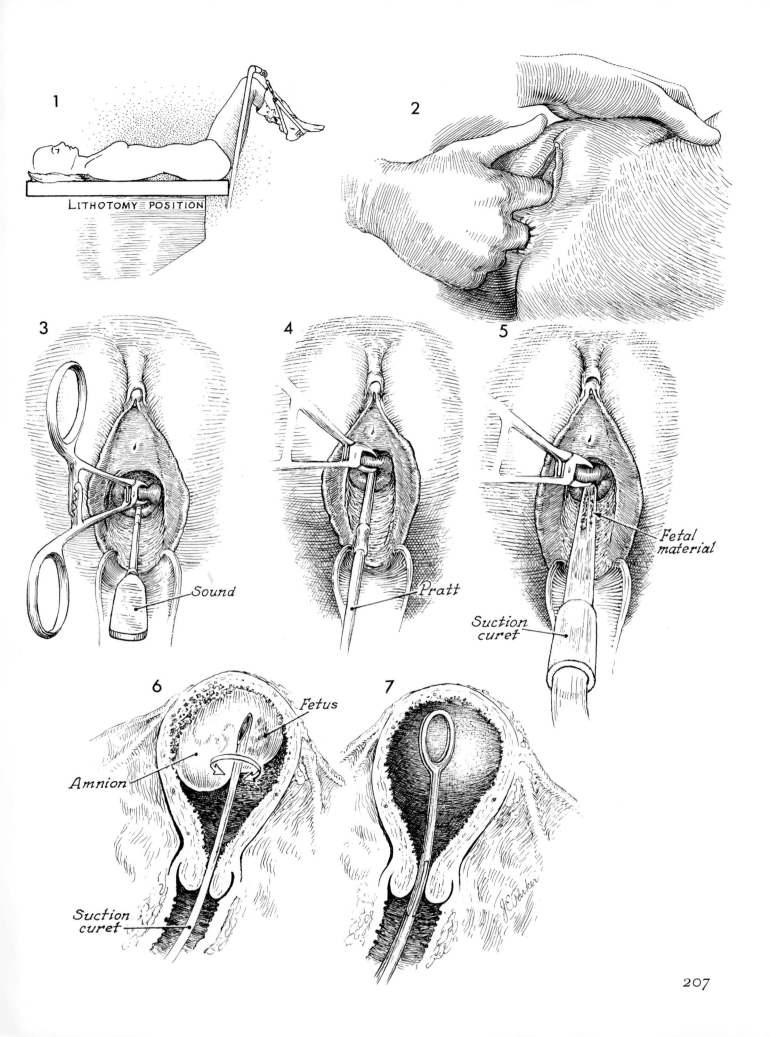

1

LITHOTOMY POSITION

2

3

Sound

4

Pratt

5

Fetal material

Suction curet

6

Fetus

Amnion

Suction curet

7

207

# Management of Major Uterine Perforations From Suction Curet or Radium Tandem

Perforation of the uterus by the suction curettage cannula or by the tandem during radium application can cause serious complications of the small and large intestine if it is managed improperly. There is a distinct difference between the effects of these two kinds of perforation. If perforation occurs during suction curettage, the small bowel may be sucked into the eyes of the curet and pulled through the opening into the endometrial cavity and out through the cervix. Laceration of the small bowel can occur during this procedure. Although the large bowel is difficult to pull through the uterine perforation and out the cervix, the suction curet can attach itself to the wall of the large bowel and evulse a segment of it.

A different problem exists with the intracavitary radiation therapy radium tandem. If the tandem perforates the uterine wall and the perforation is not recognized, it may cause severe radiation damage to the small bowel on which it comes to rest.

In both of the above situations, the surgeon should immediately insert a laparoscope through the umbilicus and under direct vision withdraw the suction curet or the tandem back into the uterus. In the case of the suction curet, the suction should be reapplied, and the pregnancy should be completely terminated to avoid further complicating the situation by adding the sequelae of incomplete abortion.

In cases of perforation by the radium tandem, once the tandem has been replaced back into the uterus, the radium application can proceed as indicated.

**Points of Caution.** If perforation occurs during suction curettage, the suction should be turned off immediately to reduce the degree of injury to the intestine.

---

## Technique

**1** In this sagittal section of the pelvis, the suction curet has perforated the fundus of the uterus. Note that the small intestine is immediately adjacent to the suction curet. B identifies the bladder; R, the rectum; and V, the vagina.

**2** If suction is continued, the small intestine can be suctioned into the eye of the curet and pulled through the fundus down into the endometrial cavity. Frequently, the surgeon mistakes the resistance of the bowel for the adherence of fetal parts and continues to pull.

**3** If sufficient force is used, the intestine is pulled out through the cervix; occasionally, evulsion of the intestinal wall results.

**4** This sagittal section shows the laparoscope being introduced in the routine manner through the umbilicus. The suction cannula is visualized.

**5** With one surgeon viewing through the laparoscope and a second surgeon operating from below and with the suction cannula disconnected from its vacuum pump, the curet is gently withdrawn back into the endometrial cavity.

**6** With the suction cannula safely in the endometrial cavity, vacuum is reapplied, and termination of the pregnancy is completed under laparoscopic control.

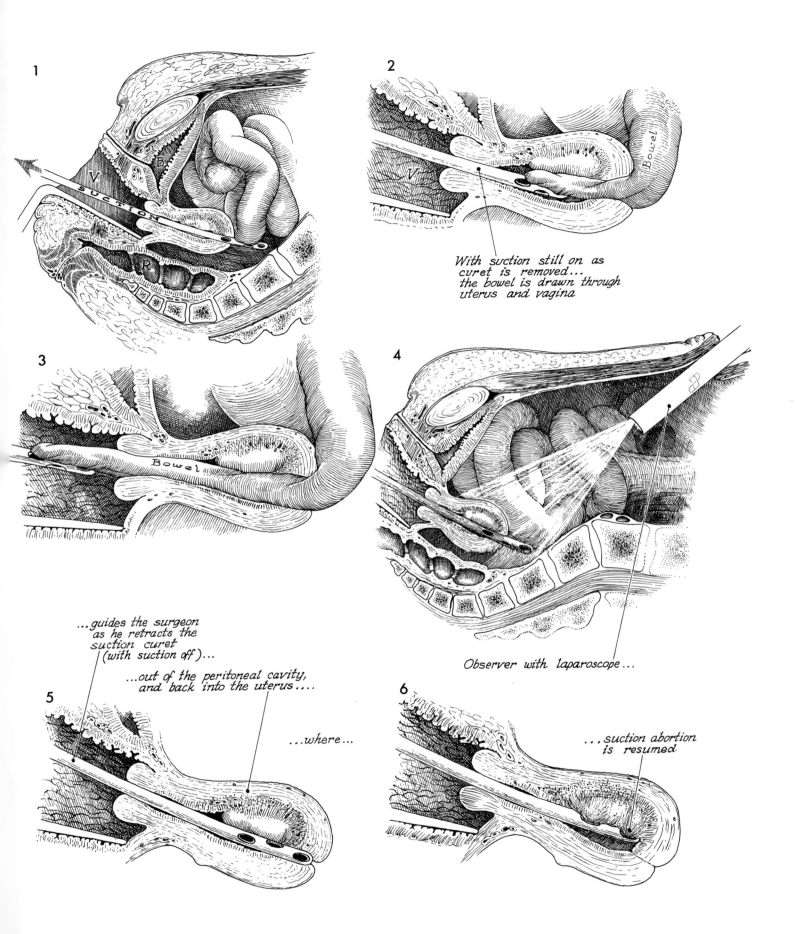

**1**

**2**

*With suction still on as curet is removed... the bowel is drawn through uterus and vagina*

**3**

Bowel

**4**

*Observer with laparoscope...*

*...guides the surgeon as he retracts the suction curet (with suction off)...*

*...out of the peritoneal cavity, and back into the uterus....*

*...where...*

**5**

**6**

*...suction abortion is resumed*

209

# Management of Major Uterine Perforations From Suction Curet or Radium Tandem

## (Continued)

**7** This sagittal section shows the intracavitary radiation therapy tandem perforating the fundus. At this point, the laparoscope is introduced through the umbilicus, and the tandem is visualized and withdrawn back into the endometrial cavity.

**8** When the tandem is safely withdrawn into the endometrial cavity, the ovoids are applied to the tandem in the routine fashion, and the intracavitary radiation therapy procedure is completed. Rarely does perforation by radium tandem result in hemorrhage severe enough to require surgical closing of the defect.

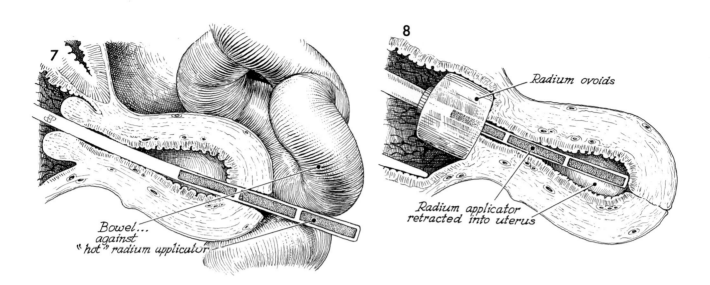

7

Bowel...
against
"hot" radium applicator

8

Radium ovoids

Radium applicator
retracted into uterus

# Cesarean Section

Cesarean section, a life-saving operation for both fetus and mother, accounts for approximately 20% of deliveries in the United States today. The lower cervical transverse incision for this operation has become the accepted technique, except in cases in which compound presentations require the classic vertical incision in the fundus of the uterus.

The purpose of the operation is to deliver the fetus through the abdomen in instances where vaginal delivery would be either impossible or dangerous to the life or health of the mother and/or fetus.

**Physiologic Changes.** There are many differences in the physiologic changes between vaginal delivery and cesarean section. Fetuses delivered by cesarean section may have a higher incidence of respiratory distress syndrome. On the other hand, vaginal delivery with dystocia can produce central nervous system damage. Further discussion involving the physiology of cesarean section is beyond the scope of this text, and the reader is referred to the obstetrical literature for additional information.

**Points of Caution.** The anesthesia for cesarean section should be selected with care. An epidural regional block is recommended, since this has the least chance of causing fetal depression.

If general anesthesia is to be used, the anesthesiologist should be consulted to ensure proper timing between the infusion of the rapid-acting barbiturates and delivery of the baby in order to minimize any depressing effect on the central nervous system of the fetus. Care should be exercised in dissecting the bladder off the lower uterine segment to prevent laceration of the bladder during the procedure. If, by chance, excessive manual stretching of the transverse incision should lacerate the uterine vessels in the broad ligament, this ligament should be opened. The uterine vessels should then be carefully dissected out and individually ligated to prevent postoperative hematoma and possible damage to the underlying ureter.

## Technique

**1** For cesarean section, a Foley catheter is placed in the bladder, and the patient is placed in the dorsal supine position. The abdomen is surgically prepped. The abdomen can be opened through a lower transverse incision or a midline incision.

**2** After opening the abdominal cavity, the vesicouterine fold is identified and opened. Moist packs can be placed in the lateral gutters on each side of the uterus to prevent blood and fluid from draining into the peritoneal cavity.

**3** When the bladder has been dissected down, a small transverse incision is made in the lower uterine segment with a scalpel.

**4** An opening is made in the amniotic sac large enough to admit two fingers.

**5** The fingers are inserted into the uterine cavity.

**6** The incision is stretched laterally.

**7** The appropriate fetal parts are grasped.

**8** Occasionally, obstetrical forceps or the hand is inserted to aid in removal of the fetus.

**9** The fetus is removed.

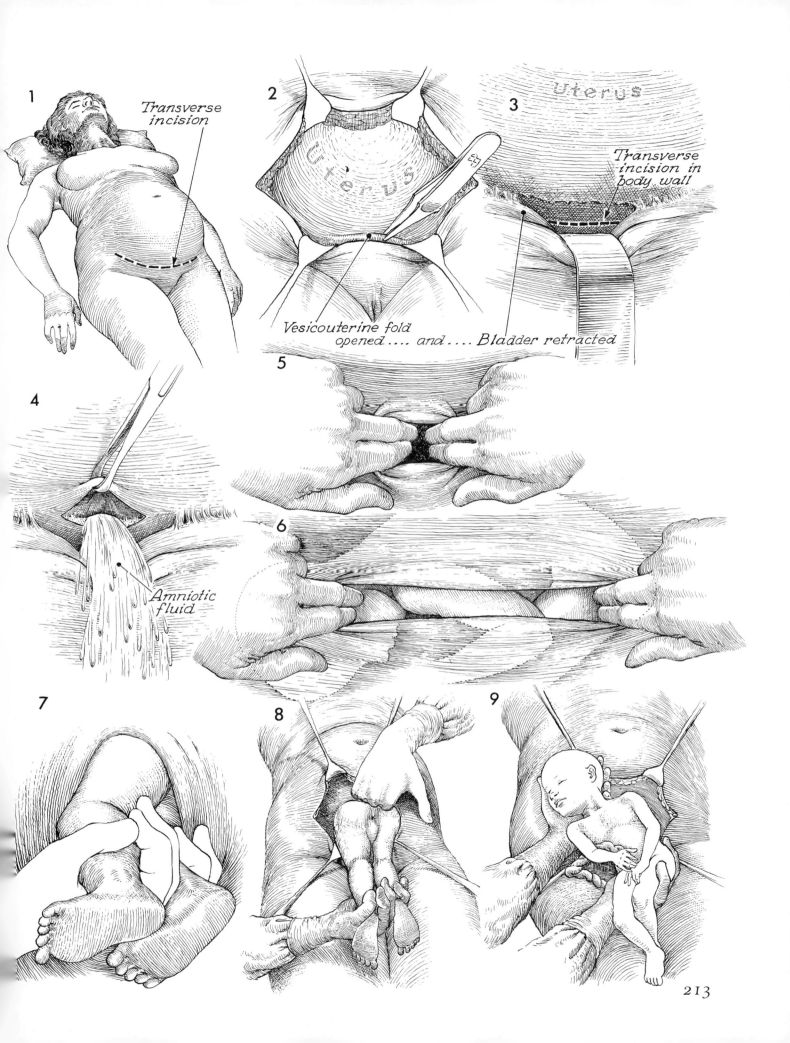

**1**

*Transverse incision*

**2**

Uterus

Uterus

*Vesicouterine fold opened.... and.... Bladder retracted*

**3**

Uterus

*Transverse incision in body wall*

**4**

*Amniotic fluid*

**5**

**6**

**7**

**8**

**9**

213

# Cesarean Section

## (Continued)

**10** The cord is doubly clamped and incised. The fetus is immediately suctioned and handed to the pediatrician.

**11** We prefer to deliver the uterus through the incision. The placenta is manually extracted.

**12** A retractor is inserted into the uterine incision. The uterus is manually explored, and any remaining placental membranes are removed under direct vision.

**13** Excess blood in and around the incision is removed by suction.

**14** The first layer of 0 synthetic absorbable suture is placed in the transverse incision as a continuous suture. A second layer of interrupted 0 synthetic absorbable suture is placed in the myometrium.

**15** The serosa of the uterus and the vesicouterine peritoneal fold are closed with continuous 3-0 synthetic absorbable suture.

**16** The parietal peritoneum is closed with continuous 3-0 synthetic absorbable suture.

**17** The rectus muscles are approximated in the midline, and the fascia is closed with interrupted 0 Vicryl suture.

**18** The remaining abdominal wall is closed in layers. The Foley catheter is left in the bladder for 24 hours.

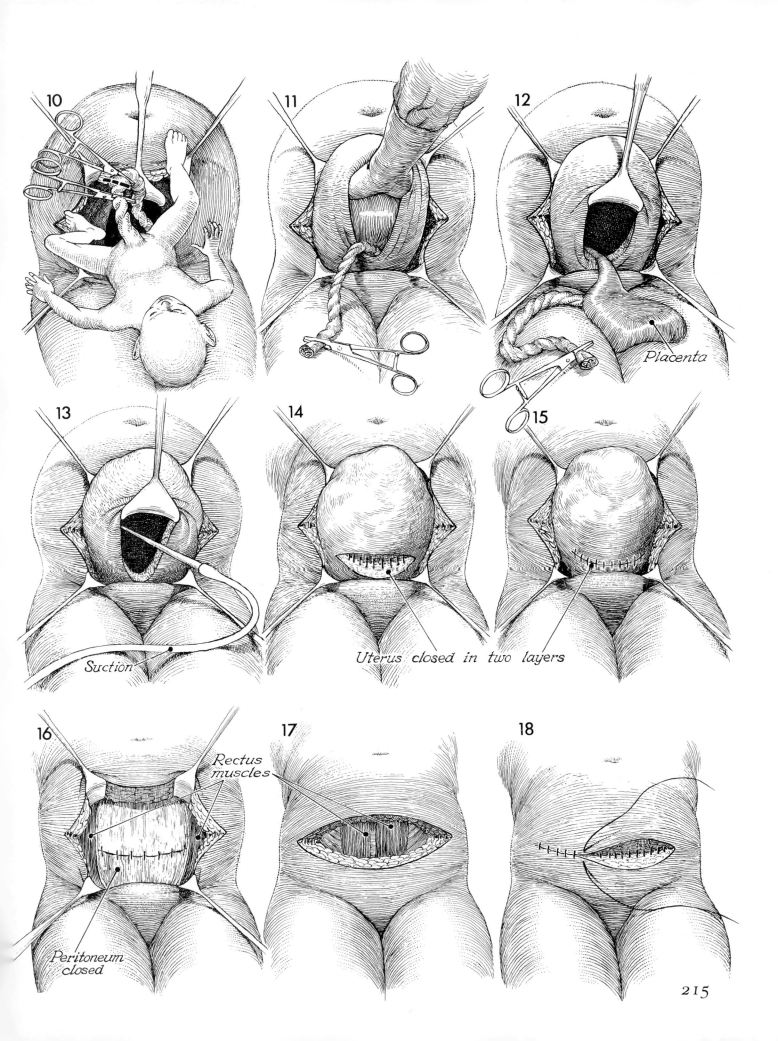

10

11

12

Placenta

13

Suction

14

Uterus closed in two layers

15

16

Rectus
muscles

Peritoneum
closed

17

18

215

# Myomectomy

When a myoma is demonstrated to be the cause of infertility in a patient who wants to have a child or when a patient is otherwise opposed to complete hysterectomy, myomectomy is indicated.

**Physiologic Changes.** When the fibroid tumor is removed from the uterus, the physiologic relationship between the endometrium and myometrium is restored, and excessive uterine bleeding should cease.

## Technique

1 With the patient in the dorsal supine position, an incision is made into the abdominal cavity, through either a midline or a Pfannenstiel approach.

2 The uterus is exposed, the bowel is packed off, and the fibroid tumor is identified.

3 With needlepoint cautery, the surgeon transects adhesions from intestine to the uterus.

4 An incision is made in the serosal surface of the uterus through the myometrium down to the myoma. An Allis clamp is applied to one edge of the incision, and the incision is elevated. A finger or hemostatic forceps is used to sweep the myometrium off the fibroid tumor.

5 A towel clip is used to grasp the fibroid tumor, and traction and/or countertraction is used to elevate the fibroid tumor out of the myometrium. A pedicle of fibrous tissue is reached. This is severed with Metzenbaum scissors or the needlepoint electrocautery, and the tumor is removed.

6 Any additional fibroids are located and grasped with a towel clip, elevated, and dissected out in a similar manner.

7 If excessive myometrium and serosa are present, these should be trimmed away.

8 The myometrium should be closed in two layers with 2-0 synthetic absorbable sutures.

9 The serosa is reapproximated with 4-0 absorbable suture.

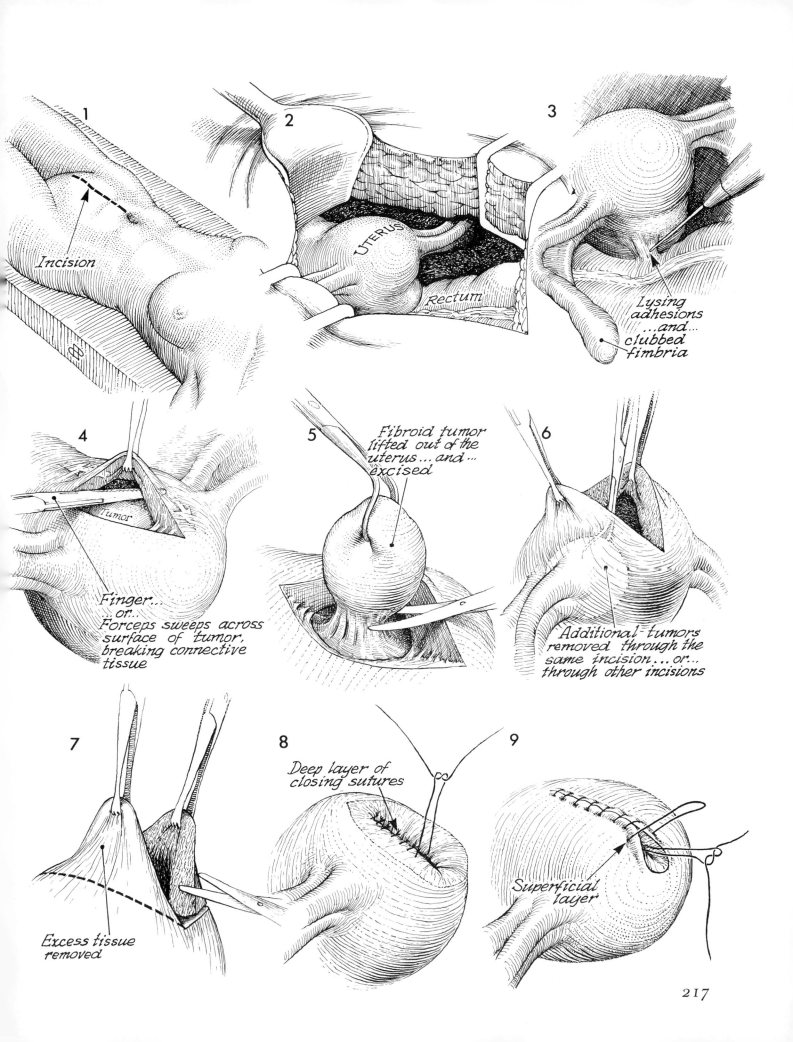

**1**

Incision

**2**

UTERUS

Rectum

**3**

Lysing
adhesions
...and...
clubbed
fimbria

**4**

Tumor

Finger...
...or...
Forceps sweeps across
surface of tumor,
breaking connective
tissue

**5**

Fibroid tumor
lifted out of the
uterus...and...
excised

**6**

Additional tumors
removed through the
same incision...or...
through other incisions

**7**

Excess tissue
removed

**8**

Deep layer of
closing sutures

**9**

Superficial
layer

217

# Jones Operation for Correction of Double Uterus

The term "double uterus" in this atlas refers to the various embryologic deformities resulting from failure of fusion of the Müllerian ducts. Most patients with a double uterus have no reproductive difficulties or fetal wastage and do not need surgical intervention. Approximately 20%, however, have habitual first- or second-trimester abortions.

Several procedures are available for correction of the double-uterus deformity (Strassman, Tompkins, and Jones operations). We have chosen to present the surgical details of the Jones operation because in our opinion it is the most physiologic approach for the correction of this deformity.

The purpose of the operation is to restore the uterus to its normal configuration by removing the fibrous septum.

**Physiologic Changes.** The fibrous septum within a double uterus makes a poor implantation site for the placenta. It lacks the proper endometrial lining necessary to support nidation and placental growth.

By removing this fibrous septum, the placenta grows on a normal, healthy endometrium.

**Points of Caution.** Many obstetricians prefer to deliver all of these patients by cesarean section at term prior to labor.

Care must be taken to ensure that parallel incisions into the fundus of the uterus are made to prevent cornual dissection of the myometrium. Cornual dissection may jeopardize the intramural portion of the Fallopian tube.

All of the fibrous septum must be removed.

# Jones Operation for Correction of Double Uterus

## (Continued)

*Technique*

**1** A frontal section of the uterus with the uterine septum is shown. The *dotted line* indicates the wedge to be excised.

**2** The patient is placed on the operating table in the dorsal position. We have found it helpful to insert a Foley catheter through the cervix into the endometrial cavity and instill 10 mL of an indigo carmine solution to stain the endometrial cavity prior to the uterine incision.

A second Foley catheter should be inserted into the bladder.

The abdomen can be opened through a midline or transverse incision. The bowel is packed away, and a self-retaining retractor is used to keep the abdominal wound open. The fundus is palpated with the thumb and index finger to locate the extent of the fibrous septum. A traction suture is placed in the midportion of the uterus. Additional traction sutures are placed lateral to the fibrous septum.

The myometrium is injected at several points with a saline-Pitressin solution (10 IU of Pitressin in 30 mL of saline solution). Injection of this solution, which produces contraction of the uterus, has been superior to applying a tourniquet to the lower uterine segment for hemostasis. Regardless of the hemostatic technique used (tourniquet or Pitressin injection), a bloodless field in the operating wound is essential for meticulous dissection and accurate placement of suture material. Brilliant green solution is used to mark the lateral extent of the fibrous septum as determined by palpation of the uterus.

**3** A scalpel is used to open the fundus along the lines marked with brilliant green solution. Traction on the three sutures is maintained by an assistant. Care must be taken at this point so that lateral dissection of the myometrium into the cornual area is avoided to prevent transection of the tube. The entire fibrous septum must be excised.

**4** A row of 3-0 Dexon sutures is placed through the endometrium, closing the endometrium and the innermost layers of the myometrium.

**5** The second row of 2-0 Dexon is used to close the myometrium with a mattress suture.

**6** Figure 6 shows three layers of sutures: those on the myometrium (*a*), those on the endometrium (*b*), and those on the serosa (*c*).

**7** The completed operation is shown. Interrupted sutures in the serosa have been placed approximately 1 cm apart from the lower uterine segment of the opposite side.

**8** This frontal section of the uterus shows the unified endometrial cavity. Sutures *a*, *b*, and *c* have been placed as described in Step 6.

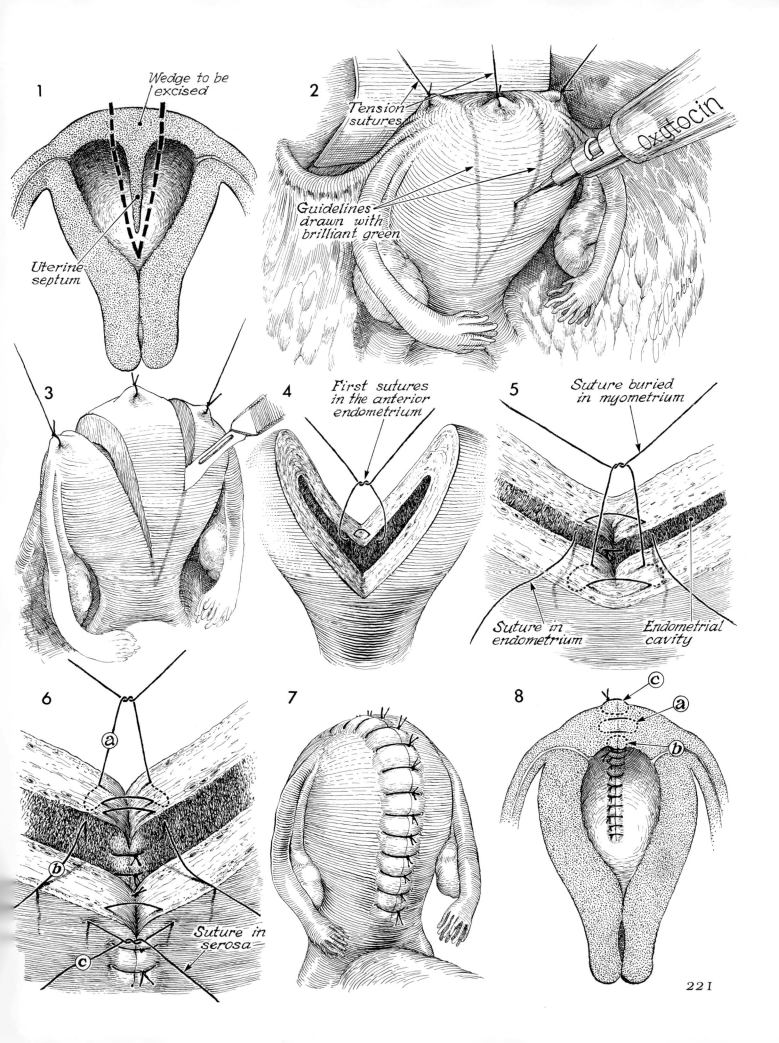

1  *Wedge to be excised*

*Uterine septum*

2  *Tension sutures*  *Oxytocin*

*Guidelines drawn with brilliant green*

3

4  *First sutures in the anterior endometrium*

5  *Suture buried in myometrium*

*Suture in endometrium*  *Endometrial cavity*

6  (a)  (b)  (c)

*Suture in serosa*

7

8  (c)  (a)  (b)

221

# Hysteroscopic Septal Resection by Loop Electrical Excision Procedure (LEEP) for Correction of a Double Uterus

A patient who is unable to carry a pregnancy to term is sometimes found, on hysterosalpingogram, to have a septate form of double uterus. In such cases, resection of the septum often corrects the problem and results in a successful pregnancy.

Before the introduction of the hysteroscopic operative instruments, this operation required a laparotomy as well as a hysterotomy with resection of the septum, i.e., Jones, Strassman, and Tompkins operations. The introduction of operative hysteroscopic instruments offers a new form of treatment that avoids a laparotomy, resulting in a shorter hospitalization and faster recovery.

**Physiologic Changes.** A septate uterus is thought to cause fetal wastage because it cannot provide sufficient endometrium, which, in turn, provides nourishment for the developing placenta. When the septum has been removed, adequate endometrium returns, and nourishment becomes available.

**Points of Caution.** Loop electrical excision can be associated with severe bleeding. Perforation of the uterus and injury to the adjacent intestine or bladder are possible but rare. Expansion of the endometrial cavity with 5% dextrose in Ringer's solution improves visualization and reduces hemorrhage, therefore allowing accurate loop electrical excision and electrocoagulation of vessels that are bleeding.

## Technique

1  The hysteroscope is inserted into the endometrial cavity after dilation of the cervix. The LEEP device is inserted down the operative channel of the hysteroscope. The endometrial cavity is expanded with 5% dextrose and Ringer's solution. The LEEP electrocoagulation machine is set on a blend between cutting and coagulation current. The hysteroscope is advanced up the uterus along the septum. The LEEP device is aimed at the fundus, where the uterine septum and endometrial tissue join. The internal os of the Fallopian tubes must be identified, and the electrical incision must be kept medial to the os of the tubes. By progressively coagulating and cutting the base of the septum with the LEEP device, the surgeon is able to resect and remove the entire septum.

2  The base of the septum has been electrocoagulated thoroughly to prevent bleeding.

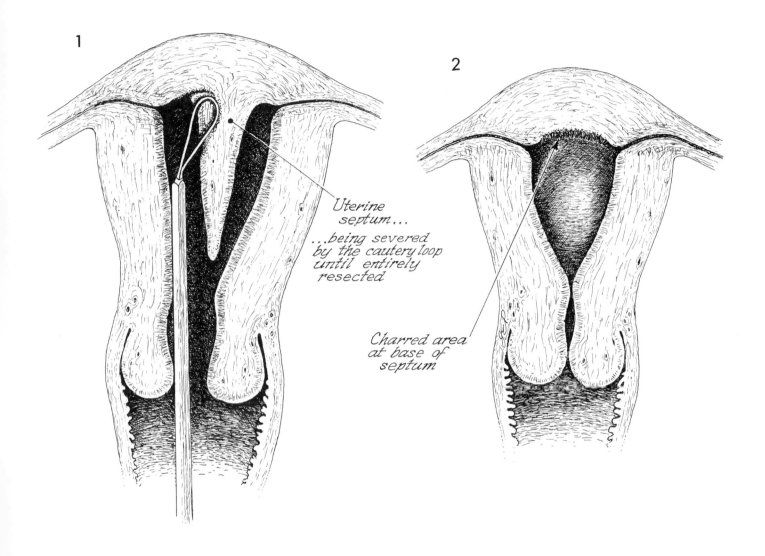

1

2

*Uterine*
*septum...*

*...being severed*
*by the cautery loop*
*until entirely*
*resected*

*Charred area*
*at base of*
*septum*

223

# Manchester Operation

The Manchester operation was designed for women with second- and third-degree uterine descensus with cystourethrocele. If stress incontinence of urine accompanies the condition, the Manchester operation can be combined with a Kelly plication of the urethrovesical sphincter. The advantages of the Manchester operation are that the surgeon does not enter the peritoneal cavity, the operating time is reduced, and the operation is not associated with a prolonged or morbid recovery. For all of these reasons, it is ideal for the elderly patient with no other uterine disease.

The purpose is to reduce the cystourethrocele and to reposition the fundus within the pelvis.

**Physiologic Changes.** The principle behind use of this procedure is to alter the angle of the uterus in the pelvis. This is accomplished by bringing the cardinal and uterosacral ligaments anterior to the lower uterine segment, which is displaced posteriorly. This rotates the axis of the uterus to bring the fundus to an anterior position.

**Points of Caution.** Injury to the bladder can be avoided by careful mobilization of the bladder off the lower uterine segment and elevation of the bladder and ureter with a right-angle retractor.

# Manchester Operation

## (Continued)

*Technique*

**1** The patient is placed in the dorsal lithotomy position. Thorough examination of the pelvis is performed. The bladder is not catheterized because it can be identified and dissected with greater safety when partially filled than when empty.

**2** The labia may be tacked to the perineum for retraction if they are redundant. A Jacobs tenaculum is placed on the anterior lip of the cervix. Downward traction on the cervix exposes the junction of the vagina and cervix where a 360° circumcision incision is made. The bladder is sharply and bluntly dissected off the lower uterine segment up to the vesicouterine fold.

**3** A right-angle retractor is placed under the bladder to expose the vesicouterine peritoneal fold. This is picked up and opened.

**4** The anterior cul-de-sac is opened, a finger is inserted, and the fundus and adnexa are explored.

**5** A right-angle Heaney retractor is placed in the anterior cul-de-sac, allowing elevation of the bladder and ureter. The cervix is rotated anteriorly, and the posterior cul-de-sac is exposed. The peritoneum of the posterior cul-de-sac is picked up and opened.

**6** The posterior cul-de-sac is opened. A finger may be inserted into the cul-de-sac, and the uterus and adnexa explored.

**7** For demonstration purposes, two right-angle retractors are shown, with the upper elevating the vagina and bladder and the lower exposing the anterior cul-de-sac. The upper retractor is removed, and the lower retractor is utilized to elevate the bladder and ureter out of the surgical field. A right-angle retractor is used to expose the lateral vaginal fornix. The cervix is retracted to the contralateral side, exposing the uterosacral and cardinal ligaments. A finger is used to explore the posterior cul-de-sac to ensure that bowel has not moved into this area prior to placing the Heaney clamp on the uterosacral and cardinal ligaments. The Heaney clamp should be placed immediately adjacent to the body of the lower uterine segment. The tips of the clamp should actually grasp a small portion of the lower uterine segment. The uterosacral ligament and a small section of the cardinal ligament are clamped and incised *(dotted line)*. The pedicle is tied with No. 1 synthetic absorbable suture.

**8** The right-angle Heaney retractors are seen in the anterior and posterior cul-de-sac, and right-angle lateral retractors have been moved to the left side of the vagina. The cervix is deviated to the patient's right and slightly anterior, exposing the uterosacral ligament on the left. The uterosacral ligament is clamped, incised, and tied with 2-0 synthetic absorbable suture.

**9** Depending on the length of the cervix, several bites may be required to remove a long cervix while the right-angle Heaney retractor is elevating the bladder and ureter. A small portion of the cardinal ligament is clamped, incised, and tied with 2-0 synthetic absorbable suture.

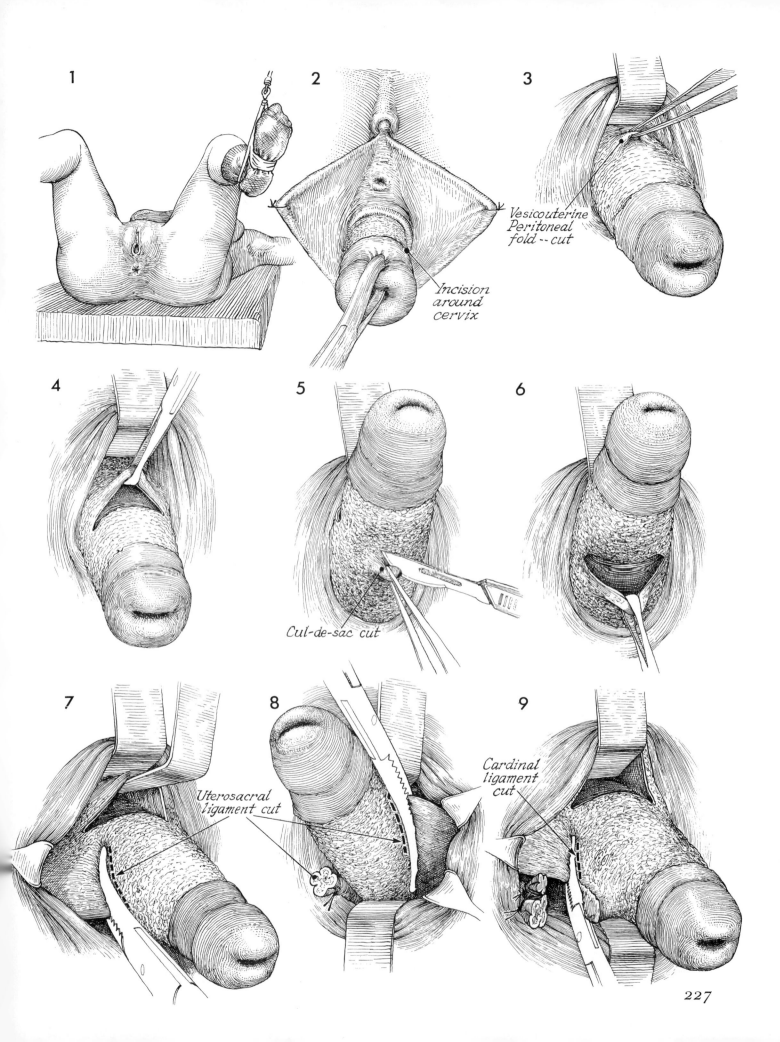

1

2 Incision around cervix
Vesicouterine Peritoneal fold -- cut

3

4

5 Cul-de-sac cut

6

7

8 Uterosacral ligament cut

9 Cardinal ligament cut

227

# Manchester Operation

## (Continued)

**10** The cardinal ligament on the opposite side is clamped, incised, and tied.

**11** It is best to remove the cervix at the lower uterine segment, and the surgeon must judge how much of the cervix should be amputated.

**12** The anterior right-angle Heaney retractor elevates the bladder and ureter, and the posterior right-angle Heaney retractor depresses the rectum. Traction is made on the cervix, and the amputation is made with a scalpel at the lower uterine segment.

**13** An attempt is made to angulate the plane of the incision in the cervix so that it is "wedged out" rather than incised perpendicular to its surface. This facilitates coverage of the lower uterine segment with vaginal mucosa. The lower uterine segment is moved posteriorly; the cardinal and uterosacral ligaments are brought across the anterior surface of the cervix and sutured to the lower uterine segment with interrupted No. 1 synthetic absorbable sutures. The bladder and ureters are elevated out of the surgical field with the right-angle Heaney retractor.

**14** The right uterosacral and cardinal ligaments have been sutured in place, and the left uterosacral and cardinal ligaments are exposed.

**15** The left cardinal and uterosacral ligaments are sutured in place, overlapping those from the right side and creating a firm ligament band in front of the lower uterine segment. The lower uterine segment is held posteriorly, bringing the fundus anteriorly. The angle of the uterus is thus changed in the pelvic canal.

**16** In most cases of second- and third-degree uterine descensus, there will be significant cystourethrocele. Therefore, the standard anterior repair as shown in Section 2, page 42, would be performed at this time.

After the anterior repair has been performed, the vaginal mucosa is closed with interrupted No. 1 synthetic absorbable sutures so that it covers the lower uterine segment with vaginal mucosa.

**17** The row of interrupted synthetic absorbable sutures closing the vaginal mucosa is extended to the opposite side.

**18** The finished procedure shows the uterine canal opened for drainage of mucus.

A Foley catheter is placed in the bladder and left in place for 4–5 days when an anterior repair and Kelly plication have been performed. If no anterior repair or Kelly plication was performed, a Foley catheter may not be necessary.

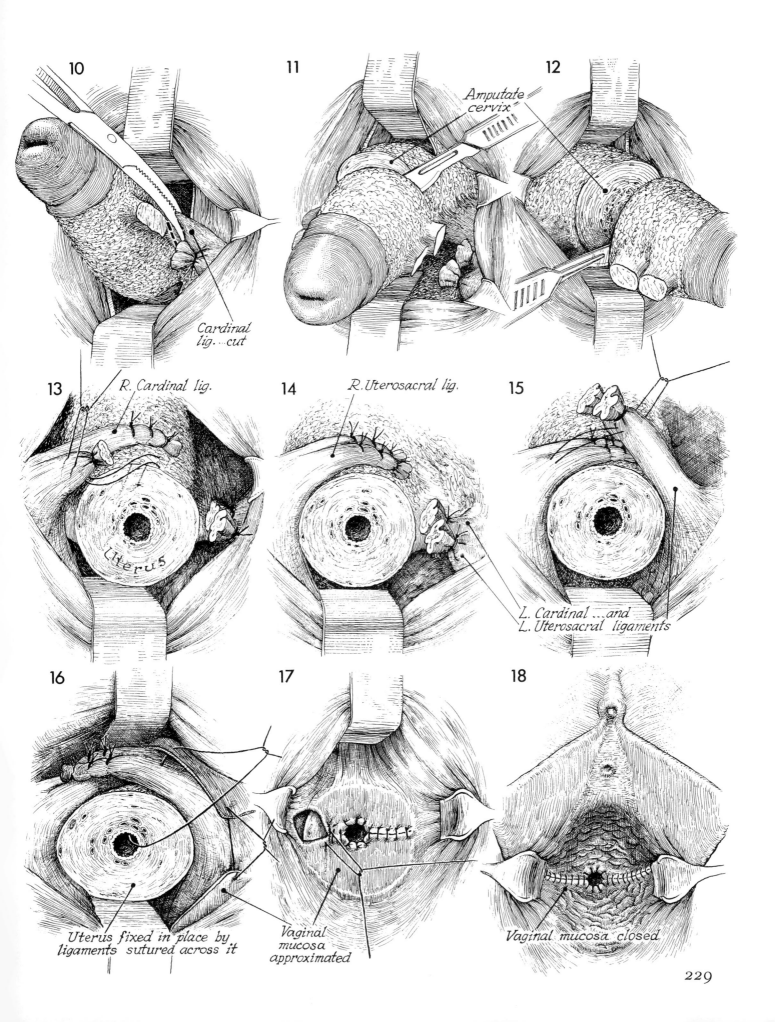

**10** Cardinal lig....cut

**11** Amputate cervix

**12**

**13** R. Cardinal lig. — Uterus

**14** R. Uterosacral lig.

**15** L. Cardinal ...and L. Uterosacral ligaments

**16** Uterus fixed in place by ligaments sutured across it

**17** Vaginal mucosa approximated

**18** Vaginal mucosa closed

229

# Total Vaginal Hysterectomy

Total vaginal hysterectomy is an excellent operation when removal of the uterus is indicated in cases of either benign disease or carcinoma in situ of the cervix. The technique described here is simple and easy and can be accomplished with a minimum of operative time. There are four basic steps involved in performing a vaginal hysterectomy: (1) entrance into the anterior and posterior cul-de-sac to expose the broad ligament, (2) progressive clamping of the broad ligament from the uterosacral cardinal ligament to the tubo-ovarian round ligament, (3) suspension of the vaginal cuff by suturing it to the uterosacral cardinal ligaments, and (4) plication of the uterosacral ligaments in the midline to obliterate the cul-de-sac and reduce the chances of enterocele. The vaginal cuff can be progressively suspended as the hysterectomy takes place rather than suspended separately at the end of the hysterectomy. There are four separate sutures that help suspend the vaginal cuff: (1) the initial suture into the uterosacral cardinal ligaments, (2) the pursestring reperitonealization suture that reinforces the uterosacral cardinal vaginal cuff suture, (3) the vaginal cuff reefing suture, and (4) the uterosacral ligament sutures tied across the midline at the end of the procedure.

The purpose of the operation is to remove the uterus via the vagina.

**Physiologic Changes.** Removal of the uterus results in the cessation of menstrual flow and causes sterility. In addition, it eliminates any existing cervical or uterine disease.

**Points of Caution.** Care must be taken to ensure that entry into the anterior cul-de-sac is made before the uterus is totally removed to avoid accidental entry into the bladder.

If the anterior and posterior cul-de-sacs can be entered, there is a significant reduction in bleeding from the pedicles of the clamped broad ligament.

The pedicles of the broad ligament should be retroperitonealized before reefing the vaginal mucosa.

The vaginal mucosa should not be closed. The edges of the vaginal mucosa should be reefed with a running locking 0 synthetic absorbable suture and left open for drainage.

# Total Vaginal Hysterectomy

## (Continued)

### Technique

**1** After appropriate general anesthesia, the patient is placed in the dorsal lithotomy position with the buttocks well off the end of the table. A thorough bimanual examination is necessary prior to performing a hysterectomy. The vulva and vagina are fully prepped with a surgical soap solution. The cervix is exposed by placing a weighted posterior vaginal retractor into the vagina. A small right-angle retractor is used to elevate the anterior vaginal wall; a second right-angle retractor displaces one lateral vaginal wall and exposes the cervix. Two Jacobs tenacula are used to grasp the anterior and posterior lips of the cervix and pull them into the vaginal introitus.

The vaginal mucosa at its junction to the cervix is being injected with a dilute solution of Pitressin. Ten IU of Pitressin are diluted with 25 mL of sterile saline solution, and 10 mL of this mixture are injected into the vaginal mucosa to aid hemostasis. This solution should not be used on patients with hypertension or cardiac arrhythmias but is most useful in healthy premenopausal patients.

**2** After the injection of Pitressin into the vaginal mucosa, the mucosa is incised with a scalpel around the entire cervix. The incision should stay above the pubovesical cervical fascia anteriorly and the perirectal fascia posteriorly.

**3** While downward traction is applied on the Jacobs tenacula, the handle of the knife is used to dissect the bladder off the anterior lower uterine segment.

**4** A sponge-covered finger dissects the bladder all the way up to the peritoneal vesicouterine fold. This step is frequently insufficiently performed for fear of entering the bladder. If dissection is not carried up to the peritoneal vesicouterine fold, entry into the anterior cul-de-sac is most difficult.

**5** A right-angle retractor is placed under the vaginal mucosa and bladder. It is used to elevate the bladder. This maneuver aids in identifying the peritoneal vesicouterine fold. The peritoneal fold appears as a white transverse line across the lower uterine segment. Strong downward traction is applied to the Jacobs tenacula on the cervix, and the peritoneal vesicouterine fold is grasped with pickup forceps and incised with sharp curved Mayo scissors.

**6** By elevating the peritoneal vesicouterine fold with the pickup forceps, a definite hole can be seen. It is advisable to insert a finger in this hole and explore the area (1) to be sure one is in the peritoneal cavity and not the bladder and (2) to uncover any unsuspected pathologic condition that was not identified during the examination. With the finger remaining in the hole, an anterior Heaney right-angle retractor is placed into the defect underneath the finger.

**7** The Jacobs tenacula are brought acutely up toward the pubic symphysis, exposing the cul-de-sac. Pickup forceps are used to retract the posterior vaginal cuff, thereby placing the peritoneum of the cul-de-sac on tension. The peritoneum of the cul-de-sac is incised with curved Mayo scissors.

**8** A finger is immediately placed into the cul-de-sac, and the area is explored as in the exploration of the anterior cul-de-sac. Approximately 75–100 mL of peritoneal fluid may be seen upon opening the cul-de-sac. A second right-angle Heaney retractor is placed into the posterior cul-de-sac.

**9** The weighted posterior vaginal retractor is removed. With the two Heaney retractors the broad ligament is exposed from the uterosacral ligament to the tubo-ovarian round ligament. A finger placed in the posterior cul-de-sac and moved laterally reveals the uterosacral ligament as it attaches to the lower uterine cervix.

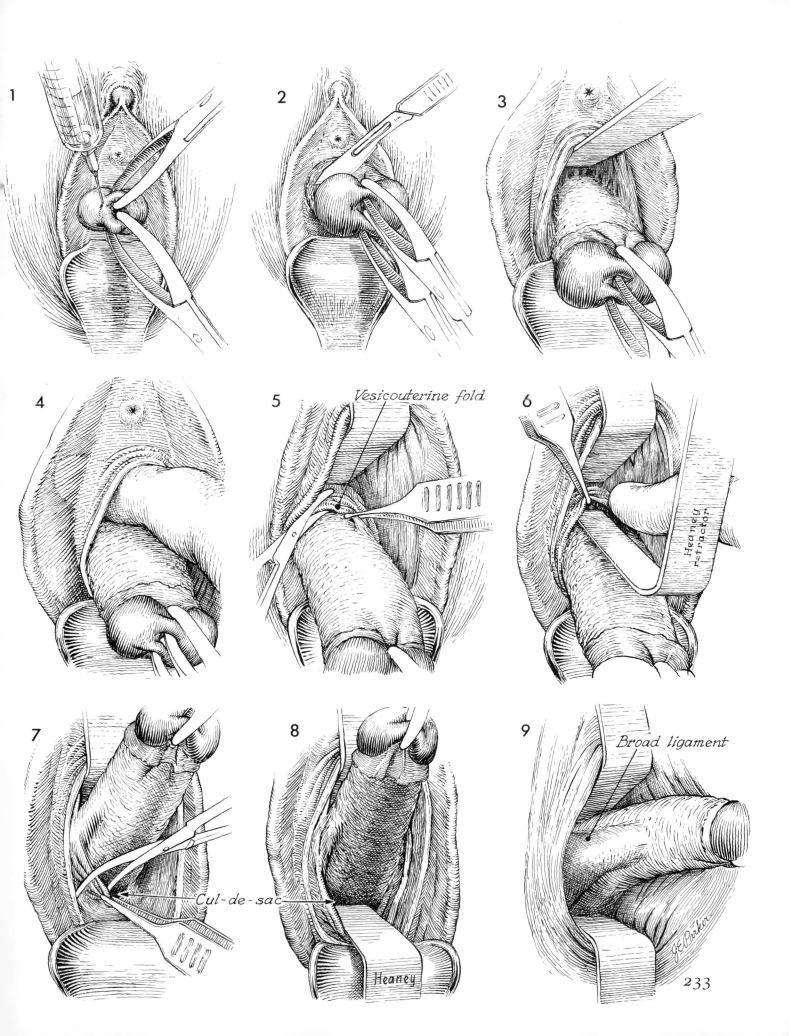

1

2

3

4

5   *Vesicouterine fold*

6   Heaney retractor.

7   *Cul-de-sac*

8   *Cul-de-sac*   Heaney

9   *Broad ligament*

J.E.Parker

233

# Total Vaginal Hysterectomy

## (Continued)

---

**10** With the cervix on upward and lateral retraction via the Jacobs tenacula, a curved Heaney clamp is placed in the posterior cul-de-sac with one blade underneath the uterosacral ligament and the opposite blade over the uterosacral ligament. The clamp is placed immediately next to the uterine cervix so that some tissue of the cervix is included in this clamp. This is done to prevent possible ureteral damage from clamping the uterosacral ligament in the lateral position.

**11** The uterosacral ligament is cut with curved Mayo scissors.

**12** A Heaney fixation 0 synthetic absorbable suture is used to suture-ligate the uterosacral ligament. In addition, the first of four steps is initiated for vaginal cuff suspension. In **A,** the suture has been placed from the inside of the uterosacral ligament at the tip of the Heaney clamp through the uterosacral ligament and brought out through the vaginal mucosa. In **B,** the suture is brought back through the vaginal mucosa and through the midportion of the uterosacral ligament underneath the Heaney clamp. This plicates the uterosacral ligaments to the angle of the vagina and aids hemostasis as well as vaginal cuff suspension.

**13** When tied, the suture is held with a Kelly clamp for traction. This suture not only ligates the uterosacral ligament but plicates that pedicle to the vaginal cuff.

**14** With the uterus on upward and lateral retraction via the Jacobs tenacula on the cervix, the cardinal ligament is clamped adjacent to the lower uterine segment and incised.

**15** The cardinal ligament is suture-ligated with 0 synthetic absorbable suture. No fixation suture is used here for fear of producing a hematoma in the vascular cardinal ligament. Before proceeding farther up the broad ligament, the lateral retractor and cervix are moved to the opposite side, exposing the opposite uterosacral and cardinal ligaments, and they are likewise clamped and suture-ligated.

**16** When the uterosacral and cardinal ligaments on each side have been clamped, incised, and suture-ligated, the remaining portion of the broad ligament attached to the lower uterine segment containing the uterine artery is clamped adjacent to the cervix. Use of a single clamp in the vaginal hysterectomy reduces the chance of damage to the ureter, whereas using two clamps will allow this portion of the broad ligament to be clamped in its lateral position, thus increasing the chance of ureteral injury.

**17** With the uterosacral ligament, the cardinal ligament, and the uterine artery pedicle on both sides now clamped, incised, and suture-ligated, the cervix is retracted upward in the midline via the Jacobs tenacula. Thyroid clamps are used to grasp the posterior uterine wall, and with a hand-over-hand "walking out" technique the fundus is delivered posteriorly.

**18** The Jacobs tenacula and the thyroid clamp are held in one hand, and the finger of the opposite hand is inserted under the tubo-ovarian round ligament, exposing the ligated portion of the lower broad ligament.

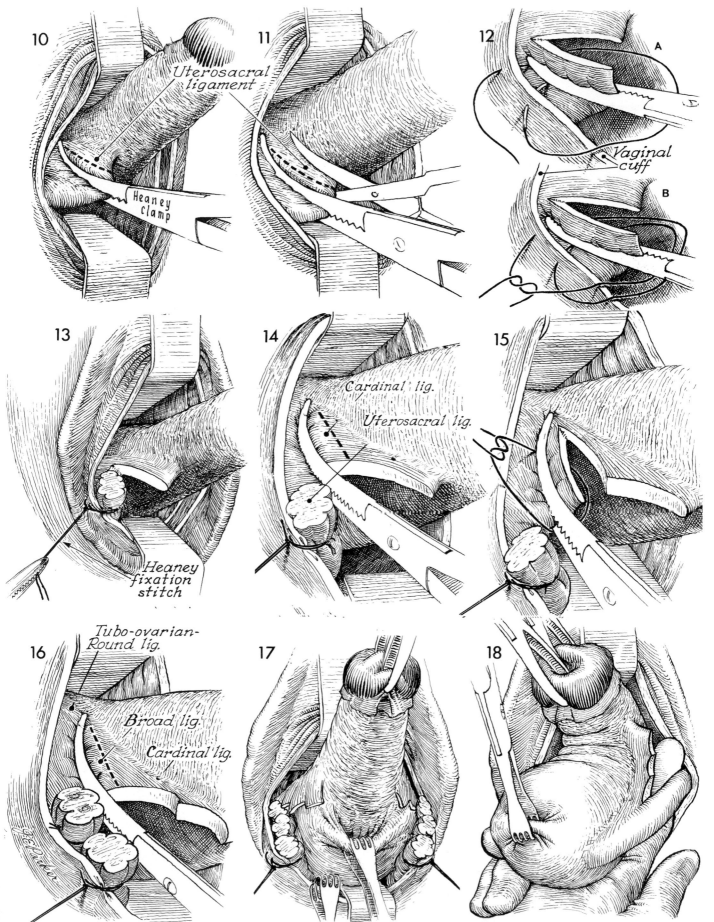

10

*Uterosacral ligament*

*Heaney clamp*

11

12
A

*Vaginal cuff*

B

13

*Heaney fixation stitch*

14

*Cardinal lig.*

*Uterosacral lig.*

15

16

*Tubo-ovarian-Round lig.*

*Broad lig.*

*Cardinal lig.*

17

18

235

# Total Vaginal Hysterectomy

## (Continued)

**19** Two Heaney clamps are applied to the tubo-ovarian round ligament, and it is incised close to the fundus.

**20** The tubo-ovarian round ligament is tied twice. In **A,** a tie of 0 synthetic absorbable suture is placed behind the second clamp. The tubo-ovarian round ligament is tied with a simple 0 synthetic absorbable suture. After the clamp at the rear of the pedicle is removed, the forward clamp is "flashed" (i.e., slightly opened and immediately closed), to allow the suture to securely ligate all the structures in this pedicle.

In **B,** a second suture ligature is tied in a fixation stitch, placing the suture in the midportion of its pedicle. In **C,** the suture is tied in front of and behind the pedicle prior to removing the first clamp. In **D,** the pedicle is tied, and the second suture is held in a straight clamp for traction.

**21** The anterior and posterior Heaney right-angle retractors are removed, and the weighted posterior vaginal retractor is placed in the vagina. The anterior vaginal wall is elevated with a short right-angle retractor. This allows better vaginal cuff exposure. The entire broad ligament and its respective pedicles are exposed from the tubo-ovarian round ligament anteriorly to the uterosacral ligament posteriorly. A free sponge is pushed into the peritoneal cavity to displace the ovaries, tubes, and bowel and give better exposure to the broad ligament structures. The tail of the sponge is used to wipe the pedicles of each of these ligaments to check for hemostasis. If there is bleeding from any pedicle or portion thereof, the bleeding points can be clamped with a curved Heaney clamp and suture-ligated. It is preferable that the suture be brought through the tip of the Heaney clamp and out through the vaginal mucosa. If the surgeon encounters a wide area of bleeding, the entire broad ligament can be suture-ligated by a running 0 synthetic absorbable suture plicating the pedicles of the broad ligament to the lateral vaginal mucosa. Care should be taken not to go deeper than the original ties on the broad ligament pedicles to prevent damage to the ureter.

The vesical peritoneal edge can be identified by grasping the anterior vaginal wall with tissue forceps. By using a hand-over-hand technique, the surgeon can progressively pull the bladder wall down into the vagina and easily identify the peritoneal edge.

**22** The reperitonealization of the pelvis, carried out with pursestring sutures, provides the second of four steps in suspension of the vaginal cuff. The suture is started on the anterior peritoneal edge and brought through the stump of the tubo-ovarian round ligament. After the stump of the tubo-ovarian round ligament is sutured, the suture ligature held for retraction can be cut. The pursestring is continued down through one or more of the pedicles and is finally brought through the uterosacral cardinal ligament pedicles and the vaginal mucosa, plicating these pedicles to the vaginal mucosa to provide additional suspension of the upper vagina. The suture is continued posteriorly across the peritoneum of the cul-de-sac with one or two stitches. The traction sutures in the uterosacral ligaments should not be cut, as they are needed in a later step. The suture is brought from the inside of the opposite uterosacral ligament out through the vaginal mucosa and carried up the pedicles of the opposite side until the tubo-ovarian round ligament on the opposite side has been sutured. The traction suture on this pedicle can be cut. The suture is passed through the anterior vesicoperitoneal edge. When this suture is tied, the pelvis is reperitonealized, and the stumps of the broad ligament are retroperitonealized.

**23** The vaginal cuff is never closed and is left open for drainage to prevent postoperative pelvic abscesses. A running locking 0 synthetic absorbable suture is started at the 12 o'clock position on the anterior vaginal cuff and is carried around the entire edge of the vagina until the cardinal and uterosacral ligaments are reached. At that point, the suture is brought through the cardinal and uterosacral ligaments, and the surgeon again plicates these ligaments to the vaginal cuff, completing the third of four steps in vaginal suspension. The same is done for the uterosacral and cardinal ligaments on the opposite side. The running locking suture is continued until the entire cuff has been sutured. The two retraction sutures held by Kelly clamps on the uterosacral ligaments are tied in the midline. This aids in obliterating the cul-de-sac and reduces the incidence of enterocele.

**24** The final step is to observe the upper vaginal area for hemorrhage. We prefer to catheterize the bladder at the end rather than at the beginning of the procedure because there may be less chance of injuring a bladder that is partially filled with urine than one that is empty. No vaginal pack is left in the vagina, and no Foley catheter is placed in the bladder. All patients undergoing vaginal hysterectomy are given antibiotics preoperatively.

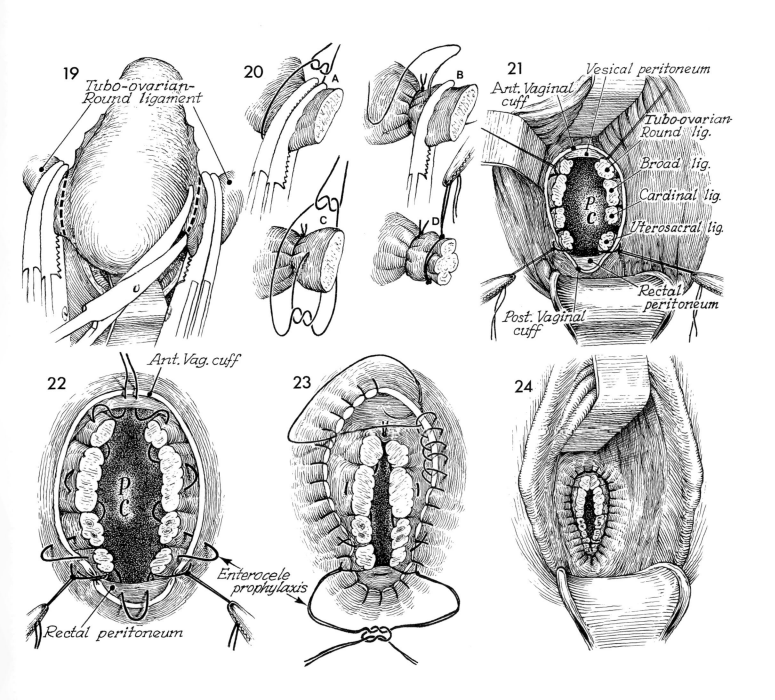

**19** Tubo-ovarian-Round ligament

**20** A B C D

**21** Ant. Vaginal cuff — Vesical peritoneum — Tubo-ovarian-Round lig. — Broad lig. — Cardinal lig. — Uterosacral lig. — Rectal peritoneum — Post. Vaginal cuff — P C

**22** Ant. Vag. cuff — P C — Rectal peritoneum — Enterocele prophylaxis

**23**

**24**

# Total Vaginal Hysterectomy

## (Continued)

VAGINAL BILATERAL SALPINGO-OOPHORECTOMY DURING TOTAL VAGINAL HYSTERECTOMY

Under certain conditions the Fallopian tubes and ovaries may be removed at the time of vaginal hysterectomy. Salpingo-oophorectomy can be performed during the hysterectomy, although it is easier to perform immediately after the uterine specimen has been removed.

If the tubes and ovaries are to be removed with the specimen, the uterus is delivered into the vagina as in Figure 18.

**25** Exposure is facilitated by clamping and cutting the round ligament on each side. The thyroid clamp on the fundus, which has been placed on traction (Fig. 18), is removed to expose the anatomy.

**26 & 27** After the round ligament has been cut and tied on each side, additional traction on the uterine fundus delivers the fundus into the vagina and places tension on the infundibulopelvic ligament. A finger can be inserted up and under this ligament. Two Heaney clamps are placed across the ligament. It is cut and doubly tied with 0 synthetic absorbable suture as demonstrated in Figure 20. The second suture on this pedicle is held in a straight clamp as seen in Figure 21 (on the tubo-ovarian round ligament). Reestablishing the peritoneum and vaginal cuff suturing are performed as in Figures 22 and 23. The infundibulopelvic ligament pedicle is used for establishing the peritoneal lining, as was the tubo-ovarian round ligament pedicle in Figure 22. The vaginal cuff is sutured with a running locking stitch and left open.

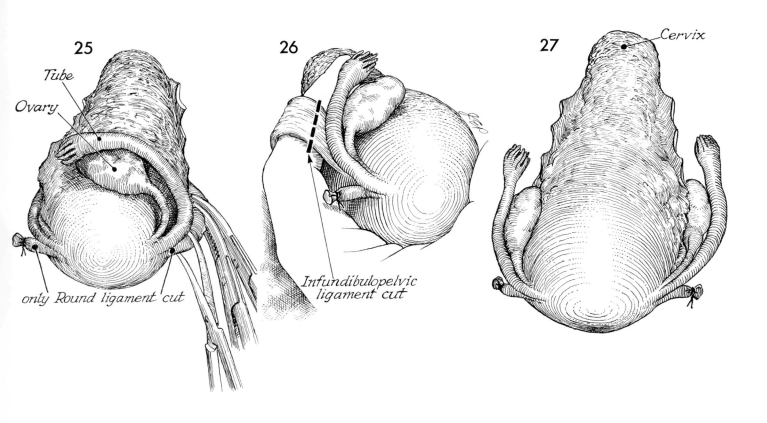

25

*Tube*

*Ovary*

*only Round ligament cut*

26

*Infundibulopelvic ligament cut*

27

*Cervix*

# Total Abdominal Hysterectomy With and Without Bilateral Salpingo-oophorectomy

Total abdominal hysterectomy is utilized for benign and malignant disease where removal of the internal genitalia is indicated. The operation can be performed with the preservation or removal of the ovaries on one or both sides. In benign disease, the possibility of bilateral and unilateral oophorectomy should be thoroughly discussed with the patient. Frequently, in malignant disease, no choice exists but to remove the tubes and ovaries, since they are frequent sites of micrometastases.

In general, the modified Richardson technique of intrafascial hysterectomy is used.

The purpose of the operation is to remove the uterus through the abdomen, with or without removing the tube and ovaries.

**Physiologic Changes.** The predominant physiologic change from removal of the uterus is the elimination of uterine disease and the menstrual flow. If the ovaries are removed with the specimen, the predominant physiologic change noted is loss of the ovarian steroid sex hormone production.

**Points of Caution.** The predominant point of caution in performing abdominal hysterectomy is to ensure that there is no damage to the bladder, ureters, or rectosigmoid colon.

Mobilization of the bladder with a combination of sharp and blunt dissection frees the bladder from the lower uterine segment and upper vagina. This reduces the incidence of damage to the bladder.

By exercising extreme care in the management of the uterine artery pedicle, the surgeon may minimize the risk of injury to the ureter. The same is true of the management of the cardinal and uterosacral ligament pedicles.

If the vaginal cuff is left open with the edges sutured, the incidence of postoperative pelvic abscess is dramatically reduced.

# Total Abdominal Hysterectomy With and Without Bilateral Salpingo-oophorectomy

## (Continued)

## *Technique*

**1** The patient is placed in the dorsal lithotomy position, and an adequate pelvic examination is performed with the patient under general anesthesia. This is extremely important because it allows the surgeon to become acquainted with the anatomy of the internal genitalia. This is frequently impossible when the patient is examined in the gynecologic clinic. The patient is then put in approximately a 15° Trendelenburg position. A Foley catheter is left in the bladder and connected to straight drainage. In general, midline incisions are preferred for malignant disease, since they allow accurate staging and exposure to the upper abdomen and aortic lymph nodes. If investigation of the upper abdomen and aortic lymph nodes is needed, the midline incision should be extended around and above the umbilicus for appropriate exposure.

For benign disease, the Pfannenstiel incision is an adequate alternative to the midline incision.

After the abdomen is entered, it should be thoroughly explored, including the liver, gallbladder, stomach, kidneys, and aortic lymph nodes.

**2** Self-retaining retractors are placed in the abdominal incision, and the bowel is packed off with warm, moist gauze packs. A 0 synthetic absorbable suture is placed in the fundus of the uterus and used for uterine traction. The uterus is deviated to the patient's right. The left round ligament is placed on stretch and incised between clamps.

**3** The distal stump of the round ligament is ligated with 0 synthetic absorbable suture. The proximal stump is held with a straight Ochsner clamp. At this point the leaves of the broad ligament are opened both anteriorly and posteriorly. This is performed by delicate dissection with the Metzenbaum scissors.

**4** While retracting the uterus cephalad, the surgeon opens the anterior leaf of the broad ligament to the vesicouterine fold. Steps 2–4 are carried out on the opposite side.

**5** The vesicoperitoneal fold is elevated, and the fine filmy attachments of the bladder to the pubovesical cervical fascia are visible. The bladder can be dissected off the lower uterine segment of the uterus and cervix by either blunt or sharp dissection. If there has been extensive lower segment disease, previous cesarean sections, or pelvic irradiation, blunt dissection of the bladder off the cervix is dangerous, and a sharp dissection technique should be performed.

**6** If the ovaries are to be preserved, the uterus is retracted toward the pubic symphysis and deviated to one side with the infundibulopelvic ligament, tube, and ovary on tension. A finger should be inserted through the peritoneum of the posterior leaf of the broad ligament under the suspensory ligament of the ovary and Fallopian tube. The tube and suspensory ligament are doubly clamped, incised, and tied with 0 synthetic absorbable suture. The distal stump of this structure is best doubly tied, first with a single tie of 0 synthetic absorbable suture and then with a ligature of 0 synthetic absorbable suture. The same procedure is carried out on the opposite side.

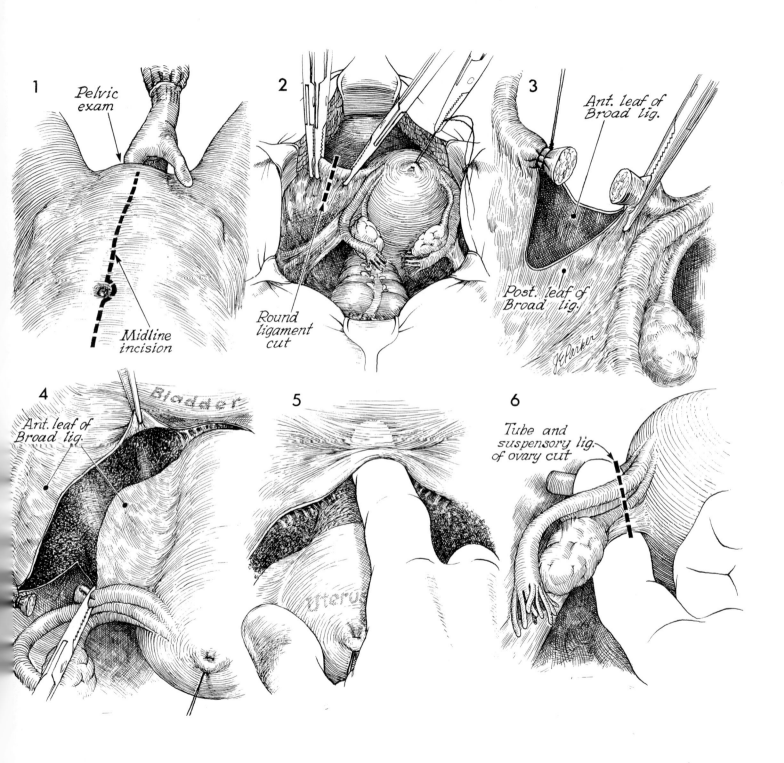

1. Pelvic exam. Midline incision

2. Round ligament cut

3. Ant. leaf of Broad lig. Post. leaf of Broad lig.

4. Ant. leaf of Broad lig. Bladder

5. Uterus

6. Tube and suspensory lig. of ovary cut

243

# Total Abdominal Hysterectomy With and Without Bilateral Salpingo-oophorectomy

## (Continued)

**7** The uterus is then retracted cephalad and deviated to one side of the pelvis with the lower broad ligament on stretch. The filmy tissue surrounding the uterine vessels is skeletonized by elevating the round ligament and dissecting the tissue away from the uterine vessels. Three curved Ochsner clamps are placed at the junction of the lower uterine segment on the uterine vessels. This is best performed by placing the tips of the curved Ochsner clamps onto the uterus and allowing them to slide off the body of the uterus, thus ensuring complete clamping of the uterine vessels. An incision is made between the upper Ochsner clamp and the two lower Ochsner clamps. This is suture-ligated with two 0 synthetic absorbable sutures, placing the first suture at the tip of the lower Ochsner clamp and tying the suture behind the base of the clamp. The middle Ochsner clamp is left in place and is similarly suture-ligated by a second ligature placed at the tip of the Ochsner clamp and tied behind the base of the clamp. No attempt is made to place a suture in the middle of the pedicle, since it contains blood vessels and a pedicle hematoma can be created.

The same procedure is carried out on the opposite side.

A delicate, transverse, curved incision is made in the pubovesical cervical fascia overlying the lower uterine segment. The separation of the pubovesical cervical fascia from the underlying cervical stroma is facilitated by placing traction on the uterus in the cephalad position.

**8** The uterus is held in traction in the cephalad position, and the handle of the knife is used to dissect the pubovesical cervical fascia inferiorly. This step mobilizes the ureter laterally and caudally.

**9** Two straight Ochsner clamps are applied to the cardinal ligament for a distance of approximately 2 cm. The cardinal ligament is incised between the two clamps, and the distal stump is ligated with 0 synthetic absorbable suture. The suture is tied at the base of the clamp; no attempt is made to place this suture within the body of the pedicle because vessels can be torn and hematomas created.

The same procedure is carried out on the opposite cardinal ligament.

**10** The posterior leaf of the broad ligament is incised down to the uterosacral ligaments and across the posterior lower uterine segment between the rectum and cervix.

**11** The uterosacral ligaments on both sides are clamped between straight Ochsner clamps, incised, and ligated with 0 synthetic absorbable suture.

**12** The uterus is placed on traction cephalad, and the lower uterine segment and upper vagina are palpated between the thumb and first finger of the surgeon's hand to ensure that the ligaments have been completely incised. The vagina is entered by a stab wound with a scalpel and is cut across with either a scalpel or scissors. The uterus is removed. The edges of the vagina are picked up with straight Ochsner clamps in a north, south, east, and west direction.

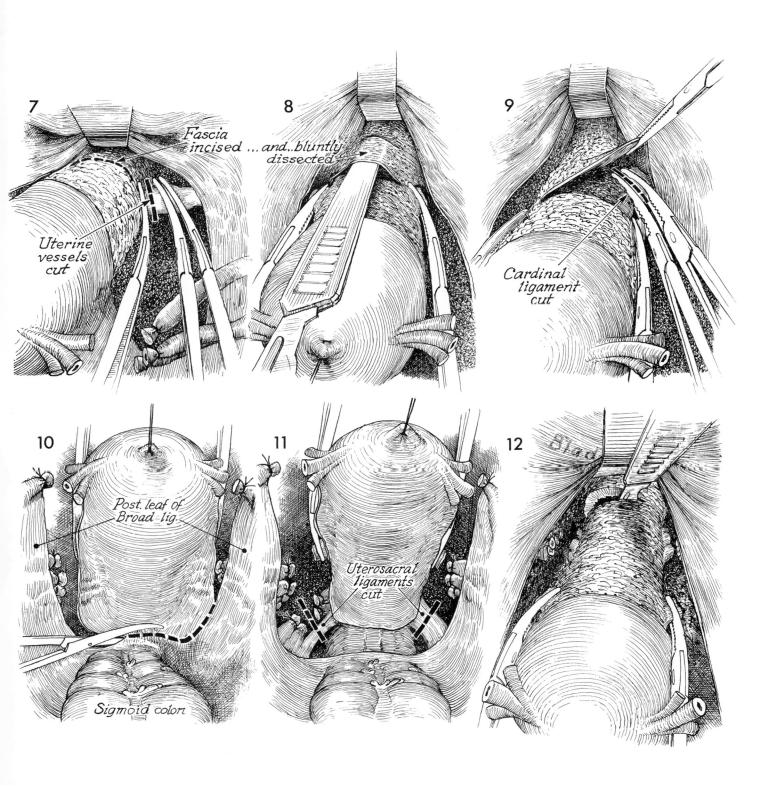

7    *Fascia incised* ... *and..bluntly dissected*

*Uterine vessels cut*

9    *Cardinal ligament cut*

10    *Post. leaf of Broad-lig.*

*Sigmoid colon*

11    *Uterosacral ligaments cut*

12    *Blad.*

# Total Abdominal Hysterectomy With and Without Bilateral Salpingo-oophorectomy

## (Continued)

**13 a.** The vaginal cuff is never closed in our clinic. This alone has accounted for a radical decrease in postoperative febrile morbidity and abscess formation. The edges of the vaginal mucosa are sutured with a running locking 0 synthetic absorbable suture starting at the midpoint of the vagina underneath the bladder and carried around to the stumps of the cardinal and uterosacral ligaments, which are sutured into the angle of the vagina.

**b.** The running locking suture is carried around the posterior wall of the vagina ensuring that the recto-vaginal space is obliterated.

**c.** The cardinal and uterosacral ligaments of the opposite side have been included in the running locking 0 synthetic absorbable suture, and the reefing process has been completed to the midpoint of the anterior vaginal wall. At this point, meticulous care should be taken to ensure that the lateral angle of the vagina is adequately secured and that hemostasis is complete between the lateral angle of the vagina and the stumps of the cardinal and uterosacral ligaments. This can be a site of hemorrhage.

At this point, the pelvis is thoroughly washed with sterile saline solution. Meticulous care is taken to ensure that hemostasis is present throughout the dissected area.

**14** The pelvis is reperitonealized with a running 2-0 synthetic absorbable suture from the anterior to the posterior leaf of the broad ligament. The stumps of the tubo-ovarian round, suspensory ligament of the ovary, and of the cardinal and uterosacral ligaments are buried retroperitoneally.

**15** Drains are rarely needed. If they are indicated, they are placed through the open vaginal cuff and carried along the lateral pelvic wall retroperitoneally.

**16** If the tube and ovary are to be removed, they are removed at Step 6 in the operation. Instead of placing a finger underneath the tube and suspensory ligament of the ovary, a finger is placed under the infundibulopelvic ligament on that side. Care is taken to ensure that the ureter is not included. In various forms of pelvic disease (endometriosis, pelvic inflammatory disease, etc.), the ureter can be deviated close to the infundibulopelvic ligament.

The infundibulopelvic ligament is doubly clamped and incised, and the distal stump of the ligament is doubly ligated with a tie of 0 synthetic absorbable suture plus a ligature of 0 synthetic absorbable suture.

For a bilateral salpingo-oophorectomy, the same procedure is carried out on the opposite infundibulopelvic ligament.

**17** The tube and ovary have been mobilized medially with the uterine specimens. The remainder of the operation is carried out as described in Steps 7–13.

**18** The peritoneum of the pelvis has been reestablished with the tube and ovary removed. The stump of the infundibulopelvic ligament is buried retroperitoneally.

Postoperatively, no vaginal packing is left in the vagina, and no Foley catheter drainage of the bladder is indicated.

The open vaginal cuff closes without difficulty. Rarely, a small bit of granulation tissue is noted in the upper vagina and is adequately treated by application of silver nitrate 4 weeks postoperatively in the clinic or office. The patient is allowed to resume sexual intercourse 4 weeks after examination in the clinic and is allowed to resume work 5 weeks postoperatively.

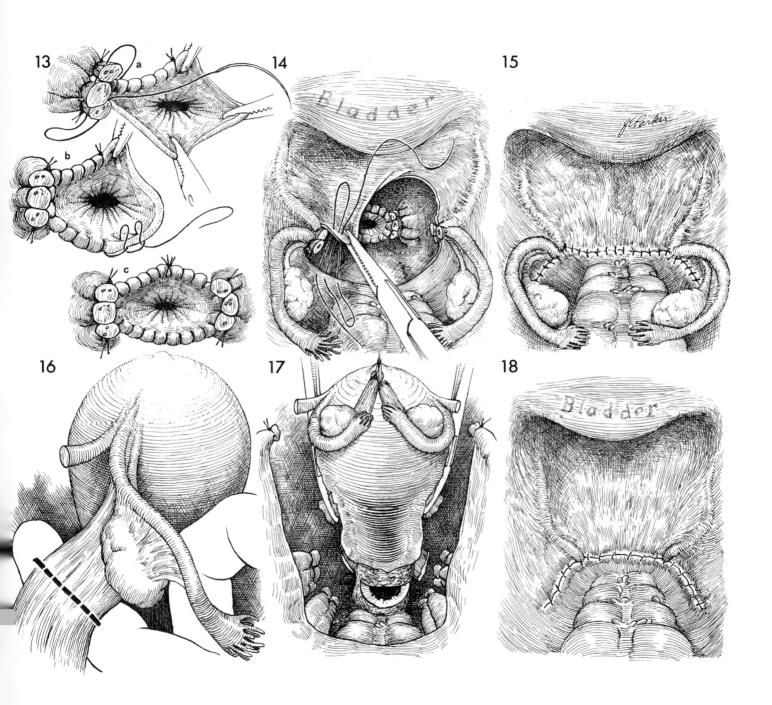

247

# Laparoscopy-Assisted Vaginal Hysterectomy

There are two reasons for performing a laparoscopy-assisted vaginal hysterectomy. The first is to attempt to make vaginal hysterectomy with its advantages available to those women whose surgeons feel uncomfortable with a regular vaginal hysterectomy and who would have a tendency toward performing the hysterectomy through the abdominal route with its disadvantages of postoperative pain, need for hospitalization, and reduced time for return to full activities and/or employment. The second is a significant reduction in length of stay in the hospital with this procedure than with an abdominal hysterectomy. It was originally thought that routine vaginal hysterectomy required 5–6 days of hospitalization. Recently, this has been shown to be untrue. It was originally thought that there would be a cost savings from laparoscopy-assisted vaginal hysterectomy compared with a regular vaginal hysterectomy. Several evaluations have shown that because of the high cost of the instruments needed and the length of operating time needed for laparoscopy-assisted vaginal hysterectomy, this procedure is more expensive than a regular vaginal hysterectomy. If the patient's surgeon feels uncomfortable with a regular vaginal hysterectomy and would convert these operations to abdominal hysterectomy, however, there is a definite advantage for the laparoscopy-assisted vaginal hysterectomy in length of stay, cost, and recovery.

The typical patient on whom a surgeon would be tempted to perform a laparoscopy-assisted vaginal hysterectomy would be one with myomata uteri, a history of pelvic inflammatory disease, a history of previous pelvic surgeries such as cesarean section, or significant endometriosis with adhesions to bowel. The hypothesis is that with laparoscopy these variables can be managed in a safer manner than with the traditional vaginal hysterectomy.

**Physiologic Changes.** The predominate physiology is the loss of the uterus and the offending signs and symptoms that require the uterus to be removed. If it is a bleeding disorder, the bleeding will stop. If it is chronic pain caused by the uterus, the pain should be eliminated. If it is an ovarian-masking problem, the ovaries would now be free and could be felt on routine examination. If there is carcinoma in situ or significant cervical intraepithelial neoplasia, then that would be removed.

**Points of Caution.** Laparoscopy is not a completely complication-free operation. Bowel injuries, urinary tract injuries, and hemorrhage are reported sequelae of laparoscopy. Clinical experience with intra-abdominal laparoscopy as well as vaginal hysterectomy must be obtained prior to initiating this procedure.

# Laparoscopy-Assisted Vaginal Hysterectomy

## (Continued)

## Technique

**1** Usually, there are five sites of puncture required for the insertion of the laparoscopic trocar and sleeves. First, a 12-mm incision is made in the inferior rim of the umbilicus for insertion of the observation laparoscope. Second, two 12-mm incisions, one in the left lower quadrant and one in the right lower quadrant, are needed. These incisions should be lateral to the rectus abdominis muscle to avoid injury to the epigastric vessels. Third, an incision is required for grasping forceps, dissection scissors, and irrigation and suction instruments. Fourth, a 5-mm suprapubic incision is needed for additional surgical instruments.

**2** This laparoscopic view of the pelvis shows the bladder (B) at the 12–1 o'clock position and the fundus at the 4–5 o'clock position with the intravaginal and cervical instrument manipulating the uterus so the infundibulopelvic ligament can be exposed. A grasping forceps has been used to remove the ovary and Fallopian tube medially, further exposing the infundibulopelvic ligament. The ureter must be clearly identified prior to placing the Endo-GIA (gastrointestinal anastomosis) stapler on the infundibulopelvic ligament. First, the size and thickness of the infundibulopelvic ligament must be known. This can best be done by placing an Endo Gauge 30-mm instrument across the infundibulopelvic ligament, measuring the thickness. This allows for the appropriate Endo-GIA stapler to be placed. The Endo-GIA stapler is placed across the infundibulopelvic ligament as well as the round ligament. Care must be taken to ensure that the ureter is not included in this grasp and is out of danger from being transected and stapled.

**3** The fundus of the uterus is at the 5 o'clock position, the tube and ovary have been moved medially by the Endo Grasp instrument, the bladder is at the 2 o'clock position, and a second application of the multiple-fire Endo-GIA 30 stapler is applied to the upper broad ligament. At the 7 o'clock position, the previously stapled and incised left infundibulopelvic ligament can be seen. The round ligament and the upper portion of the broad ligament are included in this second bite of the Endo-GIA 30 stapler.

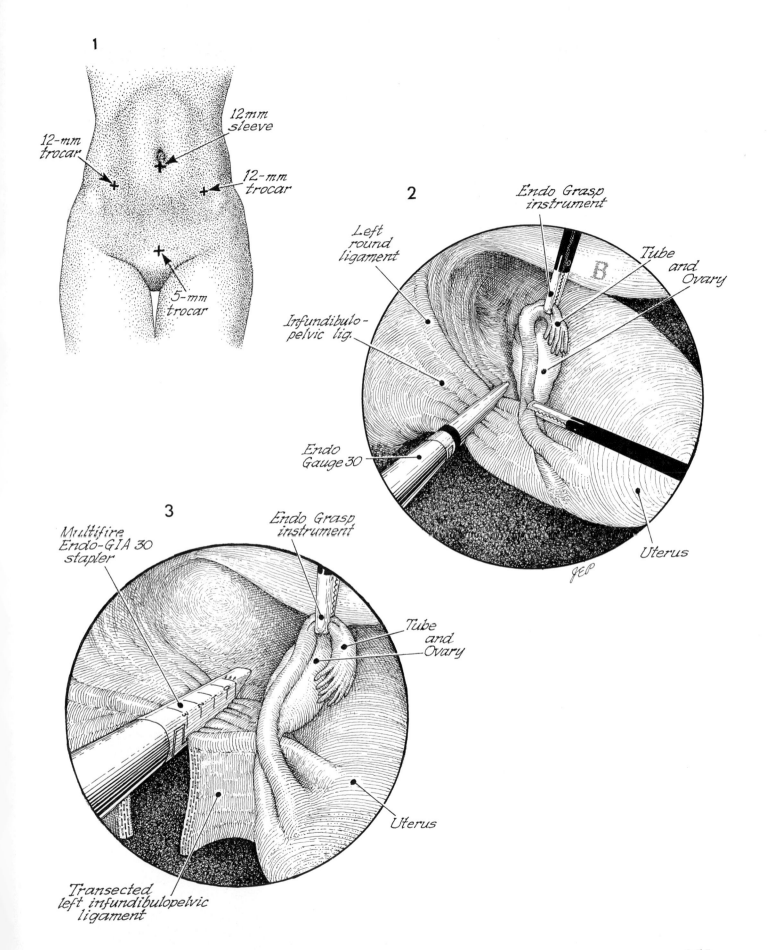

**1**

12-mm trocar

12mm sleeve

12-mm trocar

5-mm trocar

**2**

Endo Grasp instrument

Left round ligament

Tube and Ovary

Infundibulo-pelvic lig.

Endo Gauge 30

Uterus

*JEP*

**3**

Multifire Endo-GIA 30 stapler

Endo Grasp instrument

Tube and Ovary

Uterus

Transected left infundibulopelvic ligament

# Laparoscopy-Assisted Vaginal Hysterectomy

## (Continued)

**4** This endoscopic view shows the fundus of the uterus at the 9 o'clock position, the bladder at the 12 o'clock position, and the right infundibulopelvic ligament exposed by manipulating the intravaginal cervical manipulator as well as the grasping forceps, moving the tube and ovary medially. The round and infundibulopelvic ligaments can also be seen. The right ureter must be clearly identified before the Endo-GIA stapler is placed on the infundibulopelvic ligament.

**5** This laparoscopic view shows the bladder at the 12 o'clock position and the right and left infundibulopelvic ligaments stapled and transected. The round and broad ligaments have been stapled and transected down to a point approximately 0.5 cm above the ureter and uterine artery. Endo Shears are used to transect the peritoneum over the anterior uterine segment.

**6** The vesicoperitoneum is grasped with an endograsping forceps and elevated. The Endo-GIA stapler is placed adjacent to the lower uterine segment on the lower broad ligament but superior to the uterine artery.

To distinguish the anterior from the posterior surface of the uterus, the midline of the uterus from the fundus down to the lower uterine segment is slightly coagulated with electrocoagulation forceps.

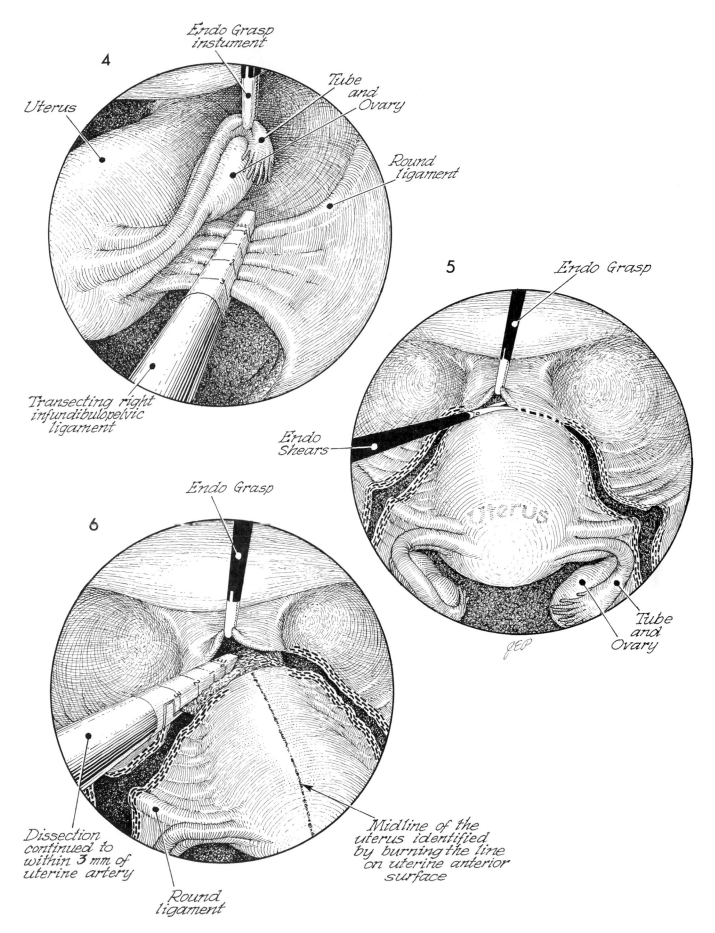

4

*Uterus*

*Endo Grasp instrument*

*Tube and Ovary*

*Round ligament*

*Transecting right infundibulopelvic ligament*

5

*Endo Grasp*

*Endo Shears*

*Uterus*

*Tube and Ovary*

gep

6

*Endo Grasp*

*Dissection continued to within 3 mm of uterine artery*

*Round ligament*

*Midline of the uterus identified by burning the line on uterine anterior surface*

253

# Laparoscopy-Assisted Vaginal Hysterectomy

## (Continued)

**7** The surgeon goes below, leaving the laparoscope in the hands of an assistant, and transects circumferentially the vaginal mucosa immediately adjacent to the cervix. The cervix is grasped with a Jacobs tenaculum, and the anterior vaginal cuff is dissected caudally until the peritoneal cavity is entered through the previous dissection of the vesicoperitoneal fold seen in Figure 5.

**8** A Lahey thyroid tenaculum is placed into the anterior cul-de-sac and pulls the uterine fundus through the anterior cul-de-sac. Traction is maintained on the cervix with the Jacobs tenaculum.

**9** The tenaculum on the cervix is released, allowing the uterus to be flipped forward; additional tenacula are placed on the anterior uterine wall, progressively pulling the fundus forward and outward as the uterus begins to emerge from the anterior cul-de-sac opening.

**10** The uterine artery on both sides is clamped, ligated, cut, and tied with synthetic absorbable suture. The uterus and adnexa are delivered through the anterior cul-de-sac wound.

**11** The posterior surface of the uterus from the fundus to the lower uterine segment can be identified because it lacks the burn stripe previously applied to the anterior surface. The vaginal mucosa is identified on both sides, clamped, and incised. The clamp is placed slightly above the uterosacral ligaments. The line of amputation of the cervix and uterus is shown.

**12** The vaginal cuff has been reefed with running 0 synthetic absorbable suture.

**13** The vagina is closed and returned to its proper position. The ties are seen on the uterosacral ligaments. They are plicated in the midline for enterocele prophylactic and vaginal cuff suspension.

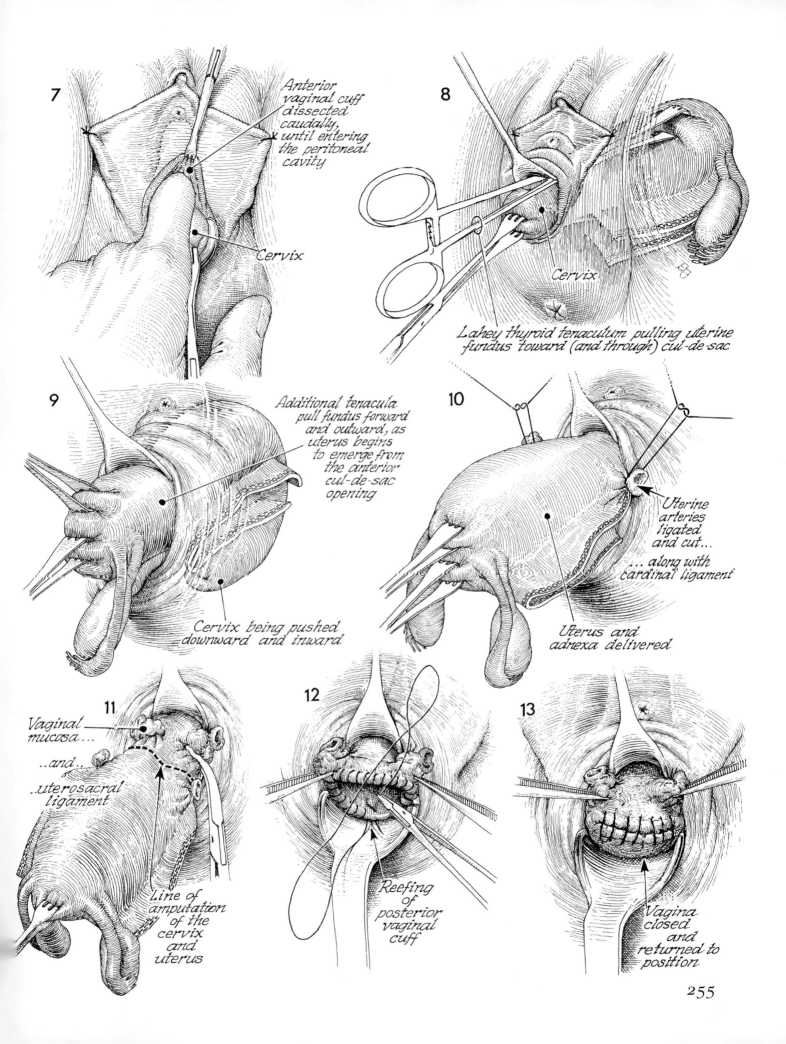

**7**

Anterior vaginal cuff dissected caudally, until entering the peritoneal cavity

Cervix

**8**

Cervix

Lahey thyroid tenaculum pulling uterine fundus toward (and through) cul-de-sac

**9**

Additional tenacula pull fundus forward and outward, as uterus begins to emerge from the anterior cul-de-sac opening

Cervix being pushed downward and inward

**10**

Uterine arteries ligated and cut...

...along with cardinal ligament

Uterus and adnexa delivered

**11**

Vaginal mucosa...

...and...

...uterosacral ligament

Line of amputation of the cervix and uterus

**12**

Reefing of posterior vaginal cuff

**13**

Vagina closed and returned to position

255

# 6

Fallopian Tubes
and Ovaries

# Laparoscopy Technique

The basic procedures for laparoscopy are the same whether this form of surgery is used for diagnosis or surgical treatment. Either a single- or a multi-incision technique may be employed. For the former, the operative laparoscope is used. For the latter, the laparoscope without operative channels is passed through the first incision, and one or more operative instruments are inserted through the other incisions as required. The operative scope is attached to a video monitor to enlarge the operative field and allow the operating room team to observe the procedure. In simple diagnostic or surgical procedures, the operative laparoscope has an advantage over the diagnostic laparoscope in that it allows an operative instrument to be passed down its channel either to stabilize structures or to aspirate blood or fluid from the operative field.

The operation is a simple, safe, cost-efficient way of diagnosing and treating problems within the female pelvis.

**Physiologic Changes.** Physiologic changes occur when laparoscopy is used to lyse adhesions, fulgurate endometrial implants, biopsy ovaries, remove ectopic pregnancies, and relieve obstruction in the Fallopian tube or obstruct the tube for sterilization by electrocauterization and/or the application of a Silastic ring or clip.

**Points of Caution.** Care must be taken to ensure that the needle for pneumoperitoneum is within the peritoneal cavity. The trocar should always be kept sharp, or a disposable trocar should be used. Electrocauterization should proceed with extreme caution.

# Laparoscopy Technique

## (Continued)

## Technique

**1** The surgeon who is knowledgeable about all aspects of laparoscopy should position the patient in the lithotomy position modified to conform to the special requirements of the procedure. The legs are not placed in the standard 90° flexion, as in the classic dorsal lithotomy position, but are positioned at 45° flexion from the hip. It is extremely important to have the buttocks at least 4 inches off the end of the operating table to facilitate manipulation of the cervical and intrauterine instruments into an advantageous position for maximum visualization of the internal genitalia. The operating table should be slanted to a 15° Trendelenburg position to displace the intestines out of the pelvis and into the upper abdomen. It is more comfortable for the operating surgeon to have the patient's arms down at her sides than extended on an arm board. We frequently insert the needle for intravenous infusion into the forearm, then place the arm at the patient's side and secure it with a draw sheet that has been previously placed underneath the patient.

**2** Anesthesia for laparoscopy can be either general or local. If general anesthesia is used, it should be administered by the same standard techniques as used for major abdominal operations. One should not attempt to achieve surgical planes of anesthesia with tranquilizers and narcotics.

If local anesthesia is used, it should be accompanied by intravenous sedation prior to the operative procedure. We prefer to sedate the patient with 50 mg meperidine (Demerol) and 10 mg diazepam (Valium) after she is placed on the operating table. In general, we limit our use of local anesthesia to laparoscopy sterilization procedures and other short diagnostic procedures that do not require extensive intraperitoneal manipulation of the tubes or ovaries.

**3** A bimanual pelvic examination should precede all laparoscopy procedures.

**4** The procedure is started by grasping the anterior lip of the cervix with a wide-mouthed Jacobs tenaculum attached to a Rubin intrauterine cannula. Exposure of the cervix should be obtained with a narrow curved Sims posterior retractor rather than a wide, flat, posterior vaginal retractor. The larger retractors produce pain, sometimes initiating a cycle of pain and anxiety that may make local anesthesia ineffective.

**5** If local anesthesia is used, the inferior rim of the umbilicus is thoroughly infiltrated with a 1% Xylocaine solution in a semicircular manner from the 9 o'clock position around to the 3 o'clock position on the umbilicus. The first injection of Xylocaine should be given at the 6 o'clock position on the inferior rim of the umbilicus, and the needle should be advanced underneath the skin as shown. In addition, approximately 2 mL should be infiltrated into the rectus fascia and muscles.

**6** Adequate countertraction on the anterior abdominal wall is necessary. Although some rely on a large pneumoperitoneum to provide adequate countertraction, we elevate the lower midline of the abdomen for this purpose. We have found that placement of the two towel clips, one each at the 5 and 7 o'clock positions on the inferior rim of the umbilicus, offers the best method of countertraction for insertion of the pneumoperitoneum needle and the trocar. After the towel clips have been placed, a 2-mm incision is made in the inferior rim of the umbilicus.

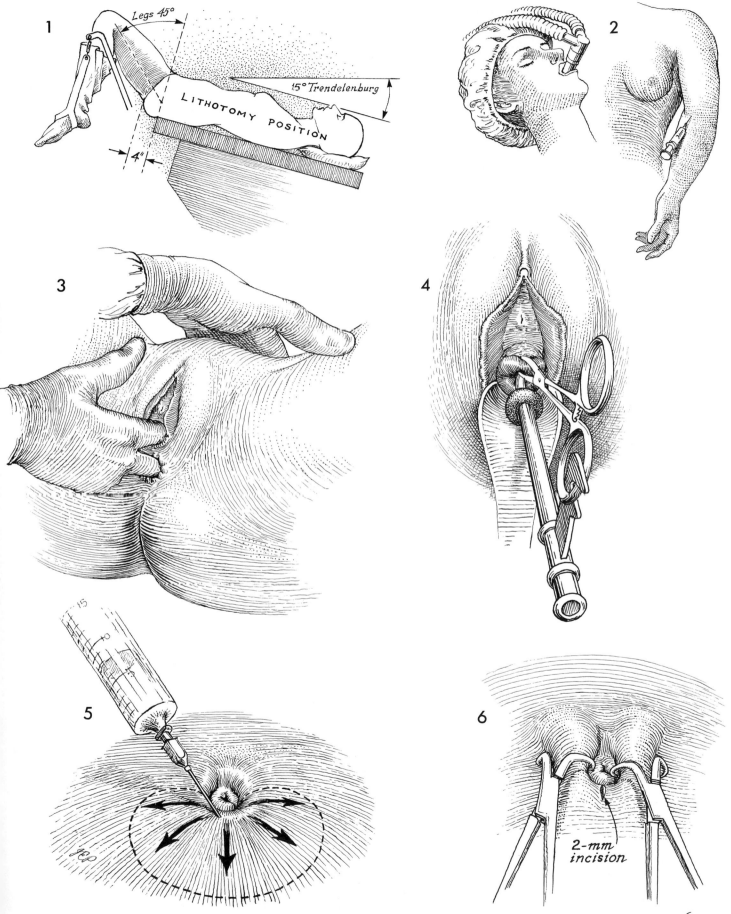

1

Legs 45°

15° Trendelenburg

LITHOTOMY POSITION

4"

2

3

4

5

6

2-mm
incision

261

# Laparoscopy Technique

## (Continued)

**7** The towel clips are elevated slightly, and a 17-gauge Tuohy epidural needle is advanced through the 2-mm incision down to the fascia.

**8** No attempt is made to penetrate the fascia with the initial insertion of the Tuohy needle.

**9** The needle is tapped against the fascia several times at a 90° angle to the plane of the body. The towel clips are further elevated for countertraction, and the needle is pushed through the rectus fascia with a short quick motion that advances the needle through the peritoneum. This technique reduces the possibility that the needle will slide off the rectus fascia and into the subcutaneous space.

**10** The pneumoperitoneum needle is immediately attached to the gas line from the carbon dioxide machine. The gas is allowed to flow and the pressure is observed to ensure that it is approximately 15 mm Hg. We have found the gas pressure method to be the most accurate way to determine proper placement of the pneumoperitoneum needle. Other techniques are the water-drop test and the saline-syringe test. With the gas pressure method, using a large-bore 17-gauge needle, a pressure greater than 15 mm Hg is an indication that the pneumoperitoneum needle is not in the free peritoneal space but is either up against a piece of bowel, in the omentum, or in the supraperitoneal space. It should be further adjusted by advancing it, twisting the bore 180° or withdrawing it slightly until such time as the pressure manometer indicates a pressure of less than 15 mm Hg. There are times when the gas line or the needle itself has an intrinsic obstruction that results in elevated false gas pressure readings. In these cases, one would accept a gas pressure of 10 mm Hg above the baseline pressure. Generally, for sterilization procedures such as the Silastic band operation, no more than 2 liters of carbon dioxide are needed. In electrocoagulation of the Fallopian tubes or other surgical procedures, however, a higher volume of gas is needed in order to obtain a larger displacement of bowel away from the pelvic organs to reduce the possibility of gastrointestinal burns. For diagnostic procedures, it is better to use at least 4–5 liters of gas for maximum displacement of the bowel. Therefore, it is better to perform diagnostic and more extensive surgical procedures under general anesthesia, as few patients can tolerate 5 liters of gas in the peritoneal cavity under local anesthesia.

**11** The 2-mm incision is extended to 1 cm.

**12** The laparoscope trocar and sleeve are inserted through the umbilicus incision in a twisting corkscrew technique that involves pushing the trocar down to the rectus fascia; with a short twisting corkscrew motion, the trocar is pushed through the rectus fascia while pulling up on the towel clips for countertraction. By using the short thrust and corkscrew motions, the surgeon advances the instrument progressively through the rectus fascia, avoiding a sudden thrust that might abruptly slip and contact the intra-abdominal or retroperitoneal organs.

**13** The trocar is removed from the sleeve, the gas hose is connected to the gas port on the trocar, and the laparoscope is advanced down the trocar sleeve into the pelvis. The angle of the insertion of the laparoscope through the sleeve and through the abdominal wall should be approximately 15–20° to the plane of the patient and not at a 90° angle, to avoid touching the lens against the surface of the bowel and the omentum. Such contact produces a pink or yellow blur instead of the recognizable abdominal structures. By holding the laparoscope in the right hand and moving the left hand between the patient's legs and grasping the Jacobs tenaculum and Rubin cannula, the uterus can be manipulated to either side or in the anterior-posterior plane for maximum visualization of all the internal genitalia.

**14** By depressing the Rubin cannula and Jacobs tenaculum, the surgeon can move the uterus into an anteflex position, thereby making the cul-de-sac, broad ligament, tubes, and ovaries visible. When maximum visualization of the structures is achieved, a nurse or assistant holds the Rubin cannula and Jacobs tenaculum in the desired position while the laparoscopist moves his left hand up to support the operating laparoscope and his right hand to perform the surgery (obviously, the reverse is true for those surgeons who are left-handed).

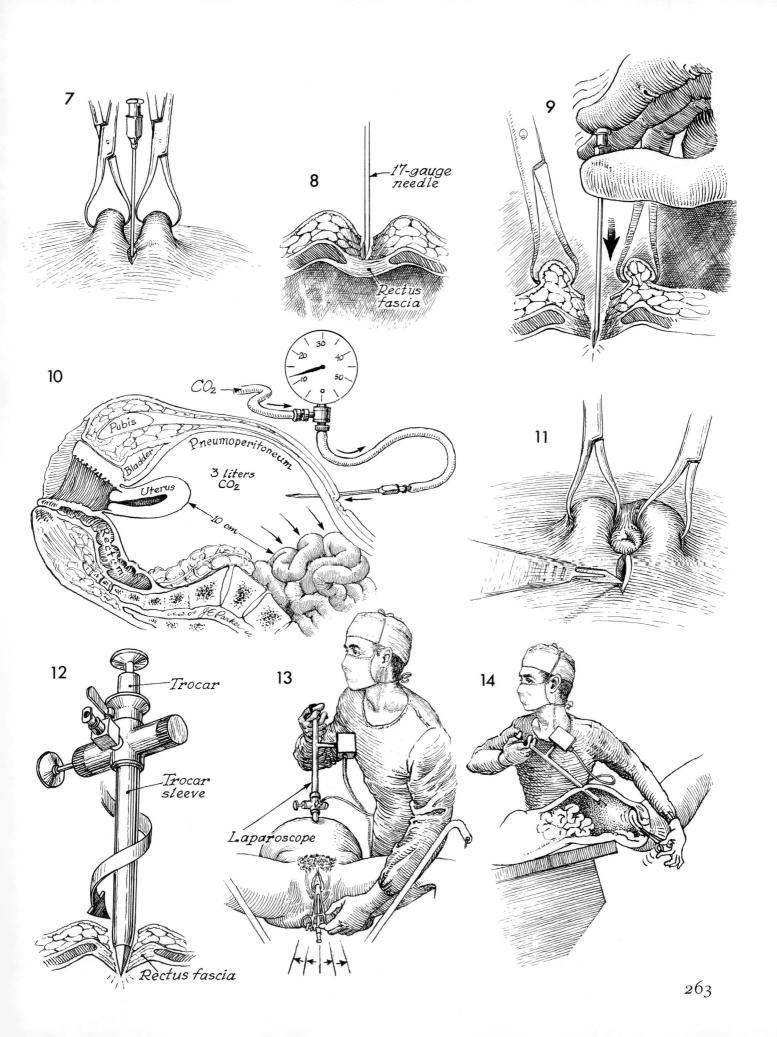

7

8

*17-gauge needle*

*Rectus fascia*

9

10

$CO_2$

*Pubis*

*Bladder*

*Uterus*

*Pneumoperitoneum*

*3 liters $CO_2$*

*10 cm*

*Rectum*

J E Parker

11

12

*Trocar*

*Trocar sleeve*

*Rectus fascia*

13

*Laparoscope*

14

263

# Laparoscopy Technique

## (Continued)

### Multi-incision Technique

Multi-incision laparoscopy is useful in most advanced surgical techniques. These cases include egg retrieval for in vitro fertilization, ovarian biopsy, extensive lysis of adhesions, extensive fulguration of endometriosis, the occasional removal of an intraperitoneal foreign body, laparoscopy-assisted vaginal hysterectomy, and resection of ectopic pregnancy.

**15** The first step in the insertion of a second instrument is to transilluminate the lower abdominal wall and select an avascular site for the incision of the second-incision trocar. We prefer the left and right lower quadrants where it is more advantageous to have the second-incision instrument at a right angle to the first-incision observation instrument. In all cases, however, an avascular area of the lower abdomen should be selected with special care to avoid the inferior epigastric artery and vein lateral to the rectus muscle.

**16** A 6-mm incision is made over the avascular area down to the fascia, and the fascia is lightly incised with the scalpel.

**17** The second-incision trocar and sleeve are held in a dagger fashion with the thumb on top of the trocar and the fingers wrapped around the trocar sleeve.

**18** The second-incision trocar and sleeve are inserted through the second-incision down to the fascia. At this point, the surgeon looks through the laparoscope or the attached video screen and slowly advances the second-incision instrument until it has perforated the peritoneum. Occasionally, it may be helpful to use the first-incision instrument as a source of countertraction by using it to elevate the anterior abdominal wall against the area where the second-incision trocar and sleeve are penetrating the peritoneum.

**19** The second-incision trocar is withdrawn from the second-incision sleeve and is now ready to receive operative instruments.

**20** The Rubin cannula and Jacobs tenaculum are held by a nurse or assistant in the most advantageous position. The surgeon holds the laparoscope with his left hand and the second-incision instrument with his right hand. Note that, as shown, an operating laparoscope is used for the first incision. This allows a second instrument to be inserted into the abdominal cavity to facilitate the desired surgery without a second incision. The ovary or Fallopian tube can be stabilized for biopsy or lysing peritubal adhesions.

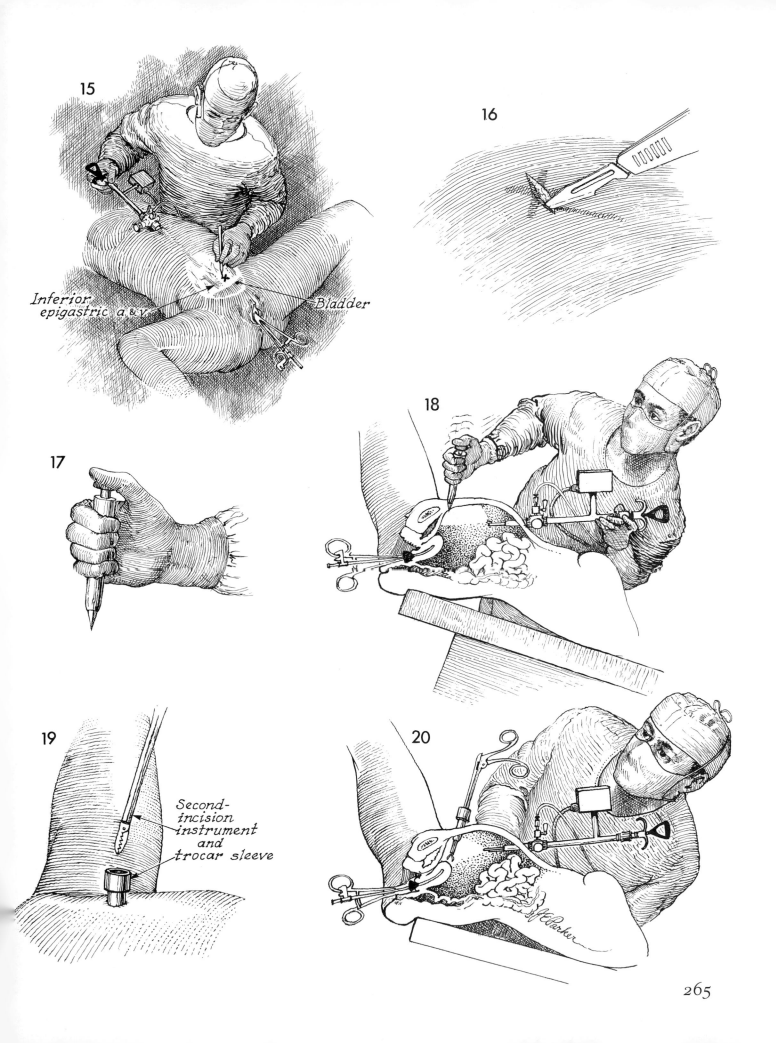

15

16

17

18

19

Second-
incision
instrument
and
trocar sleeve

20

Inferior
epigastric a. & v.

Bladder

265

# Diagnostic Uses of Laparoscopy

Laparoscopy offers the pelvic surgeon a significant advantage by providing accurate diagnostic techniques without requiring exploratory laparotomy. It is particularly useful in (1) identifying unique and unusual alterations in pelvic anatomy, (2) resolving questions about an ectopic pregnancy that is difficult to diagnose, (3) differentiating between borderline and severe cases of pelvic inflammatory disease and between pelvic disease and acute appendicitis, and (4) evaluating the pelvis and Fallopian tubes in cases of infertility.

The purpose of the operation is to visualize the lower abdomen and pelvis without performing a laparotomy.

**Physiologic Changes.** None

**Points of Caution.** Laparoscopy should not be used diagnostically where there is overwhelming evidence of pelvic disease requiring exploratory laparotomy. For example, it is unwise and contraindicated to perform diagnostic laparoscopy where there are pelvic masses greater than 14 weeks gestational size. In these cases, exploratory laparotomy should be performed. Likewise, diagnostic laparoscopy should not be performed with a gross hemoperitoneum or generalized abdominal peritonitis. Performance of laparoscopy is not excessively hazardous under these conditions, but it adds nothing to the overall diagnosis and simply delays exploratory laparotomy.

## Technique

**1** An alteration in pelvic anatomy that may be associated with a congenital anomaly of the Müllerian duct is shown. In institutions with adequate cytogenic laboratories, diagnostic laparoscopy is not required for anomalies of the internal genitalia because in most cases the anomaly can be diagnosed without operative intervention. In cases of failure in Müllerian duct fusion in which there is a rudimentary or smaller separate horn on one side and an enlarged uterine horn on the opposite side, however, the use of the laparoscope may be valuable in developing a complete treatment plan.

**2** Women with amenorrhea, abdominal pain, vaginal bleeding, and/or an adnexal mass do not need diagnostic laparoscopy to rule out the possibility of ectopic pregnancy. However, many women with ectopic pregnancy have vague symptoms and ambiguous signs. Even if a culdocentesis shows a small amount of nonclotting blood, the laparoscope is a valuable instrument in differentiating a tubular pregnancy from a bleeding corpus luteum cyst. In addition, the bleeding corpus luteum can be electrocoagulated through the laparoscope, and laparotomy may be avoided. If there is gross abdominal distention from a hemoperitoneum, however, laparoscopy only delays appropriate therapy.

Frequently, the surgeon is not able to see the dilated Fallopian tube containing the pregnancy as shown here. Often, a cornual mass is visible, consisting of clotted blood mixed with tissue.

**3** Diagnostic laparoscopy has been of great assistance in differentiating between the difficult cases of pelvic inflammatory disease and acute appendicitis. The treatment for each is quite different, and if an accurate preoperative diagnosis can be made, substantial savings in hospital costs and utilization of hospital beds can be made. In addition, purulent material can be aspirated through the laparoscope to ascertain the exact etiology of the endosalpingitis and aid in selection of appropriate antibiotic therapy. When there are signs and symptoms of generalized peritonitis, however, laparoscopy is contraindicated and only delays the exploratory laparotomy needed to correct the problem.

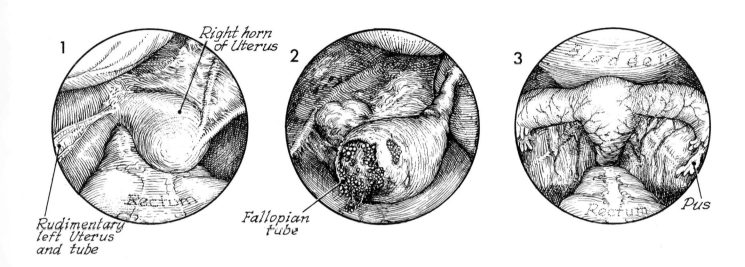

# Demonstration of Tubal Patency via Laparoscopy

Modern infertility evaluations are rarely complete without observation of the Fallopian tube and ovary for disease. Laparoscopy has replaced culdoscopy as the procedure of choice because it allows the pelvic surgeon a broader plane of observation, better manipulation of internal structures, and the ability to electrocoagulate endometrial implants (see pages 274–275).

The purpose of the operation is to inject a dye through the uterus and the Fallopian tube to demonstrate patency of the tube.

**Physiologic Changes.** None

**Points of Caution.** Care must be taken to ensure that there is a watertight seal between the acorn on the cervical cannula and the surface of the cervix to prevent the dye from leaking back into the vagina.

## Technique

**1** As with all laparoscopic diagnostic procedures, a Rubin cannula and Jacobs tenaculum are applied to the cervix prior to beginning the procedure. The patient is positioned with the buttocks at least 4 inches off the end of the operating table. This is essential if the surgeon is to have proper observation while injecting indigo carmine solution through the endometrial cavity into the Fallopian tubes.

**2** Laparoscopy is performed in the routine fashion. Generally, the one-incision technique is sufficient for adequately observing the entire pelvis. The Fallopian tubes should be grasped with a smooth 3-mm forceps and maneuvered into a position where they can be adequately observed.

**3** Ten mL of indigo carmine solution are injected through the Rubin cannula in the cervix. The solution can be observed flowing from the Fallopian tube, or the point of obstruction can be noted. It is not necessary to remove the indigo carmine from the abdomen. The instruments are withdrawn, and the laparoscopy incision is closed in a routine fashion.

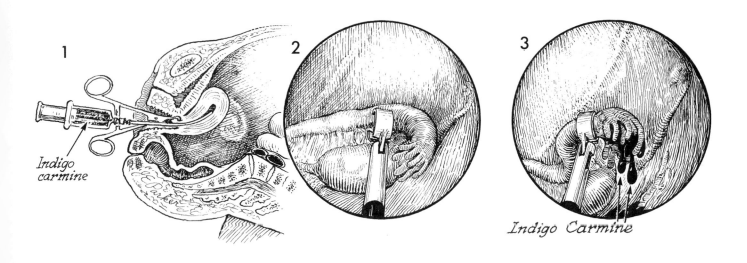

1

Indigo
carmine

2

3

Indigo Carmine

269

# Laparoscopic Resection of Unruptured Ectopic Pregnancy

The laparoscopic resection of unruptured ectopic pregnancy has become a useful and efficacious management of this problem that formally required a pelvic laparotomy with a lengthy hospital stay. These patients usually present with the triad of amenorrhea, pelvic pain, and vaginal bleeding.

The laparoscope can be an additional diagnostic aid as well as a surgical treatment.

**Physiologic Change.** The oocyte site has been impregnated with sperm, usually in the midportion of the Fallopian tube. There are some physiologic factors present that do not allow the new embryo to be taken down the tube and into the endometrial cavity. These frequently range from a history of inflammatory disease to external adhesions that obstruct the Fallopian tube.

Removal of the trophoblastic tissue from the tube immediately lowers the human chorionic gonadotropin levels in the blood.

**Points of Caution.** Laparoscopy may be difficult in patients with a large ruptured ectopic pregnancy with copious bleeding. In these patients, laparoscopy is a waste of time. These patients should be treated with laparotomy.

In certain cases, the surgeon may find that the serum chorionic gonadotropin levels have not fallen after laparoscopy. This may mean that all trophoblastic tissue has not been resected. If the patient is stable, treatment with methotrexate may be indicated.

---

*Technique*

**1** Laparoscopy has been performed in the routine manner. The ovary and the Fallopian tube with its ectopic pregnancy can be seen.

**2** The Fallopian tube is opened in a longitudinal manner.

**3** The grasping forceps enters the Fallopian tube, and the trophoblastic tissue is removed in pieces.

**4** A gauze pad is shown with the ectopic detritus.

**5** Hemorrhage control is performed with electrocoagulation of small bleeders.

**6** The wound is left open.

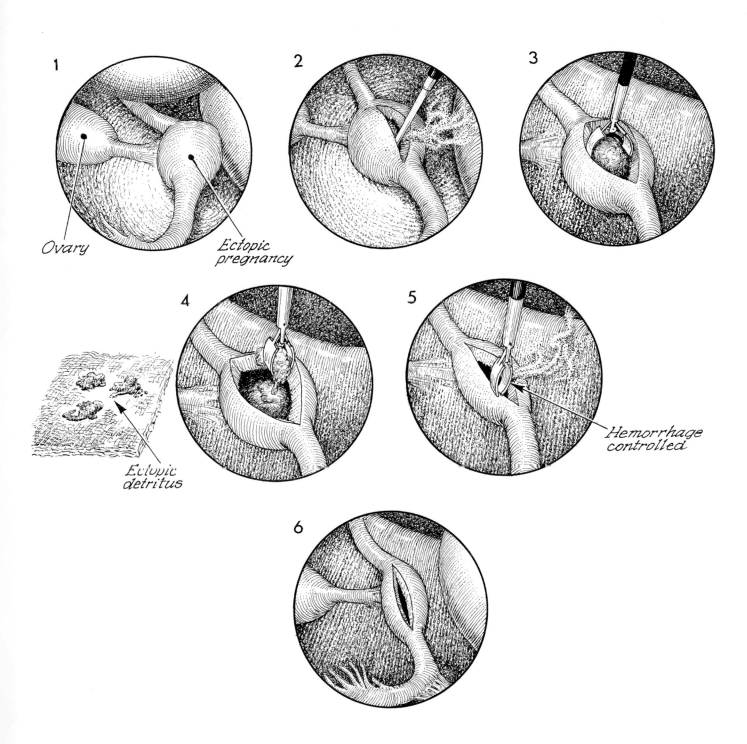

1

Ovary

Ectopic
pregnancy

2

3

4

Ectopic
detritus

5

Hemorrhage
controlled

6

271

# Ovarian Biopsy via Laparoscopy

Biopsy of the ovary is rarely necessary. Modern cytogenetic and endocrine laboratory techniques can usually ascertain whether the ovary contains oocytes. There are some cases, however, in which biopsy of the ovary may be indicated.

The purpose of the operation is to obtain an adequate biopsy of the ovary through the laparoscope.

**Physiologic Changes.** Removal of a piece of ovary can, in some cases, change the physiology of the hypo-thalamic-pituitary-ovarian axis in the same manner as wedge resection of the ovary alters the physiology in polycystic ovary disease.

**Points of Caution.** The predominant complication from ovarian biopsy is control of hemorrhage from the bed of the ovary. Thorough electrocoagulation of the entire biopsy site should be performed. The site should be observed for at least 3–4 minutes to ensure that hemostasis is complete.

## Technique

**1** Ovarian biopsy by laparoscopy requires a two-incision technique. It is preferable to use an operating laparoscope with a 3-mm grasping forceps to grasp the suspensory ligament of the ovary and anchor the ovary in a stable position.

**2** A 6-mm alligator biopsy forceps is passed through a second-incision trocar, and a large bit of ovarian capsule and stroma is taken. Bleeding from this site can be copious and must be coagulated. If bleeding obscures observation of the biopsy site, a third puncture is made in the abdominal wall. A 2-mm aspiration needle connected to a 50-mL syringe of saline solution is introduced through the puncture, and the biopsy site is irrigated with saline solution rather than suctioned.

**3** A large electrocoagulation biopsy forceps is inserted through the second-incision trocar into the biopsy wound, and the jaws of the forceps are opened. The electrical current is applied, and the ovary is coagulated thoroughly from the inside. This usually stops most of the bleeding. The site is irrigated with saline solution. The biopsy forceps can be applied to small bleeding areas with the jaws in the closed position, providing point cautery rather than widespread cautery. The ovary should be observed for at least 3–4 minutes to ensure that all bleeding is stopped prior to removing the instruments from the abdomen.

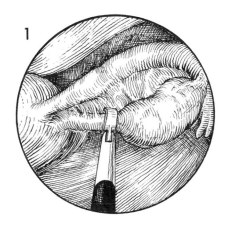

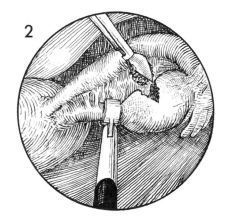

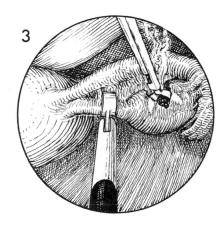

# Electrocoagulation of Endometriosis via Laparoscopy

The purpose of electrocoagulating endometrial implants found at the time of laparoscopy is to destroy the implantation site. The purpose of the operation is to eliminate endometriosis.

**Physiologic Changes.** Destruction of the endometrial implantation site in no way changes the potential of the mesothelium in the pelvis to form endometriosis. It is hoped that by eliminating the existing endometriosis, the surgeon can relieve the symptomatology (particularly in relation to infertility). In many cases, repeat surgery and treatment of endometriosis will be needed.

**Points of Caution.** Extreme care must be exercised in fulgurating endometriosis in the pelvis to avoid electrocoagulation of adjacent vital structures, such as bowel or bladder.

## Technique

**1** This view through the laparoscope shows endometrial implants on the fundus of the uterus near the junction of the round ligament and Fallopian tube.

**2** The 3-mm grasping forceps is inserted through the operating laparoscope. The forceps grasps the endometrial implant, which is thoroughly electrocoagulated. Care is taken to ensure that there is adequate insulation showing prior to performing the electrocoagulation.

**3** The electrocoagulated site is inspected to rule out hemorrhage.

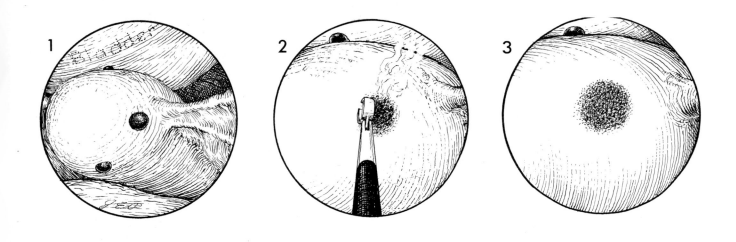

# Lysis of Adhesions via Laparoscopy

The laparoscope can be used in the lysis of intraperitoneal adhesions. The technique consists of electrofulgurating the adhesion and cutting the adhesion with scissors in the area electrocoagulated.

The purpose of the operation is to lyse intraperitoneal adhesions, utilizing the advantages of the laparoscopic technique.

**Physiologic Changes.** The Fallopian tubes, colon, and intestine are freed and are thus able to resume their physiologic functions without entrapment.

**Points of Caution.** Precise surgical judgment is needed to lyse the adhesions via the laparoscopic technique without producing injury to the organ adjacent to the adhesion. Certain kinds of adhesions are more amenable to laparoscopic lysis than others. In general, "violin-string," thin, filmy adhesions are best suited for this technique, while thick, dense adhesions that can contain a portion of a viscus should not be treated by this method.

## Technique

**1** Lysis of adhesions is best accomplished by thoroughly electrocoagulating the adhesions.

**2** After the adhesion has been electrocoagulated, it is cut with sharp laparoscopy dissecting scissors.

**3** A broad-based adhesion can be lysed in several bites by electrocoagulation, followed by sharp incision in the electrocoagulated area, followed by repeat electrocoagulation and incision.

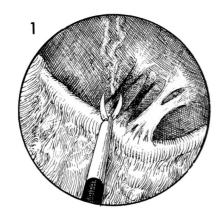

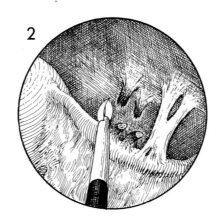

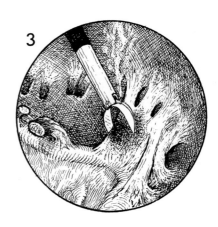

# Control of Hemorrhage During Laparoscopy

Hemorrhage secondary to laparoscopic procedures, particularly tubal sterilization, can frequently be controlled via the laparoscope with electrocoagulation and/or Silastic banding of the bleeding points.

The purpose of the operation is to control bleeding.

**Physiologic Changes.** Pelvic hemorrhage is controlled.

**Points of Caution.** If bleeding occurs adjacent to a vital structure, the Silastic band technique is preferred over the electrocoagulation technique. The electrocoagulation technique is adequate, however, for control of hemorrhage on the Fallopian tube.

Care must be taken to ensure that hemorrhage is controlled prior to withdrawing the instruments from the abdomen.

## Technique

**1** In most instances when the surgeon is using either electrocoagulation or the Silastic band technique, hemorrhage can be controlled without laparotomy. The bleeding areas are identified through the laparoscope.

**2** The laparoscopy grasping tongs of the Silastic band instrument are used to grasp the bleeding area to draw it into the Silastic band applier and to push a Silastic band over the bleeding pedicles. This band acts as a suture ligature and stops the bleeding. Two or more such bands can be applied to all bleeding areas.

**3** If the surgeon prefers electrocoagulation for control of hemorrhage, the 3-mm grasping forceps is used to electrocoagulate the bleeding stumps of the proximal or distal Fallopian tube.

After electrocoagulation or application of a Silastic band, the area should be irrigated with a small amount of sterile saline solution and observed for several minutes to be sure that all bleeding has stopped.

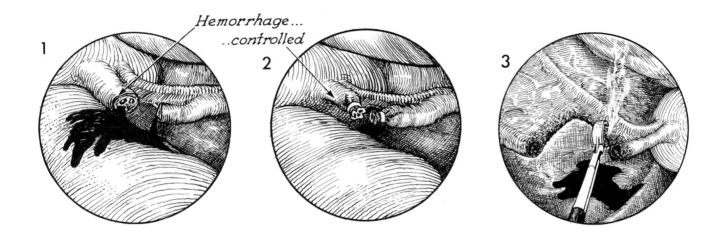

Hemorrhage...
..controlled

# Sterilization by Electrocoagulation and Division via Laparoscopy

Electrocoagulation and division of peritoneal structures via the laparoscope are facilitated if the surgeon achieves adequate displacement of the intestine out of the pelvis, maintains a clear pneumoperitoneum free of smoke, and ensures that the installation of the electrocoagulating instrument is advanced sufficiently to prevent contact between the instrument and the tip of the laparoscope. These principles are valid whether performing sterilization, fulguration of endometrial implants, biopsy of the ovary, or lysis of adhesions.

The purpose of the operation is to provide a simple method of female sterilization by electrocoagulation of the Fallopian tube via the laparoscopic technique.

**Physiologic Changes.** After the electrofulgurated and divided tube heals, migrating spermatozoa should not be transported through the Fallopian tube. Oocytes entering the distal end of the tube should not pass the point of obstruction.

**Points of Caution.** The surgeon must adhere to the points of caution noted for the laparoscopy technique described on page 272.

There is the additional risk with electrocoagulation of inadvertently burning the intestine. Even with utmost care and attention to detail, the surgeon cannot always prevent some electrocoagulation burns of the bowel. Care should be taken, however, to ensure that the insulation on the grasping forceps is well beyond the point of the metal trocar or laparoscope. In addition, the structure being electrocoagulated should be moved well away from the adjacent bowel or bladder.

---

## Technique

1 Sterilization by electrocoagulation can be achieved by either extensive electrocoagulation of the tube alone or electrocoagulation and division. Experience has shown a lower failure rate when the tube is electrocoagulated and divided. Use of electrocoagulation and division increases the possibility of hemorrhage from the mesosalpinx, however, if sufficient electrocoagulation has not been performed prior to division of the tube. The uterus is markedly anteflexed and deviated to one side, placing the tube on a slight stretch. The tube is grasped in the ischemial portion approximately 3 cm from the cornua of the uterus.

2 The tube is elevated and placed in a position that is free from contact with bowel or bladder.

3 The electrocoagulation forceps is checked to be sure that insulation is clearly visible and that the metal grasping jaws of the coagulation forceps are not in contact with the laparoscope or the trocar sleeve of the second-incision instrument. The current is turned on, and the tube is thoroughly electrocoagulated for at least 5 full seconds. Frequently, the tube will swell and make a popping noise, indicating that fluid within the lumen of the tube and tubal cells has reached the boiling point. The burn will spread over a finite area, usually 3–4 cm along the tube and 2 cm into the mesosalpinx. The burn will not spread farther because burned tissue has a greater resistance to the flow of electrical current than does normal tissue. When the tube has collapsed from its swollen state, it has been coagulated sufficiently.

4 At this point, the tube is avulsed off the mesosalpinx and from its connection to the proximal and distal tube. This is facilitated by shearing the tube against the operative port of the laparoscope. The reduced tensile strength of the burned tube has little resistance to the tearing motion of the grasping forceps.

5 Care should be taken to ensure that insulation is showing through the laparoscope at all times. It is a mistake for the metal of the grasping forceps to make contact with the metal end of the laparoscope. This may allow the electrothermal energy to flow up the shaft of the laparoscope and may produce a burn of the intestine higher in the abdomen.

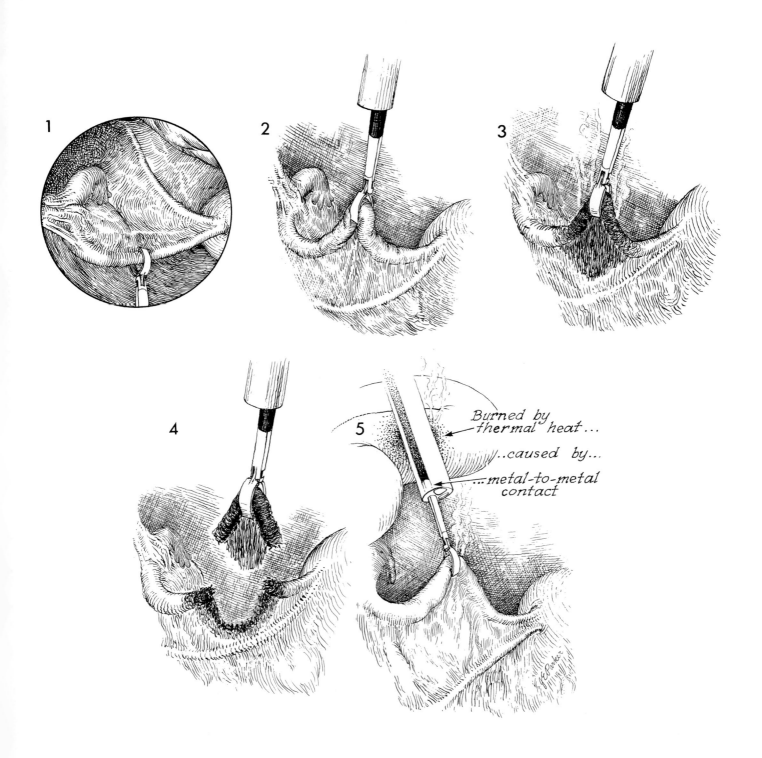

Burned by
thermal heat...

...caused by...

...metal-to-metal
contact

# Silastic Band Sterilization via Laparoscopy

The Fallopian tube can be adequately obstructed by the application of a Silastic band to a knuckle of Fallopian tube. This produces necrosis of the tube from ischemia and, thereby, causes tubal obstruction. It has an advantage over the electrocoagulation technique in that it is equally successful, statistically, preventing pregnancy and avoids the possibility of electrothermal burns.

The purpose of the Silastic band applied by laparoscopy is to obstruct the Fallopian tube to achieve female sterilization.

**Physiologic Changes.** The Fallopian tubes are obstructed.

**Points of Caution.** Care must be taken not to bring an excessively large knuckle of Fallopian tube into the housing of the banding scope. If a large mass of Fallopian tube, with associated mesosalpinx, is brought into the housing of the laparoscope, the grasping tongs will lacerate the tube.

## Technique

**1** The uterus is anteflexed by manipulating the Rubin cannula and Jacobs tenaculum. The Fallopian tube is visualized and then is grasped with the tongs of the Silastic band instrument, which has been previously loaded with a Falope ring.

**2** The Fallopian tube is drawn into the Silastic band applicator, and the Falope ring is pushed off the applicator onto a knuckle of tube.

**3** The knuckle of tube is released from the grasping tongs.

**4** If Silastic band sterilization is desired by the two-incision technique, the second-incision instrument is inserted as shown on page 265, Figure 18, and the Silastic band applicator is inserted through the second-incision trocar into the lower abdomen.

**5** The Fallopian tube is again located, and the second-incision Silastic band applicator is used to draw the Fallopian tube into the applicator and push the Silastic band over a knuckle of Fallopian tube.

**6** When the operation has been completed, either by the one-incision or two-incision technique, the pelvic area is thoroughly inspected to see that both tubes are adequately banded and that there is no hemorrhage.

**7** The instruments are withdrawn, and the incision is closed with a single 3-0 synthetic absorbable suture.

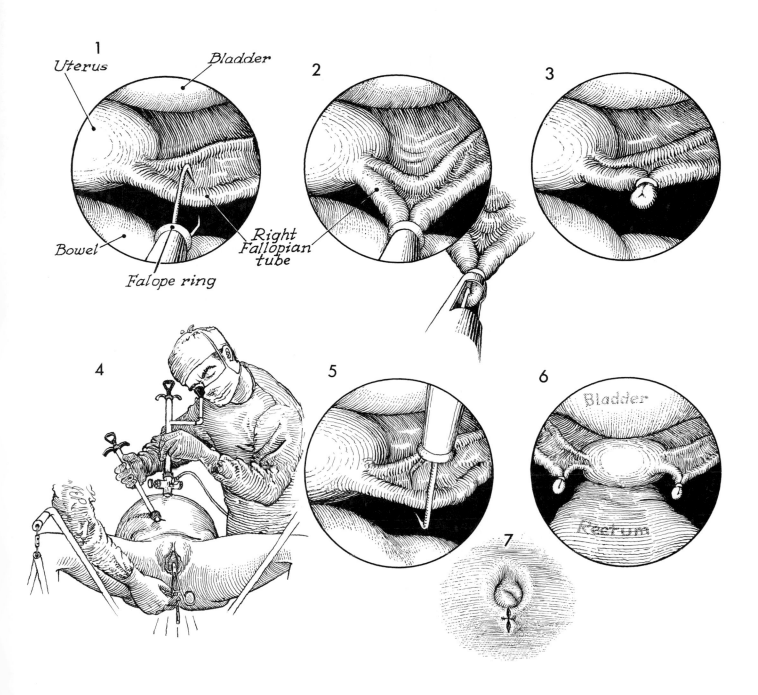

1

*Uterus*          *Bladder*

*Bowel*

*Falope ring*          *Right Fallopian tube*

2

3

4

5

6

*Bladder*

*Rectum*

7

283

# Hulka Clip Sterilization via Laparoscopy

Laparoscopic Hulka clip application for female sterilization differs from the other methods of laparoscopy sterilization in that it applies a spring-loaded Silastic clip to the Fallopian tube. It has the advantage of producing the least tissue damage to the Fallopian tube and, therefore, may prove to be the most reversible form of female sterilization. The laparoscopic technique is the same as previously described for other laparoscopic procedures.

The purpose of the operation is to effect female sterilization.

**Physiologic Changes.** The oocyte and spermatozoa are prevented from meeting in the midportion of the Fallopian tube.

**Points of Caution.** Care must be taken to ensure that the Hulka clip is over the entire Fallopian tube and that the tips of the clip grasp a small portion of mesosalpinx.

---

## Technique

**1** With a loaded clip applier next to the Fallopian tube, 2–3 mL of 1% Xylocaine solution are pushed through the clip applier and sprayed on the Fallopian tube for local anesthesia.

**2** The surgeon opens the clip by activating the shaft retractor at the end of the clip applier. The same mechanism is used to close the clip and lock it into position with its metallic spring.

**3** The clip has been applied to the Fallopian tube. It is released from the clip applier when the surgeon withdraws the shaft to the extreme position.

The same procedure is performed on the opposite tube. The surgical instruments are withdrawn, and the gas is released through the remaining trocar sleeve. The incision is closed with single 3-0 synthetic absorbable suture.

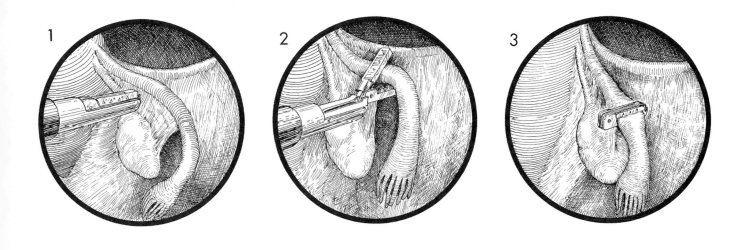

# Sterilization by the Pomeroy Operation

The Pomeroy operation is the most popular and widespread operation performed for female sterilization. It can be performed postpartum, at the time of cesarean section, or at interval sterilization through either mini-laparotomy or vaginal colpotomy.

The purpose of the operation is to obstruct the female Fallopian tubes and prevent pregnancy.

**Physiologic Changes.** All methods of tubal sterilization have a reported incidence of menometrorrhagia. This varies with different series. The exact physiologic changes that produce the menometrorrhagia are unknown at this time. The theory that ligation of the Fallopian tube reduces or alters ovarian blood supply remains to be proven.

**Points of Caution.** A 0 synthetic absorbable suture is preferable to permanent suture for ligating the knuckle of Fallopian tube. If the two ends of the Fallopian tube are permanently held in approximation, there may be a greater chance of recanalization than if they are allowed to separate when the suture is absorbed.

## Technique

**1** The patient is placed in the supine position, and the abdomen is opened in the transverse or midline direction. The Fallopian tube is grasped with the Babcock clamp and elevated.

**2** The knuckle of Fallopian tube is tied with a 0 synthetic absorbable suture.

**3** The knuckle is transected with scissors. The abdomen is closed in layers.

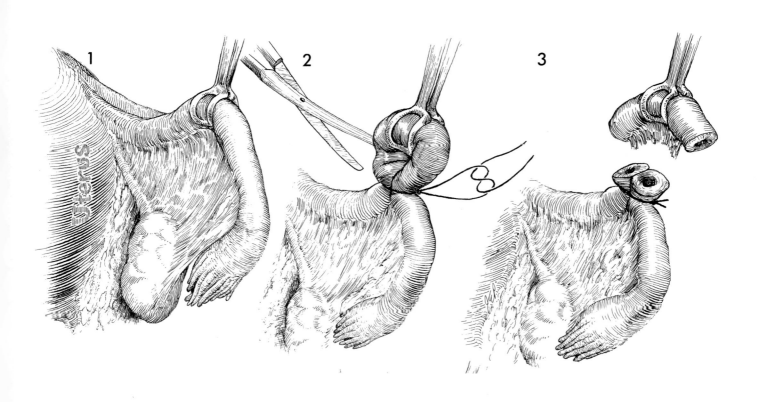

287

# Sterilization by the Modified Irving Technique

The modified Irving operation was proposed to prevent the small but persistent incidence of failures associated with the Pomeroy procedure. Although prospective randomized studies are unavailable at this writing, this operation is regarded as one of the most effective for prevention of pregnancy.

The purpose of the procedure is to prevent pregnancy by obstructing the Fallopian tubes by burying their proximal portions back into the myometrium.

**Physiologic Changes.** The physiologic changes with the modified Irving technique are similar to those associated with the other methods of tubal obstruction and ligation. In addition, the proximal portion of the Fallopian tube is buried within the myometrium. This makes recanalization or the development of a tuboperitoneal fistula extremely unlikely.

**Points of Caution.** An adequate opening in the myometrium must be made with the straight mosquito clamp if the Fallopian tube is to be pulled within the myometrium.

## Technique

**1** The abdomen is opened through a transverse or lower midline incision. The Fallopian tube is grasped with an Allis or a Babcock clamp. A small Halsted hemostat is used to open the mesosalpinx.

**2** Two 0 synthetic absorbable sutures are passed through this opening.

**3** The sutures are tied, and the segment of Fallopian tube is transected and removed. The tie on the distal segment of the proximal portion of Fallopian tube is threaded onto two French eye needles.

**4** A mosquito hemostat is used to open a 6-mm defect in the posterior wall of the uterus in the cornual region.

**5** The French eye needles are passed through this defect, one after another, and the suture is tied, pulling the proximal portion of the Fallopian tube into the defect.

**6** The completed operation shows both proximal portions of the Fallopian tube buried within the myometrium. The distal portions of the Fallopian tube are ligated and left in place.

The abdomen is closed in layers.

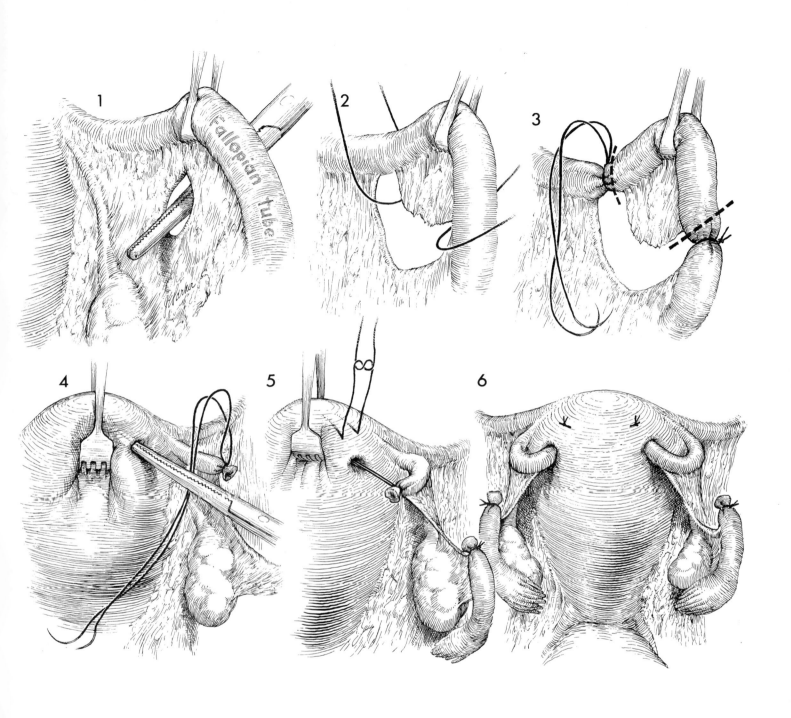

# Sterilization by the Minilaparotomy Technique

Minilaparotomy is ideal for thin women with no pelvic disease or adhesions. The procedure is difficult to perform in obese women or in women who have had inflammatory disease of the Fallopian tubes.

In thin, small patients it has the advantage of being performed with instruments less costly than those for laparoscopy. When patients are given a choice, however, they usually prefer laparoscopy because recovery is faster and less painful and they can resume their activities much sooner.

The purpose of the procedure is to obstruct the Fallopian tubes.

**Physiologic Changes.** The Fallopian tubes are obstructed.

**Points of Caution.** The bladder must be empty, or cystotomy can result. If more than 4 cm are needed to enter the abdomen—the width of 2 adult fingers—the patient is too obese for this operation, and a laparotomy should be performed with the patient under general anesthesia.

---

## Technique

**1** The patient is placed in the dorsal lithotomy position, and a thorough examination of the pelvis is performed to rule out the presence of adnexal disease. The vagina is surgically prepped. A Rubin cannula and Jacobs tenaculum are inserted into the cervix and through the cervical os, respectively. The abdomen is opened with a 4-cm transverse incision above the mons pubis.

**2** A small self-retaining retractor is inserted through the abdominal wall into the peritoneal cavity. The surgeon manipulates the previously placed Rubin cannula and Jacobs tenaculum on the cervix so that the fundus and cornua become readily visible through the small abdominal incision.

**3** A Babcock clamp is used to reach through the incision and grasp the Fallopian tube.

**4** The Fallopian tube is pulled up, and a piece of 0 synthetic absorbable suture is placed around a knuckle of tube, which is excised with scissors.

The Rubin cannula is manipulated to the other side, and a similar procedure is performed on the opposite Fallopian tube.

**5** The abdominal wall incision is closed in layers. The skin can be closed with either subcuticular or through-and-through sutures.

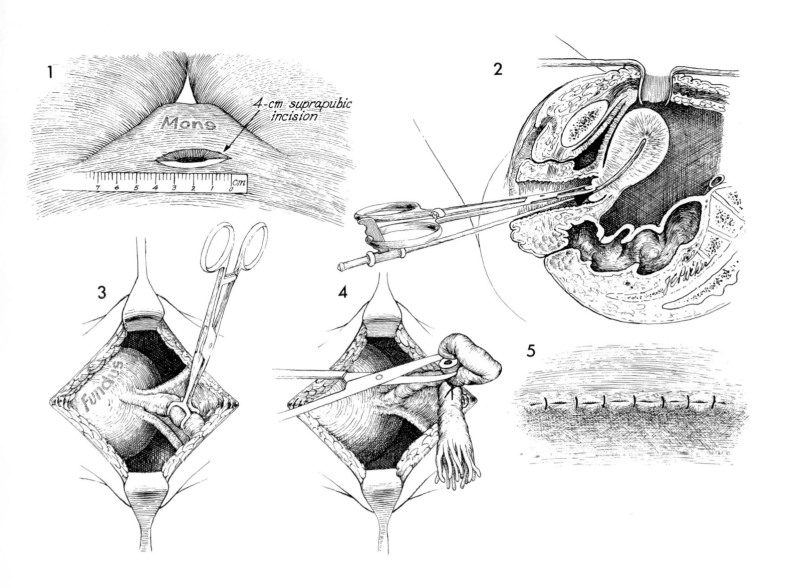

1

Mons

4-cm suprapubic incision

7 6 5 4 3 2 1 0    cm

2

3

Fundus

4

5

# Salpingectomy

The most frequent indication for salpingectomy is ectopic pregnancy, but the operation is also performed in isolated cases of inflammatory disease with a unilateral hydrosalpinx.

The purpose of the operation is to remove the Fallopian tube while leaving the uterus and ovary intact.

**Physiologic Changes.** The Fallopian tube is removed.

**Points of Caution.** The cornual portion of the Fallopian tube and mesosalpinx are extremely vascular areas. Hemostasis must be ensured.

## Technique

**1** A laparotomy is performed through a transverse or midline incision. The diseased tube is identified and freed of all peritubal adhesions. The cornual portion of the tube is clamped with a Kelly clamp, and the remainder is grasped with a Babcock clamp and elevated into a convenient position. Repeated fenestrations in the mesosalpinx are performed with a straight Halsted clamp. These should be clamped between small hemostats, and the tube can be excised from the cornual portion across the mesosalpinx to the fimbria.

**2** Each of the pedicles in the hemostats should be tied with interrupted 3-0 synthetic absorbable suture. The peritoneal lining is reestablished, and the cornual portion of the tube is buried with an interrupted 3-0 mattress suture in the broad ligament into the posterior segment of the uterine cornu.

**3** The mesosalpinx is reperitonealized with a running 3-0 synthetic absorbable suture.

**4** The mesosalpinx has been closed with a running 3-0 synthetic absorbable suture. The procedure has been completed. The abdomen is closed in routine fashion.

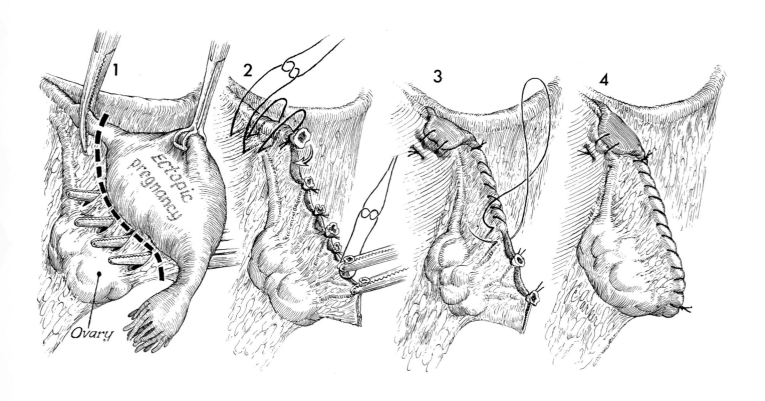

1    Ovary    Ectopic pregnancy

2

3

4

# Salpingo-oophorectomy

Salpingo-oophorectomy is needed when the disease process has invaded the Fallopian tube and ovary in such a manner that salvage of the ovary is undesirable or technically impossible. This occurs in both benign and malignant disease, particularly where the benefits derived from leaving the uterus and other adnexa in place outweigh the risks associated with the primary disease.

The purpose of the operation is to remove the tube and ovary.

**Physiologic Changes.** Although removal of one ovary may reduce the total hormone output, there is little clinical physiologic change.

**Points of Caution.** The infundibulopelvic ligament must be dissected clear to the ureter if the ligament is to be clamped in the area of the pelvic brim.

The infundibulopelvic ligament should be doubly tied because the venous network within this ligament tends to retract, producing hematomas that dissect up to the renal vessels. Transecting the round ligament and thus opening the broad ligament is not always necessary; however, it provides the most anatomic approach to this procedure and often allows a clean dissection of a tubo-ovarian mass without rupture.

## Technique

**1** A laparotomy is performed through a midline or transverse incision. The round ligament on the affected side is tied and transected. The posterior leaf of the broad ligament is then opened. The anterior leaf of the broad ligament can be seen through the opened posterior leaf, although in most cases there is no reason to open the anterior leaf.

**2** The infundibulopelvic ligament is undermined with finger dissection. Care should be taken to identify the ureter on that side. The infundibulopelvic ligament is triple-clamped and incised between the first and second clamps.

**3** The proximal side of the infundibulopelvic ligament is tied with a 0 synthetic absorbable suture, then sutured again.

**4** A defect is made in the mesosalpinx of the Fallopian tube adjacent to the cornual area. A Kelly clamp is placed across the suspensory ligament of the ovary and the Fallopian tube. The mesosalpinx of the Fallopian tube is penetrated as shown on page 293, and the mesosalpinx is clamped between the open portions. The tubes, suspensory ligament, and mesosalpinx are transected, and the tube and ovary are removed.

**5 & 6** The distal portion of the round ligament is reapproximated to the cornu of the uterus with a 0 synthetic absorbable mattress suture. The proximal stump of the round ligament is buried within the broad ligament. The defect in the broad ligament and the peritoneal lining of the mesosalpinx are reestablished with a running 3-0 synthetic absorbable suture starting at the cornu of the uterus and extending to the stump of the infundibulopelvic ligament.

The abdomen is closed in layers.

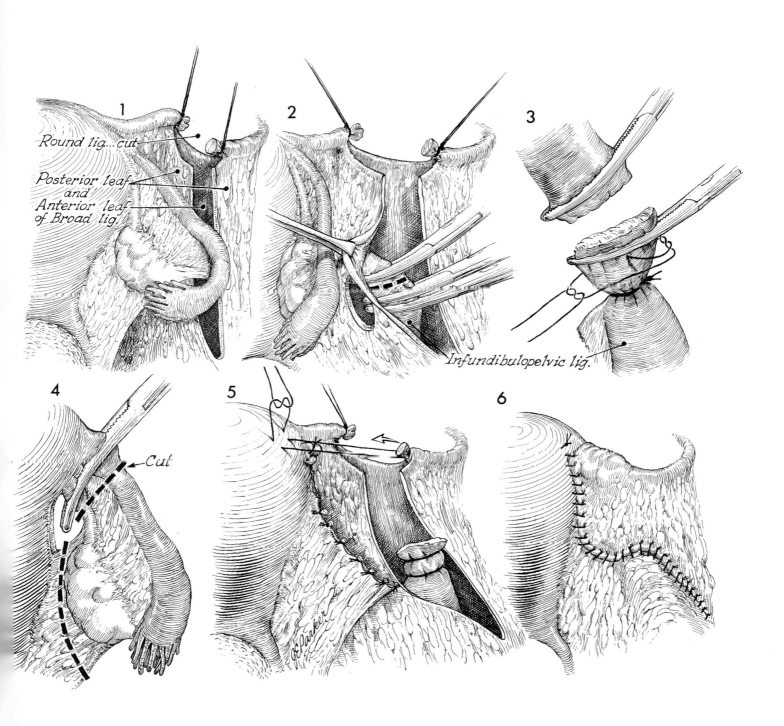

1

Round lig...cut

Posterior leaf
and
Anterior leaf
of Broad lig.

2

3

Infundibulopelvic lig.

4

Cut

5

J. Parker

6

295

# Fimbrioplasty

Fimbrioplasty is one of several reconstructive procedures designed to correct infertility.

The term fimbrioplasty is preferred over salpingostomy or simply opening the Fallopian tube, since salpingostomy does not address the important role of the fimbriae. Reconstruction, with care taken to preserve and release the multiple delicate fimbriae, is vital to making pregnancy possible. The operation should not be performed until a complete infertility evaluation of the couple has been made.

The purpose of the operation is to open the obstructed Fallopian tube and salvage enough function of the fimbriae to allow successful entrapment and transport of the oocyte.

**Physiologic Changes.** The Fallopian tube is opened, and the fimbriae are restored.

**Points of Caution.** Meticulous hemostasis is absolutely essential if this procedure is to succeed. Care must be exercised not to jeopardize the vascularity of the Fallopian tube by excessive dissection of the mesosalpinx from the ovary. In addition, irrigation, suction, and needlepoint electrocautery should be used to control hemostasis rather than sponging, clamping, and tying of bleeding blood vessels.

## Technique

1
Before fimbrioplasty, the surgeon should perform a diagnostic laparoscopy.

For diagnostic laparoscopy, the patient is placed in the dorsal lithotomy position with the hips flexed 45°, the knees flexed 90°, and the buttocks extended at least 4 inches beyond the edge of the operating table. The patient is placed in approximately a 15° Trendelenburg position.

2
A thorough bimanual pelvic examination is performed.

3
The laparoscopic instruments are introduced as recommended on page 263, and the pelvis is thoroughly inspected. If there is a gross hydrosalpinx or gross damage to the Fallopian tubes on both sides, it may be wise to abandon the procedure. The ideal patient for fimbrioplasty has a Fallopian tube that is normal except for the fimbriae, which are agglutinated or clubbed. The clubbed end of the tube is slightly distended by the injection of indigo carmine solution through the uterus during laparoscopy. The laparoscopic instruments are withdrawn; the small umbilical incision is closed with a 3-0 subcuticular suture.

4
Two positions can be useful for fimbrioplasty. One, as shown here, is the dorsal supine lithotomy position in which the legs are lowered in obstetrical stirrups so that the hips are extended 10° rather than flexed and the knees are flexed approximately 90°. The legs are abducted approximately 15°, exposing the vulva and perineum. This position is preferable when a surgeon wishes to apply instruments to the cervix and a cannula in the endometrial cavity during the procedure. It allows injection of indigo carmine solution through the cervix by means of a cervical cannula. In addition, the uterus can be elevated into the appropriate operative position without using traction sutures on the fundus or packing the cul-de-sac with gauze.

5
A Pfannenstiel incision is generally preferred in these cases. Dye marks have been placed to aid closure of the abdomen for a better cosmetic appearance.

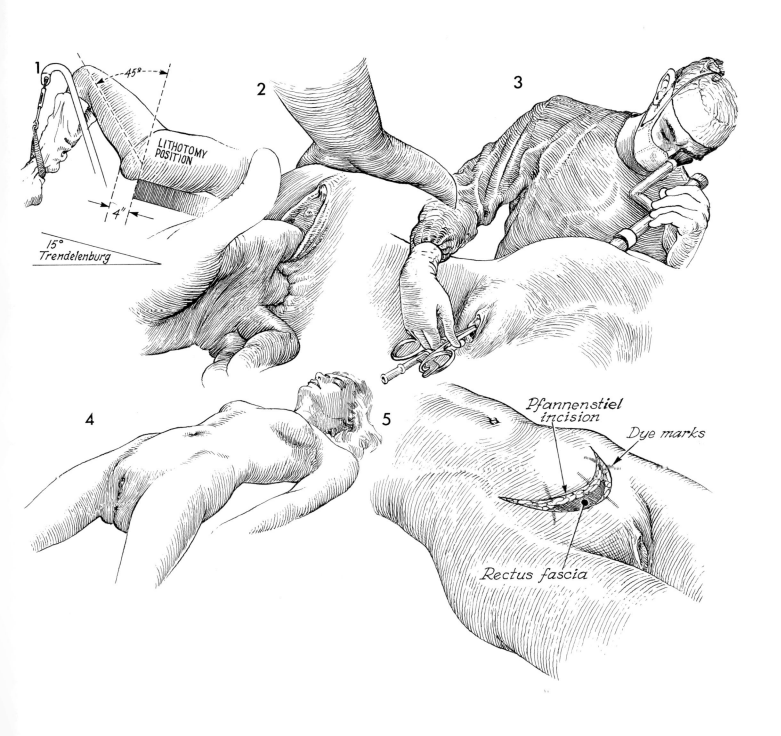

1

45°

LITHOTOMY
POSITION

4"

15°
Trendelenburg

2

3

4

5

*Pfannenstiel incision*

*Dye marks*

*Rectus fascia*

# Fimbrioplasty

## (Continued)

**6** The abdomen has been opened through the Pfannenstiel incision. Adhesions are found between the Fallopian tube, ovary, and round ligament. The bladder is on the right; the fundus is in the middle. An occlusive Buxton-type clamp is applied to the lower uterine segment, and a 21-gauge needle on a 10-mL syringe filled with indigo carmine solution is inserted through the fundus. The endometrial cavity is filled with the dye. This dye should spill into the Fallopian tubes and slightly distend the clubbed ends of the Fallopian tube that requires a fimbrioplasty.

**7** Moist packs have been placed in the cul-de-sac to elevate the uterus, tubes, and ovaries into the incision. The microtip cautery is used to remove adhesions. Visual magnification and a source of excellent light are essential if this step is to be performed. The principle of traction/countertraction on the structures is essential to safely demonstrate the adhesions.

**8** When the adhesions have been completely removed, the clubbed end of the Fallopian tube can be identified; it should be opened with the cautery on a low setting. Bright light and visual magnification will aid the surgeon in performing this delicate task.

**9** A microforceps is used to elevate the serosal layer over the end of the clubbed Fallopian tube. Small vessels are coagulated prior to opening the clubbed end of the fimbriae with the microtip electrical cautery. When the scar tissue over the clubbed end of the tube has been transected, indigo carmine dye will be observed spilling from the Fallopian tube.

**10** Microforceps and microscissors are used to pick up the scar tissue and transect the scarred serosal layer covering the fimbriae beneath. It is important to identify the fine blood vessels in the scarred covering of the fimbriae; the incisions into scarred serosa should be tailored to transect as few of the blood vessels as possible. Hemostasis is controlled with the microelectrode.

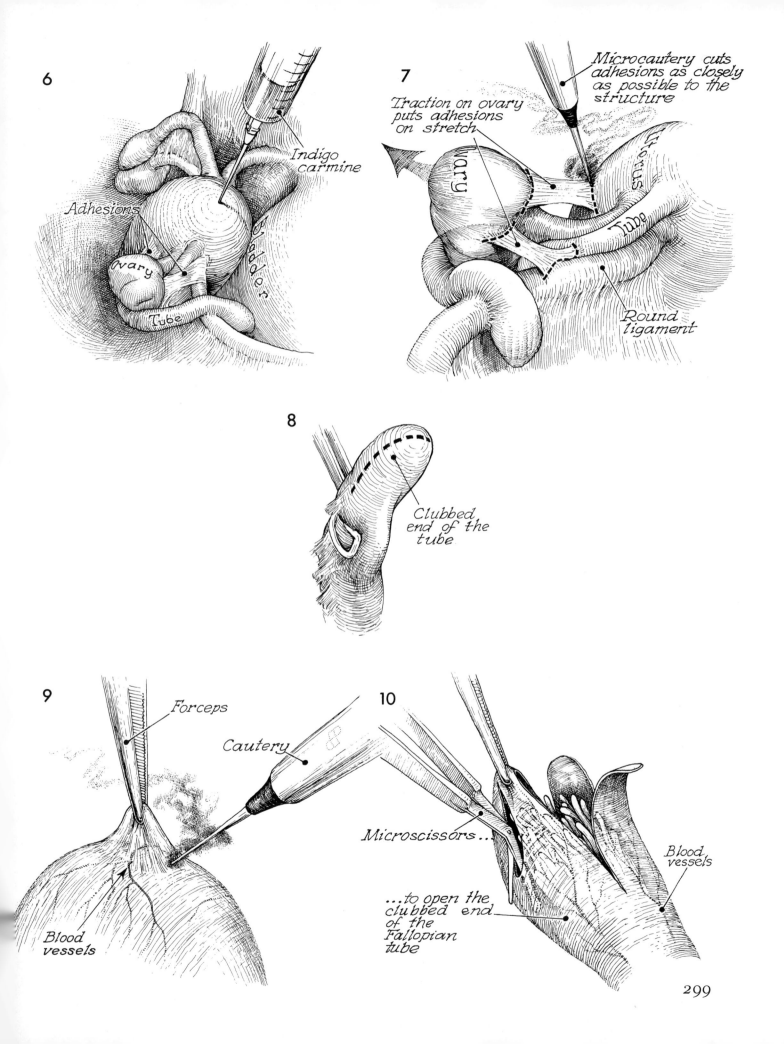

6

Indigo
carmine

Adhesions

Ovary

Tube

Bladder

7

Traction on ovary
puts adhesions
on stretch

Microcautery cuts
adhesions as closely
as possible to the
structure

Ovary

Uterus

Tube

Round
ligament

8

Clubbed
end of the
tube

9

Forceps

Cautery

Blood
vessels

10

Microscissors..

...to open the
clubbed end
of the
Fallopian
tube

Blood
vessels

# Fimbrioplasty

## (Continued)

**11** The scarred serosal covering of the clubbed Fallopian tube has been opened, and when it is folded back, the fimbriae should prolapse out of the Fallopian tube.

**12** Irrigation with warm saline solution can be used to separate the fimbriae and identify the lumen of the ampullar portion of the Fallopian tube.

**13** With 7-0 Prolene suture on a microneedle, the scarred serosa is sutured back to the serosa of the Fallopian tube in such a manner as to free the fimbriae and keep the Fallopian tubes patent.

**14** To check the patency of the Fallopian tubes, the lower uterine segment is pinched between the thumb and first finger or held with an atraumatic clamp, and a 10-mL syringe on a 21-gauge needle is inserted through the fundus to inject 10 mL of indigo carmine into the endometrial cavity. The dye should fill the Fallopian tubes and spill from the fimbriae.

**15** Hydrotubation should be performed every other day for 2 weeks. A solution containing a broad spectrum antibiotic, cortisone, and saline is injected through the cervix with a Rubin cannula.

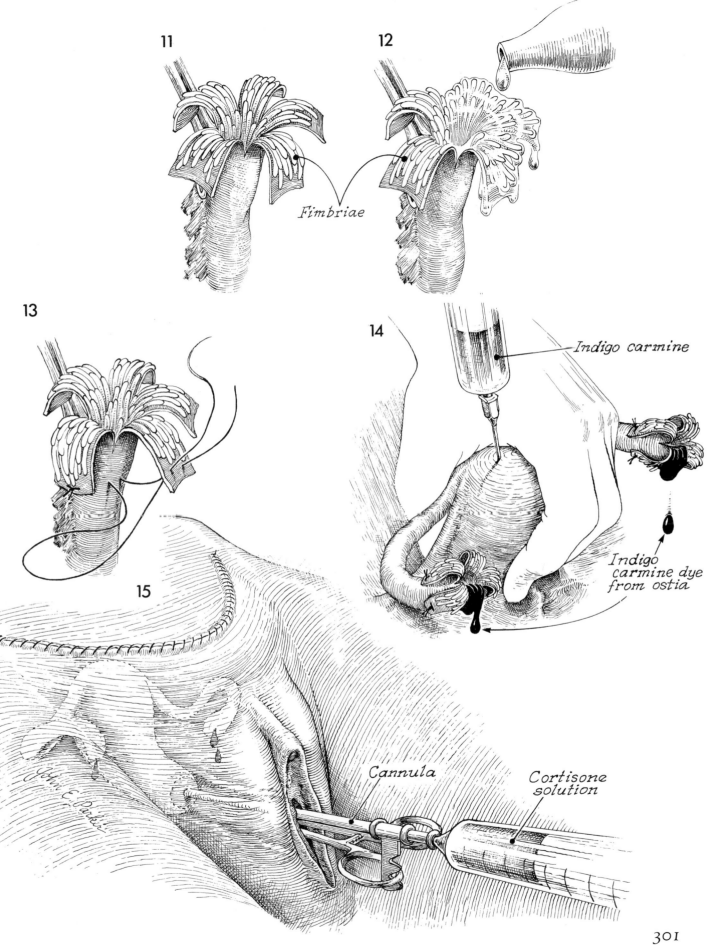

11

12

Fimbriae

13

14

Indigo carmine

Indigo carmine dye from ostia

15

Cannula

Cortisone solution

# Tuboplasty—Microresection and Anastomosis of the Fallopian Tube

Microresection and anastomosis of the Fallopian tube are indicated in those cases of infertility where tubal obstruction has been diagnosed by hysterosalpingography and confirmed by laparoscopy. In recent years, this procedure has been performed by a microtechnique, utilizing fine suture and magnification with ocular loupes or an operating microscope. If careful hemostasis and microtechniques can be used, excessive postoperative scarring and peritubular adhesions can be reduced. Scarring and stricture formation at the site of the anastomosis can also be minimized. This allows greater motility of the Fallopian tube, giving it a greater chance of receiving the oocyte, which is transported down the Fallopian tube to meet spermatozoa emerging from the proximal end of the tube.

**Physiologic Change.** The Fallopian tube is restored to its normal function.

**Points of Caution.** Meticulous hemostatic technique is essential. To ensure that a proximal portion of tube is patent, indigo carmine dye is injected via a fine-gauge spinal needle placed through the fundus into the endometrial cavity, with the lower uterine segment obstructed with a clamp.

The stent used to aid in performing the anastomosis is removed immediately after the operation.

---

## Technique

1 A double-headed operating microscope with both surgeons focusing on the intra-abdominal pelvic contents is shown. Microsurgery of the Fallopian tube requires magnification to this level. Special eyeglasses and loupes are also helpful in this technique

2 After the abdomen is entered, peritubular adhesions are totally excised, not lysed, with a microneedle cautery or fine microscissors. The uterus is elevated into an ideal operative position by packing off the cul-de-sac with wet gauze.

3 The proximal end of the scarred, distal segment of Fallopian tube is transected. A fine probe is inserted through the fimbriae and passed through the open Fallopian tube. A notch in the probe has been designed to accept a 2-0 Prolene or nylon suture.

4 The 2-0 Prolene suture is pulled through the distal segment of the Fallopian tube.

5 The proximal segment of tube is picked up and transected with microscissors.

6 The lower uterine segment is occluded with a Buxton clamp, and indigo carmine dye is injected via a 21-gauge spinal needle through the fundus into the endometrial cavity. Observation of spill from the stump indicates patency of the cornual portion of the tube.

7 A 2-0 suture is threaded through the proximal stump of Fallopian tube into the endometrial cavity where it is allowed to coil.

8 A similar procedure is performed on the opposite tube.

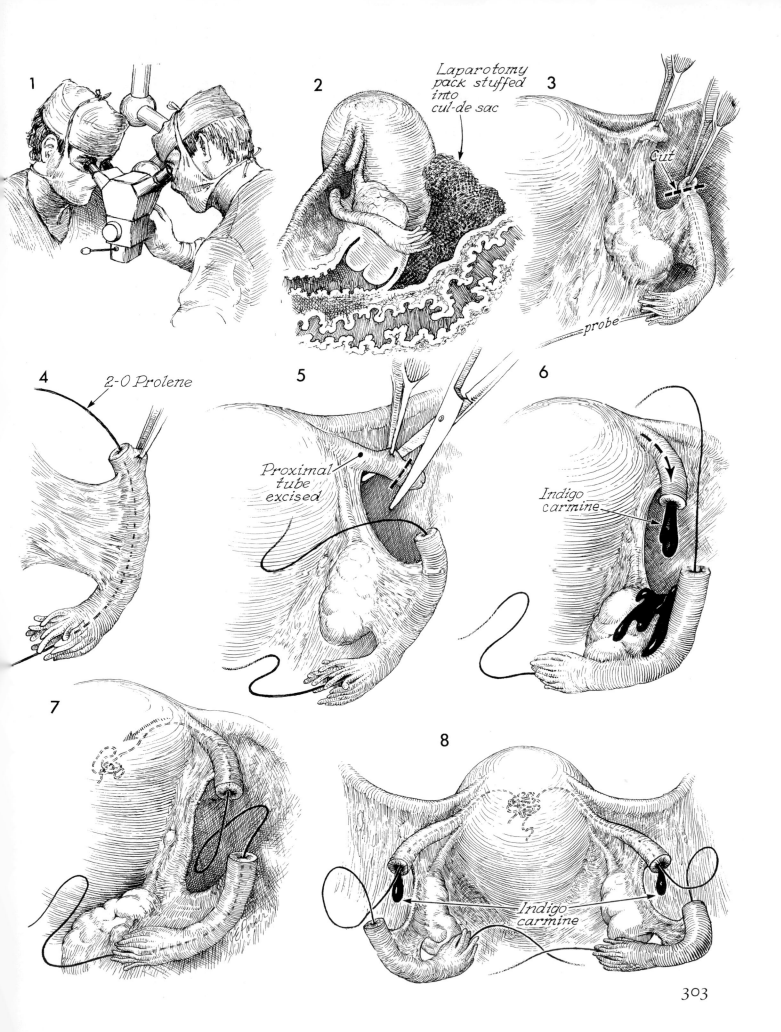

**1**

**2** *Laparotomy pack stuffed into cul-de sac*

**3** *Cut* *probe*

**4** *2-0 Prolene*

**5** *Proximal tube excised*

**6** *Indigo carmine*

**7**

**8** *Indigo carmine*

303

# Tuboplasty—Microresection and Anastomosis of the Fallopian Tube

## (Continued)

**9** The mesosalpinx of the Fallopian tubes is anastomosed with interrupted 8-0 Dexon suture via the microtechnique.

**10** After the mesosalpinx has been closed, the first layer of 8-0 Vicryl suture is placed in a north, south, east, and west position. Care is taken to place the microsuture in the submucosa layer of the tube and avoid the tubal mucosa when possible.

**11** Approximately 4 or 5 of these sutures are placed until the tube is completely closed.

**12** A second layer of 8-0 Dexon suture is placed through the serosa and outer portion of the muscle of the Fallopian tube. When tied, the tube is anastomosed in such a manner that an indigo carmine solution injected into the fundus will flow through the Fallopian tube. The same procedure is carried out on the opposite tube.

**13** In this sagittal section of the pelvis after completion of surgery, the pelvis is filled with Hiscon (low-molecular-weight dextran) to reduce adhesion formation following microsurgery by creating intra-abdominal ascites, which keeps the various tissue surfaces separated until mesothelialization is complete. *R* indicates the rectum.

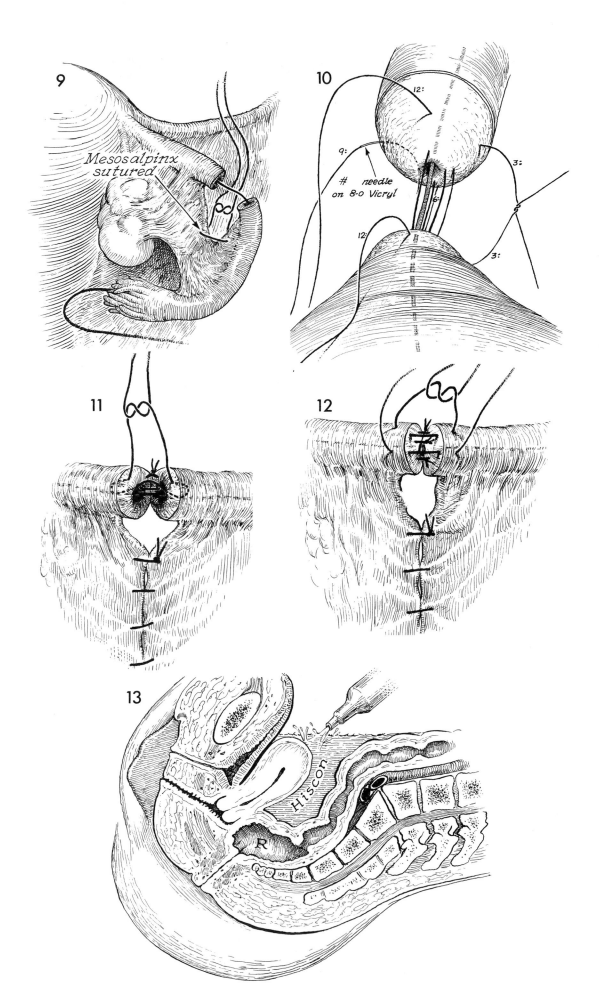

305

# Wedge Resection of the Ovary

Wedge resection of the ovary is most often performed in the treatment of polycystic ovary syndrome (Stein-Leventhal). After appropriate gynecologic and endocrinologic evaluation and after all possible medical therapy with estrogen antagonists has failed, wedge resection may be the procedure of choice to induce ovulation and regulation of menstrual periods.

**Physiologic Changes.** The precise mechanism for the induction of ovulation by wedge resection of the ovary is not known at this time. There are two possible explanations for this physiologic change: (1) the hyperplastic ovarian capsule is removed, thereby mechanically allowing ovulation, and (2) the mass of ovary is reduced, thus shifting the ratio between the level of pituitary gonadotropin and the mass of the ovary in such a way as to favor induction of ovulation.

**Points of Caution.** There are two important points of caution in this operation: (1) the control of hemorrhage from the biopsy site in the ovary and (2) the reduction in peritubular adhesion formation associated with wedge resection of the ovary. Therefore, fine meticulous technique must be utilized if peritubular adhesion formation is to be avoided.

## Technique

**1** The patient is placed in the supine position. The bladder is emptied with a Foley catheter, and a Pfannenstiel or lower midline incision is made. The abdominal cavity is entered. The uterus is retracted caudally against the pubic symphysis. The polycystic ovary should be large with a smooth oyster-like capsule.

**2** A Babcock clamp is placed on the suspensory ligament of the ovary. An additional Allis clamp may be placed on the inferior pole of the ovary to stabilize the structure so that adequate wedge resection can be performed. A scalpel is used to incise the ovary down to and including the hilum. Occasionally, a small dermoid cyst may be located in the hilum. It is also important to remove a portion of the hilum to evaluate the possibility of a hilar cell tumor that can mimic many of the signs and symptoms of Stein-Leventhal syndrome.

**3 & 4** After an adequate wedge has been taken, the ovary is closed in two layers. The first layer is closed by a running lateral mattress suture that enters the deep body of the ovary and exits through the opposite side of the ovary. The needle is reversed and reenters the body of the ovary, exiting on the opposite side. In this manner, the walls of the ovary are plicated in the midline, and dead space is eliminated.

**5** At the completion of the running mattress suture, the capsule of the ovary can be closed by continuing the fine synthetic absorbable suture through the epithelium of the ovary. Care should be taken to invert all raw edges to reduce the problem of postoperative adhesions that could have an adverse effect on future fertility. Complete hemostasis is essential if adhesions are to be avoided.

Postoperative care is similar to that for patients who have undergone pelvic laparotomy. Prophylactic antibiotics are not used.

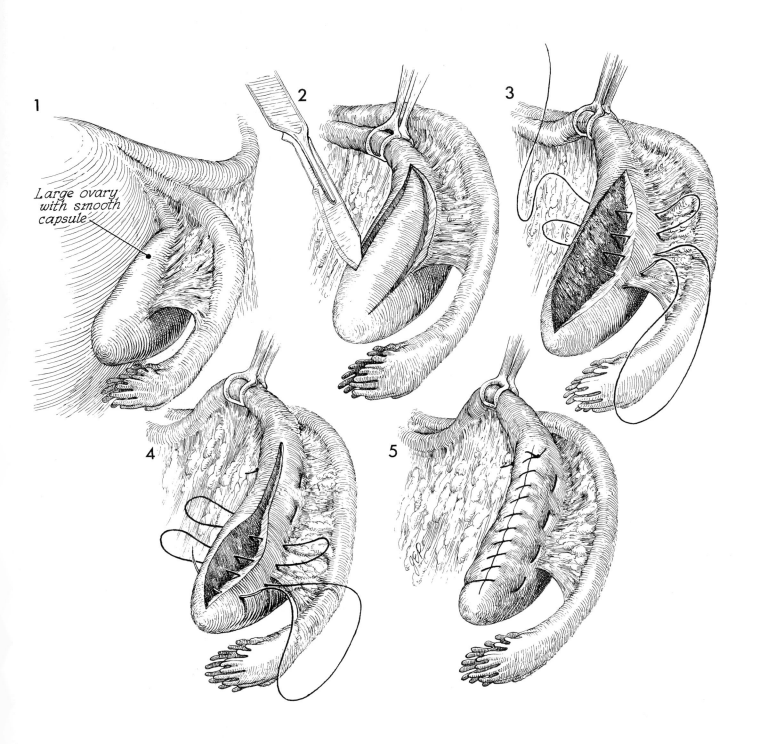

1

*Large ovary
with smooth
capsule*

2

3

4

5

307

# Torsion of Ovary

Torsion of the ovary occurs when there is some additional weight acquired by the normal ovary, usually in the form of an ovarian cyst (physiologic or pathologic). Embryologically, the ovary is a retroperitoneal structure and invaginates an envelope of peritoneum that covers it and the stalk of the ovary commonly referred to as the infundibulopelvic ligament. This arrangement allows the ovary to undergo torsion. In most cases, the torsion turns toward the midline, i.e., the right ovary twists clockwise, and the left ovary twists counterclockwise.

In the past, all such twisted ovaries were generally removed. It was accepted practice that the infundibulopelvic ligament be clamped prior to untwisting the ovary. Clamping the infundibulopelvic ligament first was said to prevent pulmonary embolism from the veins in the infundibulopelvic ligament. Very little data existed to confirm this point of view.

In younger women of the reproductive age group and those women who have completed their families but would still enjoy the benefits of a functioning ovary, salvage of this twisted ovary becomes an important issue. An ovary that has undergone torsion can be untwisted safely without pulmonary embolism. This can be done through an open laparotomy or through laparoscopy. The ovary can be safely untwisted and observed for the integrity of the vascular supply.

**Physiologic Changes.** The obvious physiologic change and the greatest threat to the ovary through torsion is loss of blood supply.

If the ovary can be salvaged, it can become a functional organ for the production of important estrogen and progesterone production as well as ovulation for those women who desire pregnancy.

**Points of Caution.** The vascular integrity of the ovary must be demonstrated prior to completing the operation. Those ovaries that have undergone gangrene should be removed. The offending ovary cyst that produced the torsion in the first place should be excised.

---

## Technique

**1** The right ovary has rotated toward the midline (clockwise).

**2** The ovary must be untwisted by hand if a laparotomy has been performed or with instruments such as grasping forceps if laparoscopy has been performed. At this point, observation should be made for vascularity of the ovary. Ovarian cystectomy should be completed at this time (see the technique for ovarian cystectomy, page 313). The performance of the ovarian cystectomy may give an excellent indication of the intact blood supply of the ovary by noting fresh arterial bleeding from the margins of the cystectomy site.

**3** If there is doubt, fluorescein dye may be injected in a peripheral vein.

**4** After 5–10 minutes, a Wood's lamp with its ultraviolet ray will cause an ovary with good blood supply to fluoresce a yellowish color. An ovary without arterial perfusion will show up as a dark purple under a Wood's lamp ultraviolet ray. These steps can assure the surgeon that the ovary has either a good vascular supply or no vascular supply. This will aid in the decision to remove the ovary or retain it.

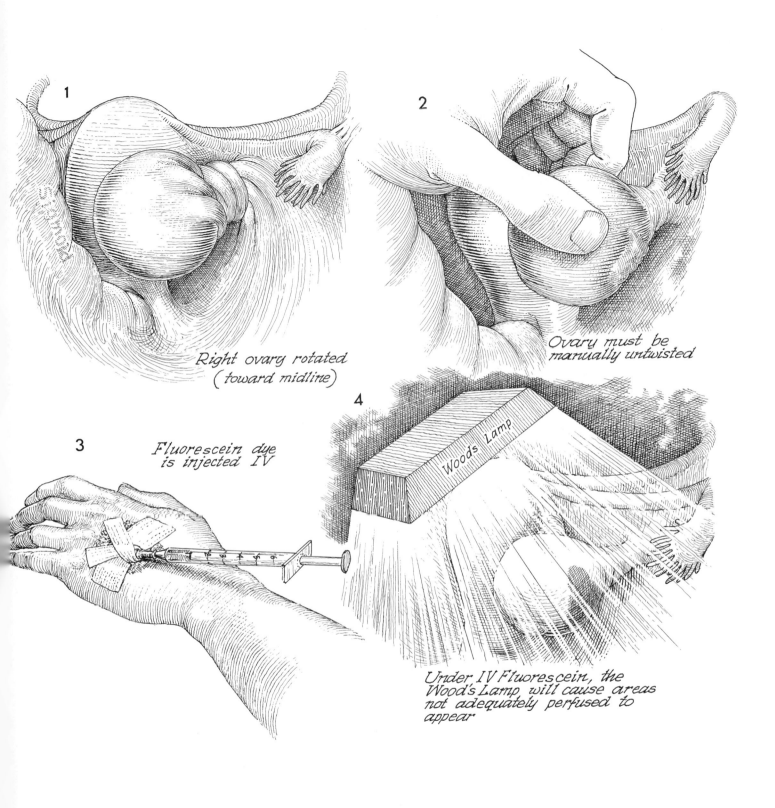

**1**

*Right ovary rotated (toward midline)*

**2**

*Ovary must be manually untwisted*

**3** *Fluorescein dye is injected IV*

**4**

Woods Lamp

*Under IV Fluorescein, the Wood's Lamp will cause areas not adequately perfused to appear*

# Ovarian Cystectomy

Ovarian cystectomy is performed in those benign conditions of the ovary in which a cyst can be removed and when it is desirable to leave a functional ovary in place. This is particularly true in women of reproductive age. Pelvic surgeons continue to be amazed at how much function remains in the smallest segment of healthy ovarian tissue. Therefore, if it is technically feasible and where one is assured that there is no malignant tissue present, it behooves those performing pelvic surgery to attempt to perform ovarian cystectomy in preference to oophorectomy, particularly in those patients who want to become pregnant.

The purpose of the operation is to excise an ovarian cyst without removing the ovary.

**Physiologic Changes.** The ovarian cyst is removed.

**Points of Caution.** The incision into the ovarian capsule must be made very carefully to prevent rupture of the cyst.

Meticulous hemostasis must be achieved to avoid ovarian hematoma. This is best performed with a running mattress suture as shown in Figures 10–12.

## Technique

**1** Patients with an adnexal mass should be placed on the operating table in the dorsal lithotomy position. A thorough examination under anesthesia is performed prior to opening the abdomen. The bladder should be emptied with a catheter. The surgeon should not be surprised to see a patient who has been referred for ovarian cyst who actually has a problem with urinary retention.

The abdomen, perineum, and vagina are surgically prepared. Although hysterectomy is rarely required, a malignancy can occasionally be encountered that will necessitate removal of the uterus. For this reason, it is best to have previously prepared the vagina with an aseptic soap solution.

**2** The patient can be changed to the supine position or to the modified dorsal lithotomy position. In general, a patient of menopausal age or above should have a lower midline incision for adnexal masses. The incidence of malignant disease is such that a lower midline incision will be required in the course of surgery, and this overrides the cosmetic advantages of a transverse incision. It is extremely difficult to adequately explore the abdomen for a malignant ovarian process through a Pfannenstiel or transverse incision. For younger patients in whom the chance of a malignant disease is quite low, a transverse or Pfannenstiel incision is acceptable. If a malignant disease is encountered in this younger age group, the transverse or Pfannenstiel incision can be closed and a midline incision can be made.

**3** A lower midline incision is made.

**4** The peritoneum is opened. The abdomen is thoroughly explored. Any suspicious tissue in the upper abdomen or along the aortic lymph nodes should be sent for a frozen section pathologic analysis.

**5** A uterine elevator or a suture is placed in the fundus of the uterus to retract it anteriorly. Bilateral cysts are shown here: the one on the left appears to be more polypoid; the one on the right appears to be involved with a significant amount of ovarian tissue.

**6** The ovary is anchored by placing Babcock clamps on the suspensory ligament of the ovary. A scalpel is used to incise the ovarian capsule near the base of the cyst.

**7** After incising the ovarian capsule with a scalpel, the surgeon uses delicate tissue forceps to elevate the capsule and small Metzenbaum scissors to dissect the alveolar tissue between the cyst and the ovarian capsule.

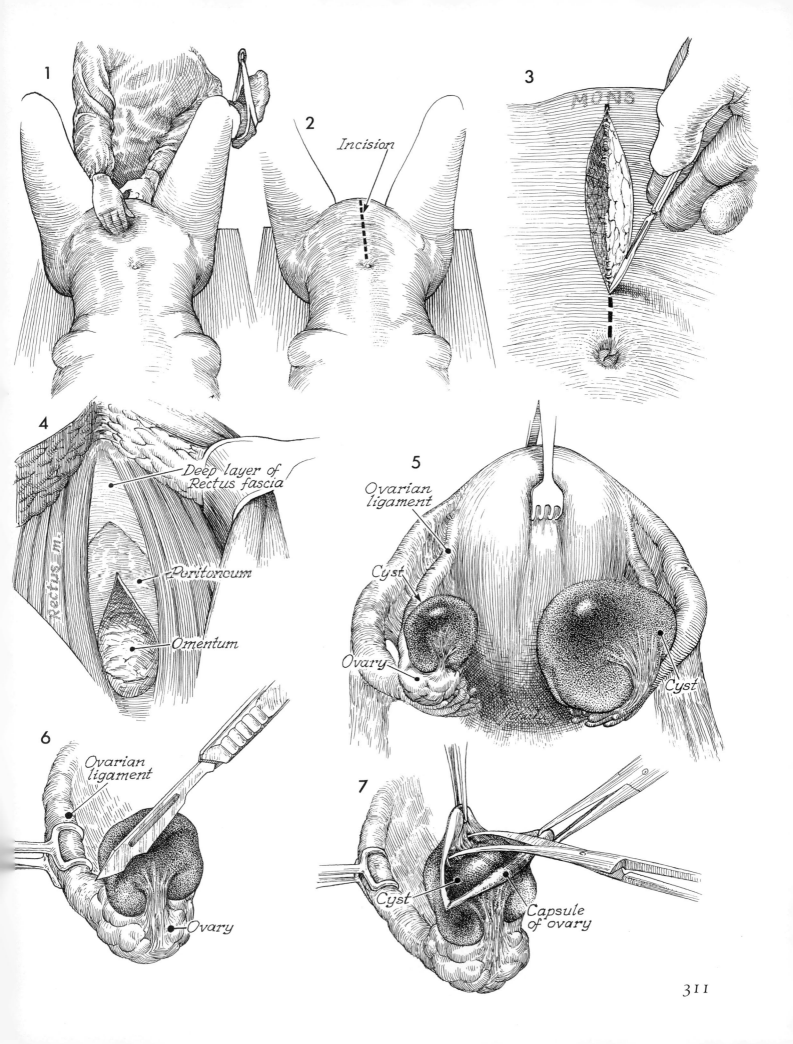

1

2

*Incision*

3

MONS

4

*Deep layer of
Rectus fascia*

*Rectus m.*

*Peritoneum*

*Omentum*

5

*Ovarian
ligament*

*Cyst*

*Ovary*

*Cyst*

6

*Ovarian
ligament*

*Ovary*

7

*Cyst*

*Capsule
of ovary*

# Ovarian Cystectomy

## (Continued)

---

**8** The margins of the ovarian capsule are held with Allis clamps. An adhesion on the cyst can be used to provide retraction, and the remaining cyst can be dissected out of the ovary with Metzenbaum scissors.

**9** The ovarian capsule and base of the ovary are shown after the cyst has been removed. Hemostasis within the bed of the ovary can be controlled by clamping and electrocoagulating small bleeders.

**10** The hemostatic running mattress suture is placed with a 3-0 synthetic absorbable suture starting at the upper pole where the suture is tied.

**11** The mattress suture of the ovary has been completed.

**12** When the lower pole of the ovary has been reached, the same suture is used to suture the edges of the ovary in a running Connell inverting suture.

**13** The completed operation is shown.

**14** Both ovarian cysts have been removed with the ovaries intact. The abdomen is closed in layers.

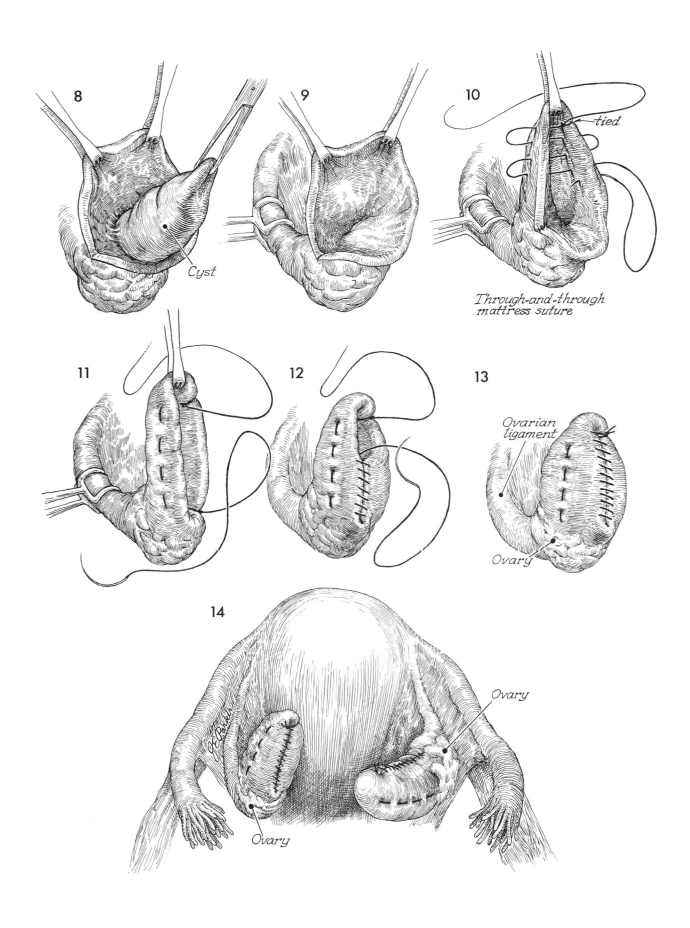

8

9

10

*tied*

*Through-and-through mattress suture*

11

12

13

*Ovarian ligament*

*Ovary*

14

*Cyst*

*Ovary*

*Ovary*

313

# Fallopian Tube Sterilization

Numerous Fallopian tube sterilization techniques are available to provide obstruction to the Fallopian tubes to prevent sperm and oocyte from fertilizing and being carried into the uterus. Obviously, with so many techniques available no one technique has satisfied all the criteria to come as close as possible to 100% effectiveness and be associated with a simple outpatient technique.

No technique has been 100% successful. In general, most techniques have had a failure rate of 4 pregnancies/1000 patients operated on. Generally, failures have occurred with two techniques: recanalization of the Fallopian tube and development of a tuboperitoneal fistula. Most failures occur within the first 2 years of surgery, although they have been reported as late as 10 years following surgery. Successful tubal reanastomosis to allow pregnancy has been directly proportional to the amount of tube destroyed. Those sterilization operations that destroy the most Fallopian tube have the least successful pregnancy rate after reanastomosis, and those techniques that have the least tubal destruction have the best pregnancy rates after reanastomosis.

**Physiologic Change.** There is little physiologic change to the patient following tubal obstruction. There has been no evidence that there is a change in sex steroid production by the ovary.

**Points of Caution.** All sterilization procedures have reported morbidity to the gastrointestinal tract and the urinary tract from entering the abdominal cavity. Very little difference can be demonstrated by one technique versus another technique.

Hemorrhage from the Fallopian tube secondary to the sterilization procedure does occur.

## Technique

1 The Pomeroy technique, introduced in 1930, involves taking a section of Fallopian tube, tying the base of the tube with a synthetic absorbable suture, and excising a knuckle of tube for pathologic confirmation that a tubal sterilization operation has been performed. It is a traditional and effective method of female sterilization. Its failure rate is in the range of 4/1000, and most failures probably occur through recanalization of the tube.

2 The Kroner operation, introduced in 1935, removes the fimbriae from the Fallopian tube. The stump of the ampullar portion of the Fallopian tube is tied, and the fimbriae are removed.

3 Hulka clip sterilization, introduced in 1972, involves the placing of a locking Silastic metallic clip across the Fallopian tube. This technique is least destructive of the Fallopian tube and gives the best results for reanastomosis if the patient changes her mind. It is an ideal technique in very young women desiring female sterilization, should they have a change in their marital status and/or a change in their attitude toward further fertility.

4 In 1970, the technique of laparoscopic electrocoagulation was popularized. Various modifications to the technique have been made, e.g., bipolar, unipolar, but there have been few differences in results. The salient feature of this technique is that it provides thorough coagulation of the tube so that a section of evulsed tube will not have bleeding from the proximal or distal end of the remaining tube nor from the bed of the mesosalpinx.

5 The Falope ring, introduced by In-Bae Yoon, M.D. in 1974, is a simple, inexpensive technique in which a Silastic band is placed around a knuckle of Fallopian tube. The knuckle is not excised as in the Pomeroy technique. The Silastic band stays in place and creates the obstruction.

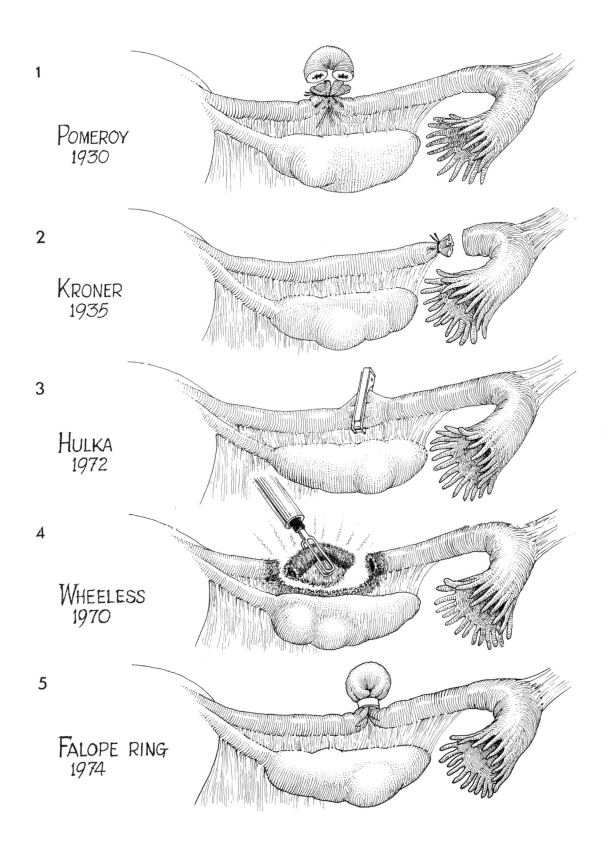

1

POMEROY
1930

2

KRONER
1935

3

HULKA
1972

4

WHEELESS
1970

5

FALOPE RING
1974

# 7
## Colon

# Appendectomy Using the Linear Dissecting Stapler

Incidental appendectomy is frequently performed in association with other pelvic surgical procedures. It must be performed when there is clinical evidence of acute appendicitis.

The purpose of the operation is to remove the appendix prior to rupture in cases of acute appendicitis or where the appendix interferes with another operation, such as a right-colon continent urostomy.

**Physiologic Changes.** Although the appendix may be associated with the immune response, its exact function remains unclear. Generally, no obvious clinical physiologic change can be demonstrated after its removal.

**Points of Caution.** Hemostasis and aseptic removal of the appendix are keys to the success of this operation. Although the appendiceal stump has been inverted in some clinics, there are excellent studies showing no apparent sequelae from not inverting the stump.

## Technique

**1** A laparotomy is performed through a McBurney or a lower midline incision. If the diagnosis is uncertain and pelvic inflammatory disease is a possibility, the incision should be a lower midline rather than a McBurney incision.

Identification of the teniae coli on the cecum facilitates location of the appendix, which may be retrocecal. The appendix should be placed on traction. Adhesions in the area of the appendix are lysed with Metzenbaum scissors.

**2** The mesoappendix is identified, and small hemostat clamps are used to open avascular sections in the mesoappendix between blood vessels. The LDS (linear dissecting) stapler (United States Surgical Corp.) is used to simultaneously staple and transect these blood vessels.

**3** Figure 3 shows enlargement of the LDS placed on a blood vessel in the mesoappendix.

**4** The appendix is transected with the LDS.

**5** The completed operation shows the stapled appendiceal stump. Care should be taken to inspect the vascular staples on the mesoappendix blood vessels for bleeding.

The area should be irrigated with normal saline solution prior to closure of the abdominal wall. No drain is used.

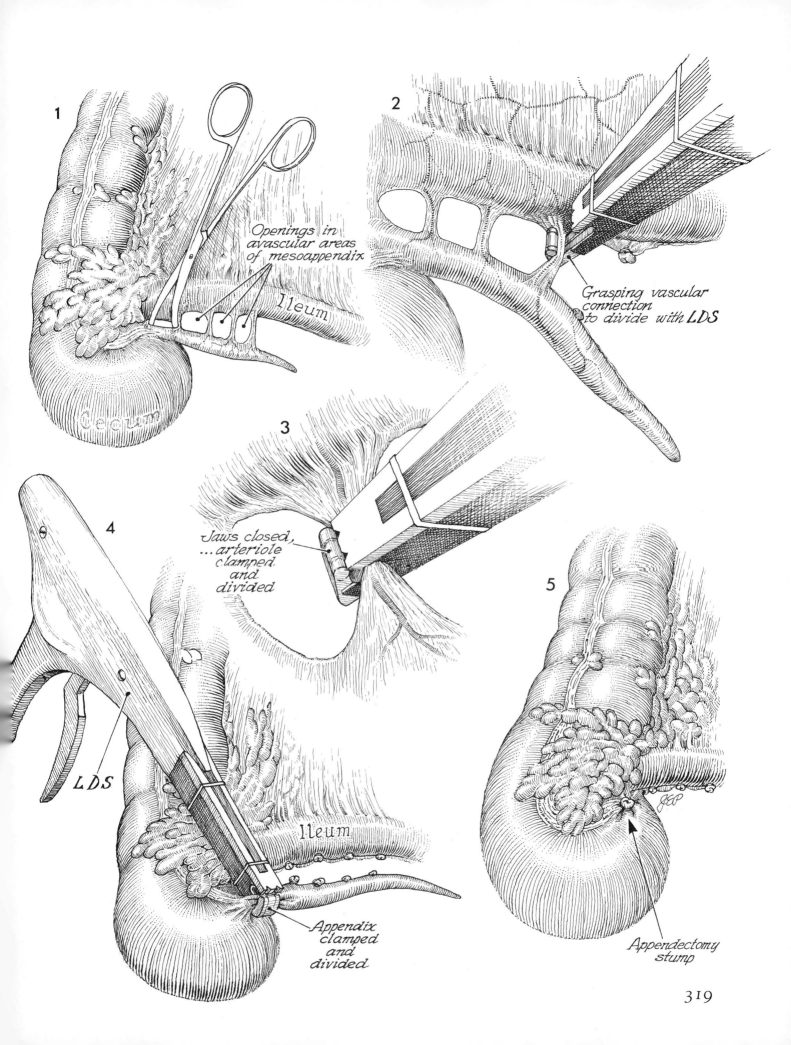

**1**

*Openings in avascular areas of mesoappendix*

*Ileum*

*Cecum*

**2**

*Grasping vascular connection to divide with LDS*

**3**

*Jaws closed, ...arteriole clamped and divided*

**4**

*LDS*

*Ileum*

*Appendix clamped and divided*

**5**

*Appendectomy stump*

319

# Transverse Loop Colostomy

Transverse loop colostomy is a simple, fast, and relatively easy procedure used for those patients with pelvic disease in whom a temporary fecal diversion is needed and who are not candidates for an end sigmoid colostomy because of medical or technical reasons.

In general, transverse colostomies related to gynecologic malignancies should be performed on the left rather than the right transverse colon. A left transverse colostomy has the advantage of additional length of colon for fecal fluid absorption and allows the right transverse colon to remain available for small bowel bypass if needed in the future.

The purpose of the transverse loop colostomy is to divert the fecal stream.

**Physiologic Changes.** The fecal stream is diverted. Stool from the transverse colostomy will contain a larger volume of water than stool from a sigmoid colostomy. Therefore, a transverse colostomy may be more difficult to regulate.

**Points of Caution.** The incision for the colostomy should be well designed. The site for the stoma should be marked the night before surgery while the patient is in the standing position so that the stoma for the colostomy is not on the underside of the abdominal panniculus. The stoma site should be selected so as not to interfere with the waistline of clothing. The incision should be long enough to ensure adequate exposure of the bowel.

The three anatomic characteristics of the colon should be identified prior to performing the operation: the teniae coli, haustral markings, and the colonic relationship to the omentum. Closure of the abdominal wall around the colostomy should be tight enough to prevent hernia but should allow enough space to prevent strangulation and ischemia of the colonic loop.

## Technique

**1** The patient is placed in the dorsal position. A transverse incision is made left of the midline and approximately 6 cm above the umbilicus.

**2** The colon is identified by the three anatomic characteristics: haustral markings, teniae coli, and omentum. A Metzenbaum scissors is used to lyse the fine filmy adhesions of the omentum for a distance of 8–10 cm.

**3** The colon is rotated, and the posterior leaf of the omentum is likewise dissected from the surface of the bowel. This leaves a defect in the omentum.

**4** The defect in the omentum is seen with the colon lying underneath. The mesocolon with its vessels is identified.

**5** An avascular portion of the mesocolon is opened for a distance of approximately 3 cm. This is performed by placing the index finger of one hand under the colon and tenting up the avascular portion of the mesocolon.

**6** The index finger of one hand is inserted through the opening in the mesocolon. The colon is elevated through the defect in the omentum. A rod is passed through the mesocolon. The omentum acts as a seal around the colon to reduce spillage into the peritoneal cavity when the colon is opened.

**7** The colon is brought through the incision in the abdominal wall. If a large incision was needed to perform the procedure, a portion of the abdominal wall including the skin is closed with interrupted sutures. The wound is left open 1 finger width to ensure against strangulation. A rubber hose is connected to each end of the glass rod, or the rod is attached to the ring of a contemporary colostomy bag. The colon is ventilated by opening the anterior colonic wall in the longitudinal plane if the bowel has been prepared before surgery. The colostomy should be sutured with a 3-0 synthetic absorbable "rosebud" stitch.

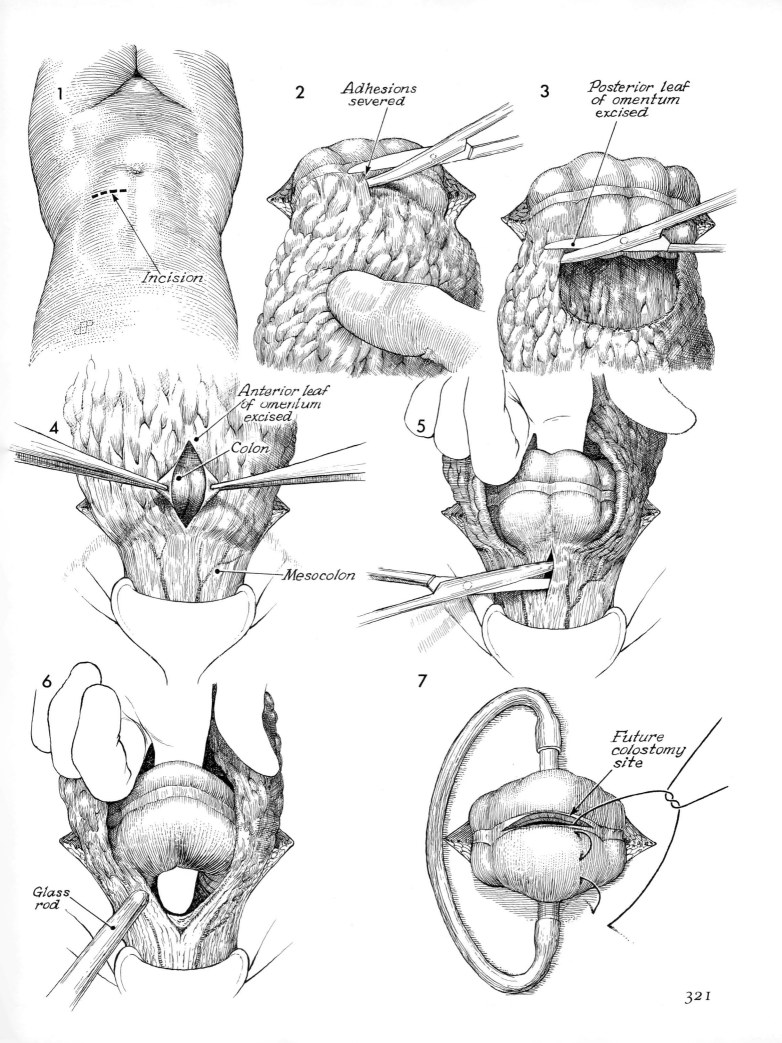

**1** Incision

**2** Adhesions severed

**3** Posterior leaf of omentum excised

**4** Anterior leaf of omentum excised
Colon
Mesocolon

**5**

**6** Glass rod

**7** Future colostomy site

# End Sigmoid Colostomy With Hartmann's Pouch

End sigmoid colostomy with a Hartmann's pouch is the procedure of choice when permanent fecal diversion is required. In some clinics, the distal portion of the rectosigmoid colon is exteriorized as a mucous fistula in lieu of a Hartmann's pouch. The need for this in colonic problems related to gynecologic oncology is rare.

**Physiologic Changes.** In this operation, the fecal stream is diverted from the rectum and anus. Compared with transverse colostomy, end sigmoid colostomy gives additional length to the colon for absorption of fecal fluid. Therefore, the stool is similar to that passed per anum. End sigmoid colostomy offers an opportunity for colostomy regulation that is generally not available in transverse colostomies. A single stoma improves the fit of the colostomy bag and reduces skin excoriation.

**Points of Caution.** An adequate incision is needed to identify, mobilize, and open the mesentery of the sigmoid colon. The incision should be selected to fit the needs of the individual patient, ensuring proper placement of the colostomy stoma. The stoma should not be placed in the patient's waistline, where clothing will interfere with it, and should never be placed on the underside of a large abdominal panniculus in obese patients. Several sutures placed from the serosal surface of the bowel to the peritoneum will reduce herniation and prolapse of the colon through the stoma.

---

## Technique

**1** The patient is placed in the supine position. The abdomen is opened through a left paramedian or midline incision. The sigmoid colon is identified, mobilized, and elevated. The site for transection of the bowel is made on consideration of the pathologic diagnosis. The mesentery is opened for approximately 8 cm. Often, the superior hemorrhoidal branch of the inferior mesenteric artery must be clamped and divided, but the inferior mesenteric artery itself is generally preserved. The gastrointestinal anastomosis (GIA) autosuture stapler is placed across the colon and activated.

**2** With the GIA stapler, the proximal end of the distal segment of the colon (Hartmann's pouch) is adequately closed. No further surgery to this segment is needed.

**3** The appropriate site for the colostomy stoma has been marked on the patient's abdomen with indelible ink prior to surgery. An Allis clamp is placed on the skin at this site and elevated.

**4** While the skin is held on traction, a knife is used to remove a disc of skin and subcutaneous tissue of appropriate diameter.

**5** The skin disc has been removed.

**6** The subcutaneous fat is elevated with an Allis clamp.

**7** With the fat elevated, a knife is used to remove the remaining fatty tissue, exposing the rectus fascia.

**8** The rectus fascia is exposed.

**9** The rectus fascia is elevated with an Allis clamp. A knife is used to remove a disc of rectus fascia 4 cm in diameter.

**10** A large Kelly clamp is inserted through the peritoneum, bluntly penetrating the fibers of the rectus muscle. This incision is expanded with the Kelly clamp and fingers until two fingers (4 cm) traverse the defect from the skin to peritoneum without difficulty.

**11** A Babcock clamp is inserted through the abdominal wall defect. The distal segment of the descending colon is grasped.

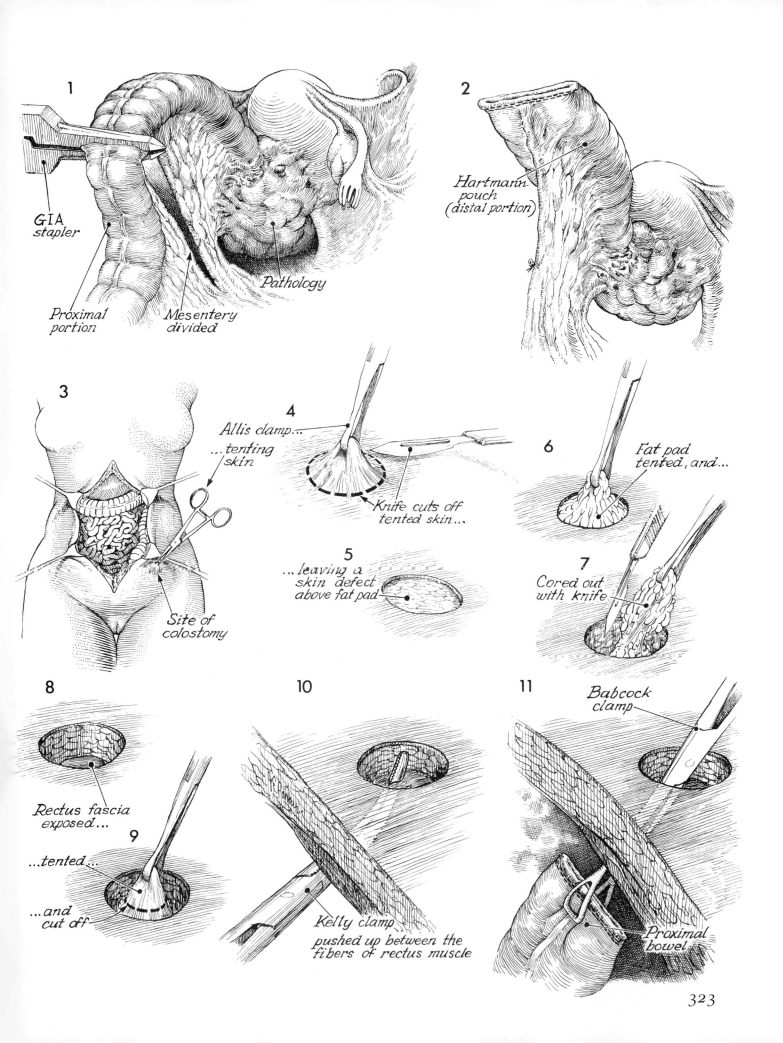

1

GIA stapler

Proximal portion

Mesentery divided

Pathology

2

Hartmann pouch (distal portion)

3

...tenting skin

Site of colostomy

4

Allis clamp...

Knife cuts off tented skin...

5

...leaving a skin defect above fat pad

6

Fat pad tented, and...

7

Cored out with knife...

8

Rectus fascia exposed...

9

...tented...

...and cut off

10

Kelly clamp pushed up between the fibers of rectus muscle

11

Babcock clamp

Proximal bowel

323

# End Sigmoid Colostomy With Hartmann's Pouch

## (Continued)

**12** This distal segment of the descending colon is pulled through the defect for a distance of approximately 7 cm. Excess fatty tissue on the mesenteric side of the colon is clamped and tied up to but not exceeding 3 cm.

**13** The excess fatty tissue is removed. The blood supply of the colon is such that up to 5 cm of colon can be nourished from the point of ligation of vessels in the mesentery. Colon in excess of this amount may become ischemic and necrose.

**14** The stapled end of the proximal colon is elevated with a forceps and resected with curved Mayo scissors.

**15** A "rosebud" stitch is utilized to evert the colon onto the skin, thereby elevating it off the skin edge by 1½ cm. Elevating the stoma protects the skin from fecal spillage. The stitch is started on the surface of the skin 1 cm from the edge, goes through the epidermis and dermis, is passed through the serosa and muscularis of the bowel wall, and then traverses the edge of the bowel.

**16** When tied, the stoma is inverted and raised off the level of the skin.

**17** The mesentery of the large bowel is sutured or stapled to the peritoneum to prevent internal hernia.

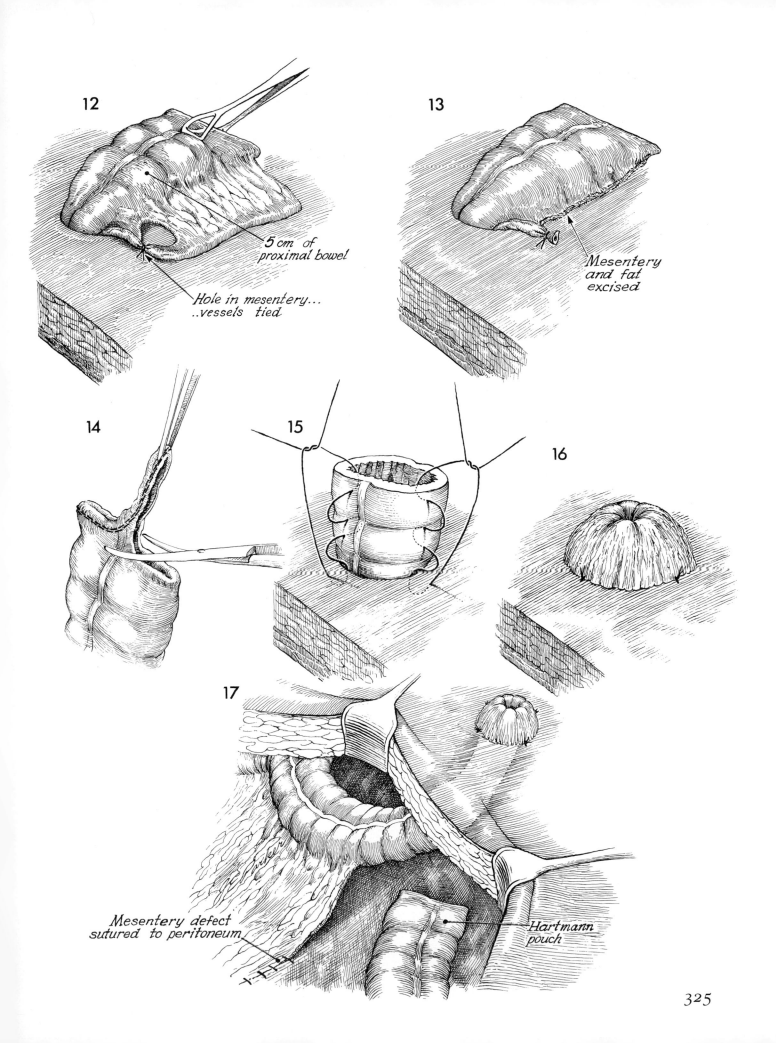

**12**

5 cm of
proximal bowel

Hole in mesentery...
...vessels tied

**13**

Mesentery
and fat
excised

**14**

**15**

**16**

**17**

Mesentery defect
sutured to peritoneum

Hartmann
pouch

# Closure of a Loop Colostomy

Closure of a loop colostomy is facilitated if the posterior wall of the colon has not been transected. If it has been transected, a classical colocolostomy is required.

The purpose of this operation is to close the colostomy and reestablish continuity of the colon without stricture at the site of the anastomosis.

**Physiologic Changes.** After this procedure, the patient may resume defecation per anum. In addition, the patient will receive more nutritive value from food because the additional colonic surface will allow greater absorption of water and nutrients from the intestinal contents.

**Points of Caution.** Care must be taken to prevent stenosis at the anastomotic site. If the diameter of the anastomosis is less than 2 cm, the anastomosis should be taken down and resected. A classic end-to-end anastomosis should then be performed to ensure adequate diameter to the intestine. If the posterior wall of the colon has been preserved, care should be taken to close the colostomy prior to opening the peritoneal cavity. This will reduce intraperitoneal contamination from the stoma site.

Copious irrigation of the wound should be made prior to primary closure. If gross contamination has occurred, delayed closure of the wound should be considered.

## Technique

1 The patient should have a thorough surgical bowel prep prior to closure of the colostomy. This should consist of a clear liquid diet, a nonabsorbable antibiotic (such as neomycin and Sulfathalidine), and a thorough mechanical cleansing of the bowel.

The patient is placed in the supine position, and adequate anesthesia is administered. The abdomen is surgically prepared, and an elliptical incision is made in the skin approximately 2 cm from the margin of the colostomy stoma. This incision is carried down to the rectus fascia, but no farther.

2 After the incision has been made, Allis clamps are applied to the ends of the elliptical incision, and traction is applied upward. A sharp Metzenbaum scissors is used to trim excessive skin away from the margin of the bowel. Adhesions between the serosal surface of the bowel and rectus fascia are lysed by sharp dissection.

3 The bowel has been prepared for a Gambee single-layer through-and-through anastomosis. Synthetic absorbable sutures are placed through the wall of the bowel, starting on the mucosa, exiting through the serosa, reentering the serosa on the opposite side, and exiting through the mucosa of the opposite side. Thus the knot will be tied in the lumen of the bowel (see page 331).

4 The Gambee anastomosis is near its completion with an inverting suture technique.

5 When the Gambee anastomosis has been completed, several Lembert sutures are placed north (N), east (E), and west (W) to relieve tension on the suture line and improve wound healing.

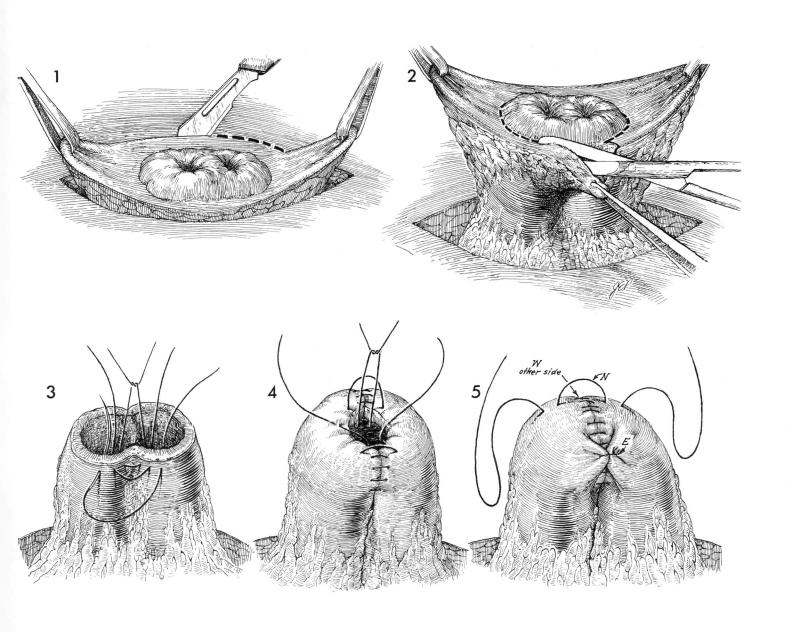

# Closure of a Loop Colostomy

## (Continued)

**6** After the anastomosis is completed, the peritoneum is entered, and adhesions are dissected with Metzenbaum scissors.

**7** The rectus fascia has been closed with synthetic delayed absorbable suture. A Hemovac suction drain is placed above the closure of the fascia and below the subcutaneous tissue.

**8** The skin is closed with stainless steel clips. Note the suction drain ghosted under the closure. This is removed in 24–36 hours.

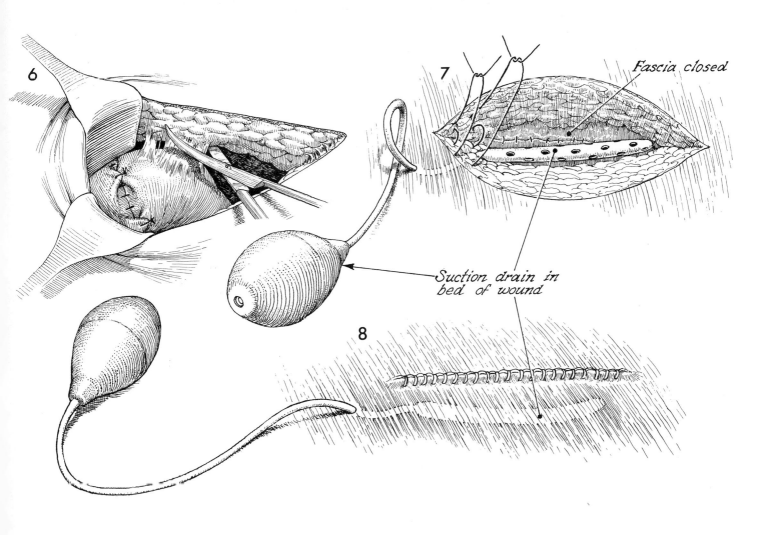

6

7    *Fascia closed*

Suction drain in
bed of wound

8

329

# Anterior Resection of the Colon With Low Anastomosis Using the Gambee Suture Technique

The purpose of this operation is to resect the rectosigmoid colon and reanastomose the descending colon to the rectum by utilizing the Gambee single-layer suture technique.

**Physiologic Changes.** The physiologic changes associated with removal of the rectosigmoid colon are minimal.

If the patient has had total pelvic irradiation, a low anastomosis should be protected by a temporary diverting colostomy for 8–10 weeks. If there has been no pelvic irradiation and an adequate preoperative bowel preparation has been performed, however, a diverting colostomy may not be required.

**Points of Caution.** Adequate mobilization of the descending colon, even if this means mobilizing the splenic flexure and transverse colon, must be made in order that the descending colon will reach the rectum without tension. Anastomoses performed under tension do not heal well.

## Technique

**1** Two positions may be used for this operation. First, if a simple anterior resection with low anastomosis of the rectosigmoid colon is to be performed and 10–12 cm of rectum are to be preserved, the patient can be operated on in the supine position. If there is a chance that the rectum may require transection below 10 cm, however, the patient should be operated on in the modified dorsal lithotomy position, exposing the perineum for anastomosis using an EEA (end-to-end anastomosis) stapler.

The abdomen, vagina, and perineum should be surgically prepped prior to the procedure, and a Foley catheter should be placed in the bladder. The abdomen should be opened through a left paramedian or midline incision.

**2** The diseased portion of the rectosigmoid colon has been identified, and the appropriate segment of colon has been selected for resection. Two linen-shod clamps are placed at each end of the section designated. The surgeon clamps the colonic vessels by opening small holes in the mesentery. If possible, the left colonic branch of the inferior mesenteric artery is preserved. The remaining portion of the mesentery is transected with scissors. The colonic segment and its mesentery are removed.

**3** After the descending colon has been sufficiently mobilized to allow approximation to the rectum without tension, a stabilizing 3-0 synthetic absorbable suture is placed at the mesenteric border (S) with a Lembert stitch.

**4** A Gambee through-and-through single-layer anastomosis is begun with interrupted 3-0 synthetic absorbable sutures. The needle is passed through the walls of the rectum and descending colon, and each knot is tied on the inside of the lumen (see Section 8, page 351).

**5 & 6** The anastomosis is continued left and right around the circumference of the lumen.

**7** The last sutures in the antimesenteric border of the bowel should be placed using a near-far inverting stitch as demonstrated in Section 8, page 351, Figure 15.

**8** A few Lembert 3-0 synthetic absorbable sutures are placed around the anastomosis to relieve tension.

**9** The anastomosis, completed with Lembert tension-relieving sutures placed east (E), north (N), and west (W) around the bowel, is shown.

Where the vaginal cuff has been reefed following a hysterectomy is a convenient site for insertion of a closed suction drain.

A Salem pump nasogastric tube is placed in the stomach and connected to low suction until bowel function is established.

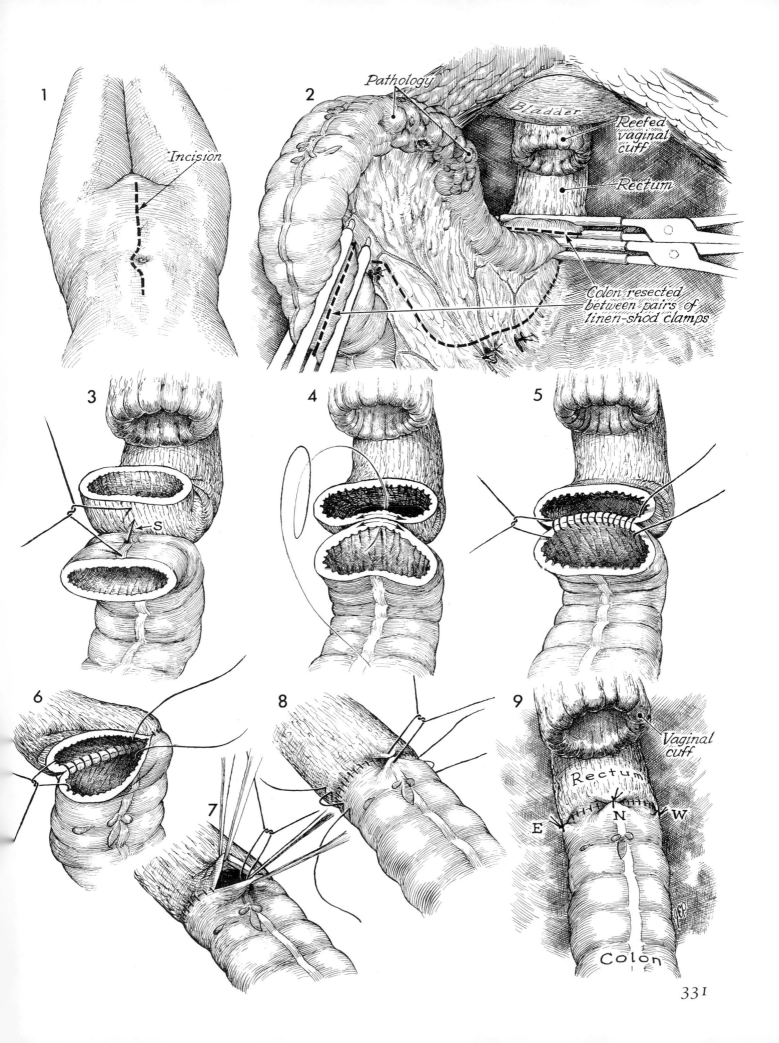

1

Incision

2

Pathology

Bladder

Reefed
vaginal
cuff

Rectum

Colon resected
between pairs of
linen-shod clamps

3

S

4

5

6

7

8

9

Vaginal
cuff

Rectum

E

N

W

Colon

331

# Low Anastomosis of Colon to Rectum Using the End-to-End Surgical Stapler Technique

There are two techniques for low anastomosis of colon to rectum: the suture technique and the EEA (end-to-end anastomosis) stapler technique.

The EEA stapler technique has allowed very low anastomoses to be performed that were previously thought to be extremely difficult with suture. Suture anastomoses below 7 cm have been associated with a high incidence of anastomotic leaks. The stapler technique offers a clean, vascular, and safe method for very low anastomoses of colon to rectum with a resultant fecal incontinence rate of less than 5% and anastomotic leak rate of less than 7%.

In gynecologic oncology, it is wise to protect these very low anastomoses with a proximal colostomy if the patient (1) has previously been irradiated, (2) has significant diverticular disease, or (3) has had no bowel preparation.

The purpose of the operation is to establish continuity of the colon and rectum.

**Physiologic Changes.** The low anastomosis performed with the EEA surgical stapler has a superior blood supply. It is associated with less tissue trauma and has a lower incidence of leaks from the anastomosis. Therefore, we feel it is a superior anastomosis, particularly in scarred ischemic bowel following irradiation therapy to the pelvis.

**Points of Caution.** Adequate mobilization of the descending colon must be made. Frequently, the splenocolic ligament must be transected and the transverse colon must be adequately mobilized to ensure that there is no tension on the anastomosis. If complete mobilization requires sacrificing the inferior mesenteric artery, extreme care must be taken to ensure that the blood supply from the middle colic artery is intact along with the marginal artery of the colon.

Care must be taken in placing the pursestring sutures. They should not be placed more than 0.5 cm from the margin of the bowel. Otherwise, too much tissue will be gathered into the anvil and jam the stapling mechanism of the EEA stapler. This will result in a defective anastomosis. The size of the EEA stapler must be carefully selected to conform with the diameter of the colon and rectum. Forcing a stapler that is too large will only split the colon and result in ischemia and necrosis.

After the EEA stapler has been fired and before the stapler is removed, it may be efficacious to place interrupted Lembert sutures with synthetic absorbable material north, south, and west around the stapled bowel to relieve tension on the staple suture line and improve wound healing.

The last step in the operation involves three tests: inspection of the anastomosis, observation of the "O" rings from the stapler, and the "bubble test." The last of these, the so-called "bubble test," is of maximum importance. Most anastomotic leaks can be diagnosed at the time of surgery, and therefore, the surgeon should not wait until the fifth to seventh postoperative day to learn that the anastomosis is leaking.

# Low Anastomosis of Colon to Rectum Using the End-to-End Surgical Stapler Technique

## (Continued)

*Technique*

**1** In this view into the pelvis after anterior resection of the colon and complete hysterectomy have been performed, the vaginal cuff can be seen to be reefed with absorbable suture. The rectal stump is shown at the level of the levator ani muscles. The descending colon has been closed with the automatic surgical stapler.

**2** In this sagittal section of the female pelvis following removal of the uterus and lower rectosigmoid colon, note that the vaginal vault has been reefed with interrupted absorbable sutures. The EEA stapler is in position to be inserted through the anus. The rectal stump has a pursestring suture of 2-0 nylon in place. The descending colon is noted at the pelvic brim. *B* indicates bladder; and *Symph*, pubic symphysis.

**3** Mobilization of the descending colon is illustrated. The peritoneum in the left lateral gutter has been incised up to the splenocolic ligament. The splenocolic ligament has been clamped and divided. When the colon can be placed into the pelvis adjacent to the rectal stump without tension, mobilization will be considered complete. Note the identification of the left ureter, which must be kept in view at all times. At the top, the EEA stapler has been placed through the rectal stump. The pursestring suture has been tied around the central rod, and the anvil of the stapler has been opened. Allis clamps are used to guide the descending colon over the anvil.

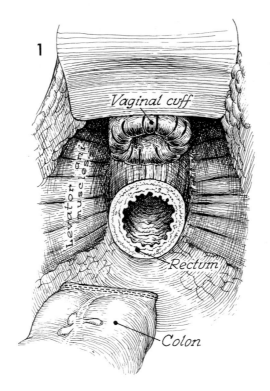

1

Vaginal cuff

Levator ani muscle est

Rectum

Colon

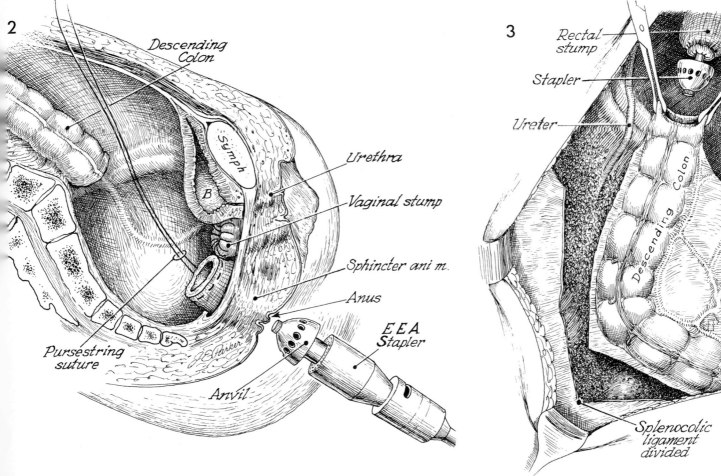

2

Descending Colon

Symph

B

Urethra

Vaginal stump

Sphincter ani m.

Anus

E E A Stapler

Pursestring suture

J.E.Parker

Anvil

3

Rectal stump

Stapler

Ureter

Descending Colon

Splenocolic ligament divided

# Low Anastomosis of Colon to Rectum Using the End-to-End Surgical Stapler Technique

## (Continued)

**4** A pelvic view shows the vaginal cuff reefed with synthetic absorbable suture. A pursestring suture has been placed in the rectal stump and tied around the central rod of the EEA stapler. The anvil of the stapler has been advanced, and the descending colon has been mobilized from above. At this point, the descending colon contains two rows of surgical staples that prevent spillage of its contents into the wound.

**5** In this view, a 2-0 nylon suture on a Keith needle passes through the eye of the special pursestring-applying clamp on the opposite side; the suture exits at the heel of the clamp, reenters the eye on the proximal side, and exits the eye at the toe of the clamp. Thus, a pursestring suture is placed 3 mm from the margin of the *dotted line* for transecting the descending colon. The colon is now transected beneath the double row of stainless steel surgical staplers at the level of the *dotted line*.

**6** The lumen of the descending colon is held open with Allis clamps. The anvil of the EEA stapler is inserted through the open lumen. Note the pursestring on the left side of the colon.

**7** The pursestring suture is tied around the central rod. By closing the wing nut on the handle of the automatic surgical stapler, the surgeon mechanically approximates the two ends of bowel.

**8** When the mechanical approximation of the two ends of bowel is satisfactorily completed, four synthetic absorbable Lembert sutures are placed north, east *(E)*, south *(S)*, and west *(W)* to relieve tension on the suture line and to give added support to the anastomosis.

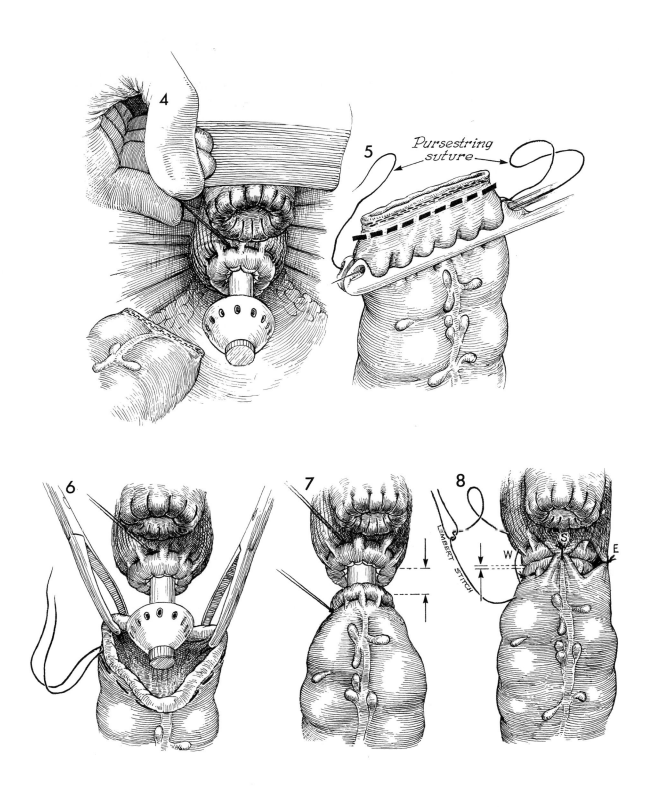

Pursestring suture

LEMBERT STITCH

S    E
W

337

# Low Anastomosis of Colon to Rectum Using the End-to-End Surgical Stapler Technique

## (Continued)

**9** In this sagittal section showing the approximated rectum and colon, the EEA stapler is loaded with a double row of staples that have passed through the inverted margins of the intestine. At the same time, the circular scalpel within the stapler cuts away excessive inverted bowel.

The surgeon reopens the stapler by turning the wing nut on the handle. The stapler is slowly brought through the fresh anastomosis with a twisting motion and is removed from the patient.

**10** If adequate omentum is available, a J flap is made and brought into the pelvis to cover the anastomosis (see Section 10, page 399).

**11** In this sagittal section of the pelvis after the EEA stapler anastomosis has been completed, the pelvic cavity is filled with sterile saline solution **(a),** and a sterile sigmoidoscope is advanced through the anus up to the level of the anastomosis **(b).** The entire anastomosis is observed. If points of hemorrhage are noted, they are coagulated. If defects are present, they are noted. A small volume of air is pumped into the rectum. The stapled anastomosis should be airtight. If there is a defect, bubbles will rise to the surface of the saline solution and can be observed by the surgeon. The EEA stapler is dismantled, and the two pieces of bowel, rectum and colon **(c),** are removed from the stapling device. In all cases they should be complete circles. If they are not complete circles, a defect in the anastomosis is indicated, and the anastomosis should be taken down and repeated, or the defect should be appropriately closed with suture.

**12** In cases where the pelvis has been previously irradiated, a protective diverting transverse loop colostomy is performed at a convenient location.

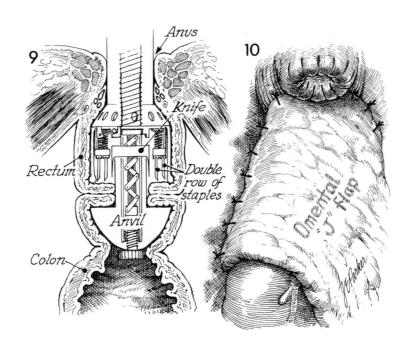

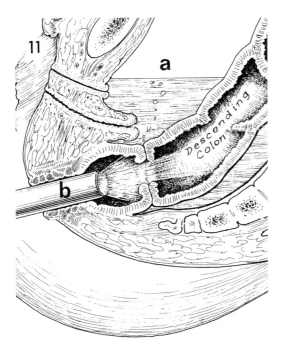

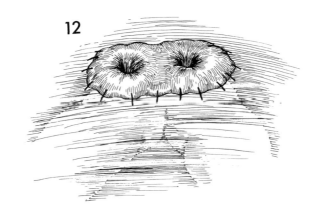

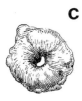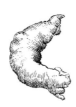

# Anterior Resection of the Colon With Low Anastomosis via the Strasbourg-Baker Technique

The Strasbourg-Baker technique allows side-to-end anastomosis of the sigmoid colon to the rectal stump without sacrificing the inferior mesenteric artery. It also usually allows preservation of the superior hemorrhoidal artery. It can be performed with the suture technique or the new EEA (end-to-end anastomosis) stapler.

When the blood supply to the proximal colon has been compromised from pelvic irradiation or inflammatory disease of the bowel, the anastomosis between the colon and rectum may be compromised by inadequate blood supply. In this procedure, it is important that the sigmoid colon be of sufficient length to perform the anastomosis without sacrificing the superior hemorrhoidal branch of the inferior mesenteric artery. If both these arteries are sacrificed, the blood supply for the descending and sigmoid colon becomes dependent on the middle colic artery and the integrity of the marginal artery of the colon; and if the marginal artery has been compromised through inflammation or radiation, a portion of the sigmoid colon may become ischemic.

**Points of Caution.** Adequate mobilization of the descending colon must be achieved to prevent tension on the anastomosis. Occasionally, the terminal branch of the superior hemorrhoidal artery may have to be sacrificed to accomplish this. Care should be taken to retain as many of the sigmoid artery branches of the inferior mesenteric artery as possible to improve the blood supply to the terminal colon and the anastomosis.

After achieving anastomosis with the EEA stapler, the surgeon should perform the three standard tests that confirm that an anastomosis is without defects: (1) the sterile sigmoidoscope should be inserted through the anus, and the anastomosis should be thoroughly inspected by visualization; (2) a small amount of air should be pumped into the rectum, and the pelvis should be filled with sterile saline solution—a stream of bubbles from the anastomosis indicates a defect; and (3) the two intact concentric rings of bowel retrieved from the anvil of the EEA stapler should be observed.

In resecting the excessive sigmoid colon distal to anastomosis by the EEA stapler, the surgeon must be careful not to inadvertently place the TA-55 stapler across the superior hemorrhoidal artery or one of its main branches.

---

## Technique

**1** The anatomy of the sigmoid colon and its mesenteric blood supply are illustrated. If possible, the proximal sigmoid should be resected below the superior hemorrhoidal artery. The disease process itself, however, must dictate the level of sigmoid resection.

**2** Anterior resection has been completed. The EEA stapler, with the anvil detached, has been inserted through the open end of the sigmoid colon, and the stapler rod has been brought through the antimesenteric border of the colon with sharp dissection. After the rod has emerged from the antimesenteric border of the colon, the anvil is reattached.

**3** Pursestring sutures are placed around the rectal stump and around the antimesenteric border of the sigmoid colon at the site where the rod has emerged.

**4** The wing nut on the EEA stapler is tightened, the stapler is activated, and the anastomosis is completed.

Care is taken to identify the terminal branches of the superior hemorrhoidal artery. A small defect is made in the mesentery with a blunt instrument. The TA-55 stapler is inserted through the defect, encompassing the redundant portion of the sigmoid colon. The TA-55 stapler is fired, and the redundant portion of colon is excised. Care must be taken to try to place the TA-55 stapler distal to the superior hemorrhoidal artery if possible. Insufficient mobilization of the colon, however, may require the sacrifice of the terminal branch of the superior hemorrhoidal artery. It is more important to have a tension-free anastomosis than to retain this branch.

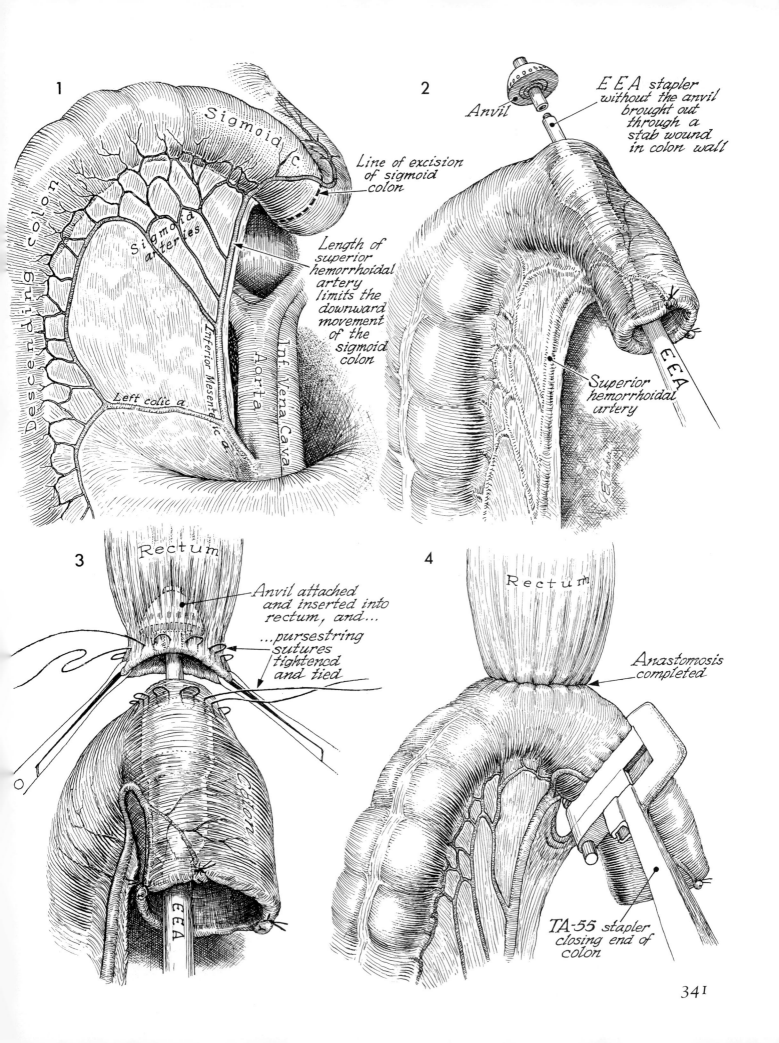

**1**

Descending colon

Sigmoid c.

Sigmoid arteries

Left colic a.

Inferior Mesenteric a.

Aorta

Inf. Vena Cava

Line of excision of sigmoid colon

Length of superior hemorrhoidal artery limits the downward movement of the sigmoid colon

**2**

Anvil

E E A stapler without the anvil brought out through a stab wound in colon wall

E E A

Superior hemorrhoidal artery

**3**

Rectum

Anvil attached and inserted into rectum, and...

...pursestring sutures tightened and tied

Colon

E E A

**4**

Rectum

Anastomosis completed

TA-55 stapler closing end of colon

341

# 8

## Small Bowel

# Small Bowel Surgery

In cases of extensive gynecologic or pelvic malignancy, particularly those associated with previous irradiation, the efficacy of small bowel bypass for obstruction, fistula formation, and stenosis is well established.

Recently, the efficacy of terminal ileectomy with right colectomy and ileotransverse colostomy (see Section 10) has also been demonstrated.

Segmental intestinal resection and anastomosis often result in numerous incidental enterotomies, with the spillage of intestinal contents increasing the danger of postoperative pelvic sepsis. The dissection required for intestinal resection leaves large, raw, irradiated areas where the new intestinal anastomoses may adhere, necrose, and produce recurrent fistulae formation. This procedure has been shown to have an abnormally high operative mortality and, therefore, should be avoided if possible.

The decision to reexplore the patient 4 or 5 months after the small bowel bypass, take down the bypass segment, and eliminate the abdominal wall intestinal mucous fistula stoma is one that requires sound, mature surgical and oncologic judgment. When in doubt, the mucous fistula stoma should be left in place.

The two most common pathologic events related to pelvic disease that occur in the small bowel are obstruction and fistula formation in the terminal ileum. These are demonstrated in Figures 1 and 2. Figure 3 shows the percentages of injuries as related to the intestine, secondary to pelvic surgery and/or disease. Approximately 85% of all intestinal problems related to pelvic disease or obstetric and/or gynecologic surgery are located in the terminal ileum. This is probably because the terminal ileum generally remains in the true pelvis and, therefore, is readily accessible to irradiation injury and/or pelvic adhesion formation.

In contrast, only about 10% of intestinal injuries are in the rectum or the sigmoid colon, and less than 2% involve either the transverse colon, jejunum, or other parts of the intestine. This is an important surgical fact in that it assists the surgeon at exploratory laparotomy, when multiple dilated loops of bowel are encountered too rapidly, to identify the diseased segment of small bowel. After identifying the cecum, the surgeon can trace the terminal ileum back for 3 feet and find the pathologic problem in 85% of cases. This is far easier than identifying the ligament of Treitz and tracing the small bowel distally toward the cecum.

Figures 1 and 2 illustrate the anatomic condition of the small bowel associated with obstruction and combinations of obstruction and fistula formation. The small intestine proximal to the obstruction will be dilated 2–3 times the diameter of intestine distal to the disease. This is helpful in identification of efferent and afferent loops of bowel.

The purpose of these operations is to radically resect or bypass a point of disease in the small bowel.

**Physiologic Changes.** The terminal ileum is responsible for absorption of fat-soluble vitamins plus vitamin $B_{12}$. Patients who have extensive loss of the ileum can be left with what has been referred to as short bowel syndrome. This consists of diarrhea, failure to absorb the fat-soluble vitamins (A, D, E, K) plus vitamin $B_{12}$, and difficulty in absorption of high-molecular-weight fats.

Many of these patients need postoperative assistance from a medical gastroenterologist to adjust their diet, control diarrhea, and generally help them to adapt to the rearrangement of their anatomy.

**Points of Caution.** The most important aspect of performing a small bowel resection or bypass is to ensure the vascular integrity of the bowel to be anastomosed. This is aided by keeping trauma to the bowel wall at a minimum.

All open mesenteric areas must be closed. Internal hernia and obstruction are serious and can be fatal complications in these heavily irradiated patients.

The advantage of small bowel bypass over small bowel resection is that it avoids extensive dissection in a heavily irradiated fibrotic pelvis. Only that dissection needed to perform the bypass should be made, and the remainder of the diseased bowel should be left impacted in the heavily irradiated pelvis. Since both procedures, resection and bypass, are required at different times in pelvic surgery, however, both are illustrated in this section.

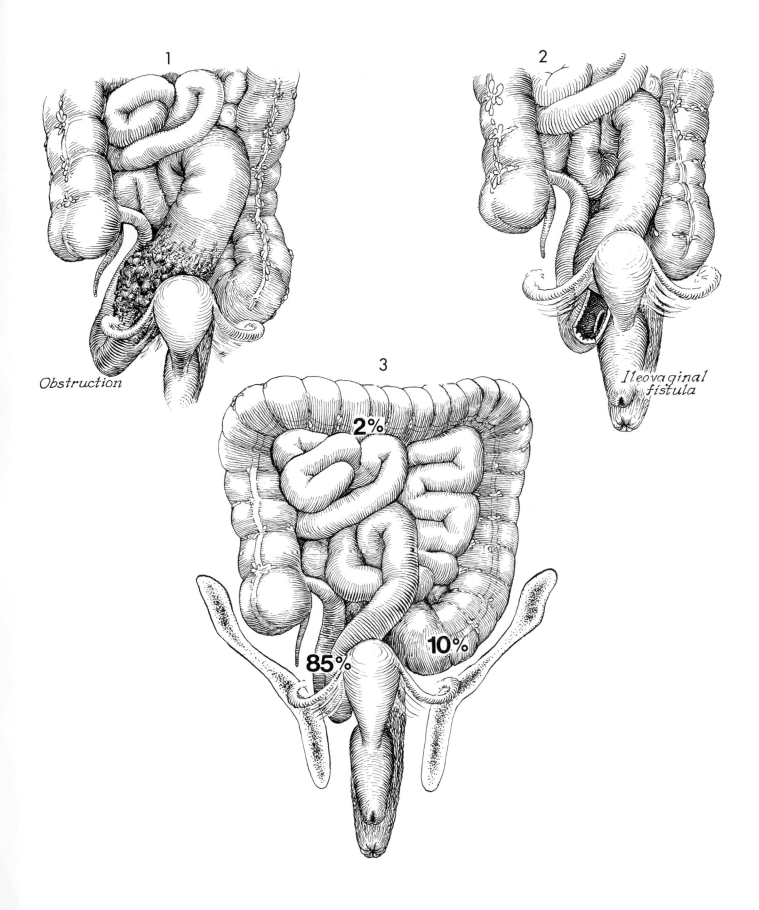

1

Obstruction

2

Ileovaginal
fistula

3

2%

10%

85%

345

# Small Bowel Resection With End-to-End Anastomosis Using the Gambee Technique

Small bowel resection is preferred over small bowel bypass in situations where the pathologic condition is confined to a segment of the small bowel that is not impacted in a dense irradiated fibrotic pelvis or where a knuckle of small bowel is involved within a pelvic tumor. Resection over bypass should also be performed in those cases where extensive dissection of the small bowel to locate and mobilize the pathologic segment is not required. If the surgeon insists on mobilization and resection of all small bowel disease, the surgeon must be willing to resect the ileum and right colon and perform a high ileotransverse colostomy. The multiple enterotomies not only spill intestinal contents into the wound but also are frequently overlooked at the time of repair. In addition, those enterotomies that are repaired become adherent to the dense irradiated fibrotic pelvic walls and break down at the suture line to form recurrent enteric cutaneous and/or vaginal fistulae. In summary, experienced pelvic surgeons have learned (usually the hard way) that small bowel resection should be confined to those few cases where the pathologic segment of the small bowel can be easily mobilized and isolated. Otherwise, small bowel bypass should be performed.

The pathologic segment of small bowel is removed, and the remaining small bowel is reanastomosed to a healthy segment of intestine.

**Physiologic Changes.** Removal of extensive segments of small bowel may produce postoperative diarrhea and failure of fat-soluble vitamin absorption.

**Points of Caution.** The predominant point of caution in resection of the small bowel is to ensure the vascular integrity of the anastomosis. The vascular supply of the terminal 10 cm of small bowel is unreliable. In heavily irradiated patients it is preferable to perform an ileoascending colostomy rather than an ileo-ileostomy for anastomosis in the terminal 10 cm of the ileum.

## Technique

Small bowel resection with end-to-end anastomosis using the Gambee technique is demonstrated here. Anastomosis using the surgical stapler technique is shown in Section 3, page 161.

1 Patients for small bowel resection are placed in the supine position. A Foley catheter is inserted into the bladder. A sump-type nasogastric tube is passed into the stomach.

2 A thorough bimanual examination is performed prior to the operation.

3 A midline incision is made, usually extending around the umbilicus. The abdomen is entered and explored. As stated on page 344, in the majority of cases, small bowel disease associated with pelvic disorders is located within 3 feet of the ileocecal bowel. This fact is of significant value to the pelvic surgeon in that it allows the surgeon to trace the small bowel back from the cecum rather than trace the bowel down from the ligament of Treitz.

At this point, the decision must be made to perform either a small bowel resection or a small bowel bypass.

If the limits of the small bowel disease are identifiable and can be mobilized without extensive dissection, small bowel resection is the procedure of choice. If, however, as in the majority of cases, the diseased segment of small bowel is embedded deep in the true pelvis, particularly after heavy pelvic irradiation, it is wiser to perform a small bowel bypass.

4 The small bowel to be resected is mobilized, and the mesentery is carefully studied for vascular arcades. A point of transection is selected sufficiently distant from the diseased portion and in the immediate vicinity of a healthy vascular arcade. The bowel should be suspended between Babcock clamps or warm moist saline gauze held between the thumb and first finger. The peritoneum of the mesentery is opened with a scalpel, using a delicate technique that does not transect the underlying blood vessels.

5 Linen-shod intestinal clamps are applied proximal and distal to the point of transection. The mesentery is opened in a V-shaped fashion. The small vessels crossing the line of transection are clamped and tied.

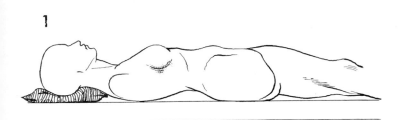

1

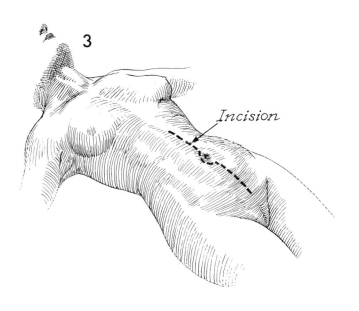

2

3

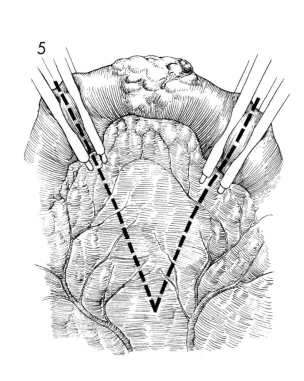

*Incision*

4

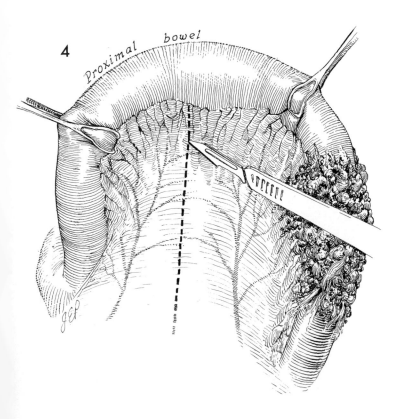

Proximal    bowel

5

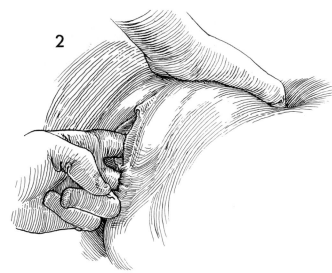

347

# Small Bowel Resection With End-to-End Anastomosis Using the Gambee Technique

## (Continued)

**6** The bowel to be resected is held by an assistant while the surgeon creates small openings in avascular segments of the mesentery along the line of transection. Small vessels are clamped and tied with Dexon suture.

Note that the line of transection in the bowel is oblique rather than perpendicular. The blood supply to the small bowel is such that the antimesenteric border of the bowel can become ischemic if the vascular arcade supplying the edge of the resected bowel is transected perpendicularly. A second reason for transecting the bowel in an oblique rather than a perpendicular line is that an oblique transection will give a larger anastomosis and reduce the incidence of stricture formation.

**7** The bowel has been transected, and the diseased portion has been stapled off with the TA-55 surgical stapler and separated from the healthy terminal ileum and cecum.

**8** The diseased portion of bowel has been removed to the side, and a healthy segment of the proximal ileum (P) is brought down to anastomose to a healthy segment of the distal ileum (D).

The first step in this anastomosis is to place a Lembert suture of 3-0 Dexon through the mesenteric border approximately 1 cm from the edge of the mucosa. The purpose of this stitch is to take tension off the future suture line and to hold the intestine in appropriate approximation for the remainder of the anastomosis.

**9** The intestine is now available for the Gambee technique of single-layer through-and-through suture anastomosis.

### Gambee Technique

The steps of the Gambee technique are outlined in Figures 10–17.

**10** The first step in the Gambee technique is to place the suture, previously noted in Figure 8, on the mesenteric border of the intestine. This is referred to here as the south (S) suture.

**11** The Gambee technique is a single-layer through-and- through anastomosis; all knots are tied within the lumen of the bowel. **b** is a cross section of **a**. Note that the initial Lembert suture (L) placed at the mesenteric border of the bowel has been tied and thus tends to invert the edges of the mucosa. The Gambee suture (G) has been placed through the mucosa; the entire wall of the bowel exits the serosa, enters the serosa of the bowel on the opposite side, passes the bowel wall, and emerges from the mucosa. When tied, it further inverts the edge of the bowel.

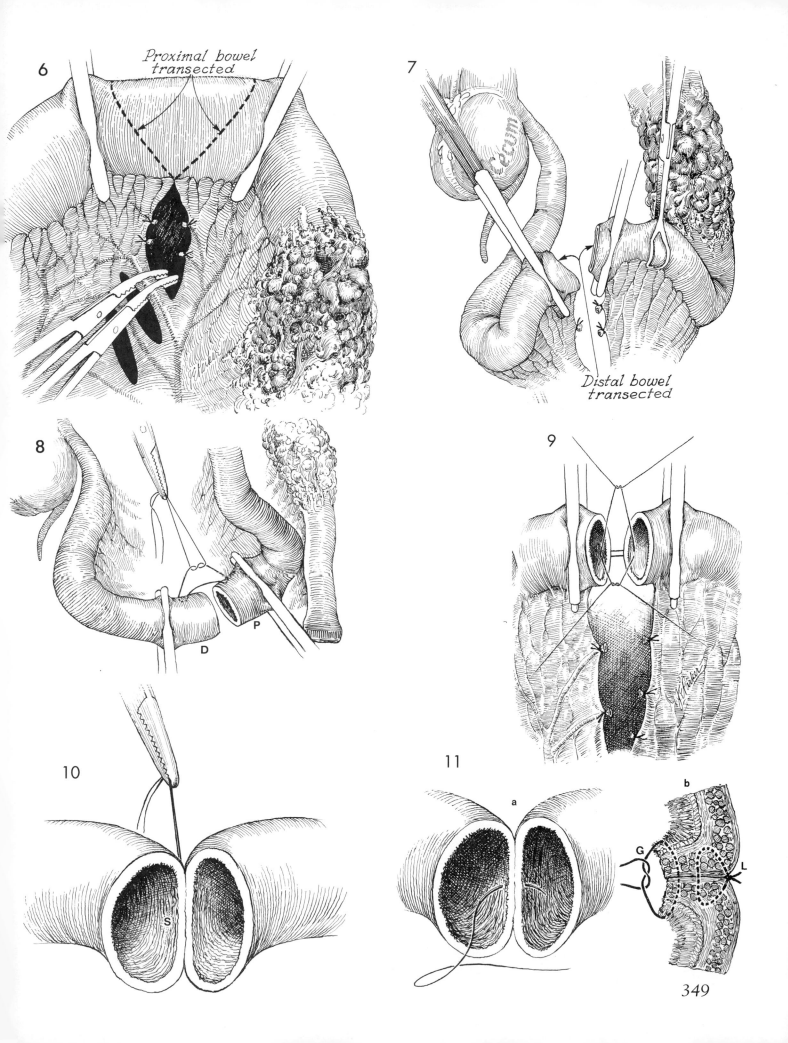

**6** Proximal bowel transected

**7** cecum

Distal bowel transected

**8** D P

**9**

**10** S

**11** a b

G L

# Small Bowel Resection With End-to-End Anastomosis Using the Gambee Technique

## (Continued)

**12** Each successive Gambee suture is placed approximately 3 mm apart around the entire circumstance of the bowel.

**13** A cross section of the Gambee suture reveals the path of the suture. In **a,** the suture enters the bowel through the mucosa, passes through the entire wall of bowel, exits from the serosa, passes back through the serosa of the opposite segment of bowel, penetrates the entire bowel wall, and exits the mucosa. In **b,** the Gambee suture is tied with the knot on the lumen side of the bowel, tending to invert the anastomosis.

**14** The process has been almost completed around the entire circumference of bowel.

**15** When all but a 5-mm defect in the bowel remains, the near-far inverting suture can be applied. **a** shows the near-far inverting suture in place. When tied, it will dramatically invert the entire suture line. **b** is a cross section of the near-far inverting suture, outlining the details of the technique. Note that the near-far inverting suture is the only stitch in the Gambee technique that is tied on the serosa of the bowel rather than the mucosa of the bowel. The stitch is started by placing the suture through the serosa of one segment of bowel approximately 1 cm from the edge. It penetrates the entire surface of bowel and exits the mucosa approximately 1 cm from the edge. The suture is immediately reversed and is passed back through the mucosa of the same segment of bowel 3 mm from the edge, penetrates the entire wall of the same segment of bowel, and exits the serosa. This is the near and the far aspect of this stitch. The suture is then placed through the near edge of the opposite segment of bowel 3 mm from the edge through its serosa to penetrate the entire wall of the intestine and exit from the mucosa. The needle is immediately placed back through the mucosa approximately 1 cm from its edge, penetrates the entire wall of the bowel, and exits from the serosa approximately 1 cm from its edge. Tying the suture dramatically inverts the entire anastomosis.

**16** Four tension-relieving Lembert sutures of 3-0 Dexon are placed north (N), east (E), and west (W) of the bowel. These sutures further invert the anastomosis and take tension off the suture line to improve healing.

**17** The mesentery of the small intestine is closed with interrupted 3-0 synthetic absorbable sutures to prevent internal hernia.

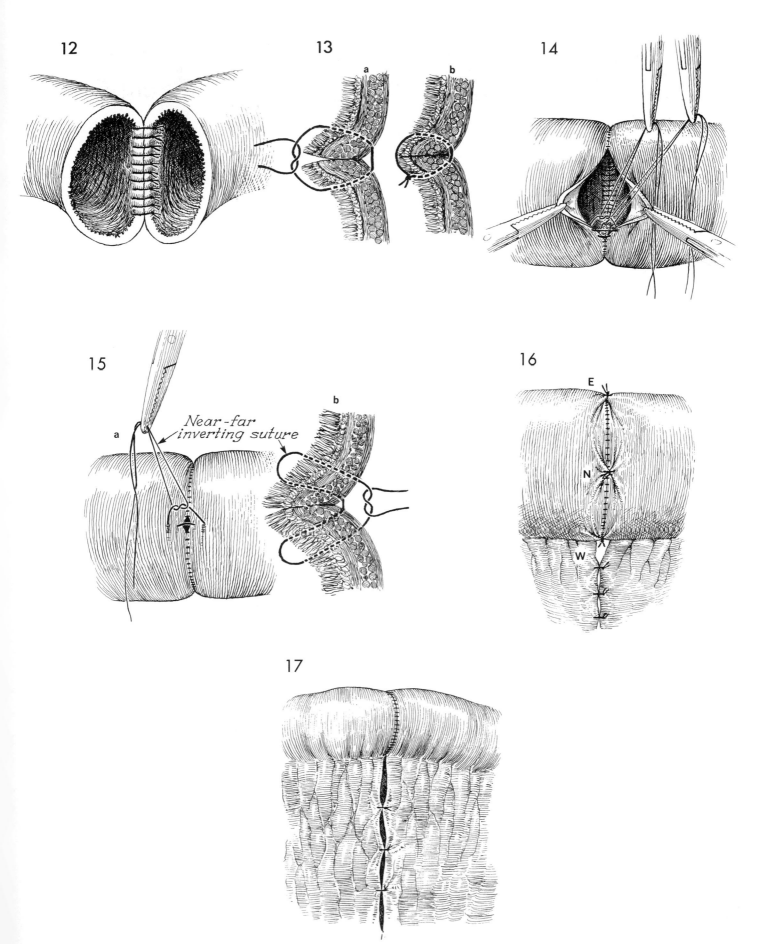

**12**

**13**

a        b

**14**

**15**

*Near-far
inverting suture*

a

b

**16**

E

N

W

**17**

# Small Bowel Bypass With Ileoileal Anastomosis and Mucous Fistula

In those cases where the small bowel is involved with obstruction and/or fistula formation following total pelvic irradiation and/or advanced malignant disease is impacted in the true pelvis, a bypass with mucous fistula rather than a bowel resection is the operation of choice. After small bowel resection, patients frequently develop (1) recurrent small bowel obstruction from adherence of the anastomosis site to the large raw dissected areas within the true pelvis, or (2) recurrent fistula formation at the site of anastomosis, or (3) breakdown of the closure of multiple inadvertent enterotomies associated with the surgery.

We have preferred bypass with an end-to-end anastomosis and mucous fistula rather than the side-to-side technique. Although the side-to-side anastomosis is more aesthetically acceptable to the patient, it is frequently associated with recurrent obstruction and persistent fistula drainage because it does not isolate the diseased portion of small bowel. The end-to-end or end-to-side technique of small bowel bypass requires a mucous fistula with an abdominal stoma that eventually contracts, produces small amounts of mucus, and has a lower incidence of recurrent obstruction and fistula drainage.

**Physiologic Changes.** In this operation, continuity of the intestine is established, and the patient is able to regain oral alimentation. With loss of the terminal ileum, however, fat-soluble vitamins and high-molecu-lar-weight fat absorption can be disturbed, and postoperative diarrhea is frequently encountered. These undesirable side effects can be reduced with modification of the patient's diet. Vitamins can be replaced either systemically, as for vitamin $B_{12}$, or by therapeutic oral supplementation, as for vitamins A, D, E, and K, which will be absorbed by the proximal intestine. The mucous fistula may drain excessively until the pathologic indication for the bypass has been relieved. One month postoperatively, mucous drainage is usually scant, and most patients wear only a small gauze dressing over the mucous fistula stoma site.

**Points of Caution.** We have found that the segment of bowel to be brought out as the mucous fistula stoma is optional. From a physiologic point of view it would seem that the peristaltic end of the segment should be used. If additional dissection is required to bring out the peristaltic end of the segment, however, the antiperistaltic end can be brought out as the mucous fistula stoma with equal effect.

Caution should be taken to ensure the vascular integrity of the terminal ileum. The blood supply to the terminal 10 cm of ileum is unreliable. This is particularly true if the patient has received total pelvic irradiation. If there is any doubt as to the integrity of the blood supply in the terminal ileum, the ileoileal anastomosis should be abandoned, and an ileoascending colostomy should be performed.

# Small Bowel Bypass With Ileoileal Anastomosis and Mucous Fistula

## (Continued)

## Technique

The first four steps in small bowel bypass with ileoileal anastomosis and mucous fistula are the same as for small bowel resection.

**1** The abdomen is opened through a lower midline incision extended around the umbilicus, and the peritoneal cavity is entered. The afferent and efferent loops of intestine associated with the diseased segment of bowel are identified. The efferent loop will generally be grossly distended because most patients have some degree of obstruction, even in ileovaginal fistula formation. The afferent loop will be smaller and can generally be traced back from the ileocecal area without significant dissection. The purpose of this entire operation can be defeated, however, if the surgeon insists on total identification of all loops prior to the bypass procedure.

The dilated efferent proximal segment of bowel is elevated with rubber-shod clamps at a sufficient distance from the diseased segment. This is usually at a site that does not require dissection of the bowel into the true pelvis. The mesentery of the bowel is opened, and the vessels are clamped and tied. The bowel is transected in an oblique manner.

**2** The distal segment or afferent loop is likewise elevated, its mesentery is opened, and the vessels are transected and tied. The bowel is transected in an oblique manner. Thus the diseased segment of bowel, impacted deep in the true pelvis, is isolated.

**3** Some surgeons prefer to exteriorize both ends of the diseased segment of bowel as a double mucous fistula. We have not found this necessary, however, and multiple abdominal wall stomata only add to the aesthetic burden for the patient. The end of the diseased segment to be left in the lower abdomen and pelvis is closed with the automatic surgical stapler or with synthetic absorbable suture in the Gambee technique. Either the peristaltic or the antiperistaltic end can be closed, and the opposite end can be exteriorized as the mucous fistula.

**4** The proximal (P) and distal (D) segments of healthy bowel are now anastomosed by either the suture technique, as described in small bowel resection with the Gambee anastomosis, or by the automatic surgical stapler technique, as described in Section 7. Note that the diseased segment of intestine has been closed with the surgical stapler and is left densely impacted within the pelvis. Thus, no large raw areas of dissection are available to which the new anastomosis might adhere. In addition, multiple inadvertent enterotomies, with their intestinal spillage, have been avoided.

**5** The ileoileostomy has been performed with either the suture technique or the stapler technique. The abdomen has been closed, and the most convenient end of the diseased segment of intestine has been exteriorized through the lower midline incision of the abdominal wall closure. Note that the opposite end of the diseased segment has been closed off and left impacted within the pelvis. For demonstration purposes, the diseased segment represented here shows the pathologic condition alone. The reader should imagine that this segment is much longer with many entangled loops of intestine dipping deep into the pelvis, as shown in Figure 1, page 345.

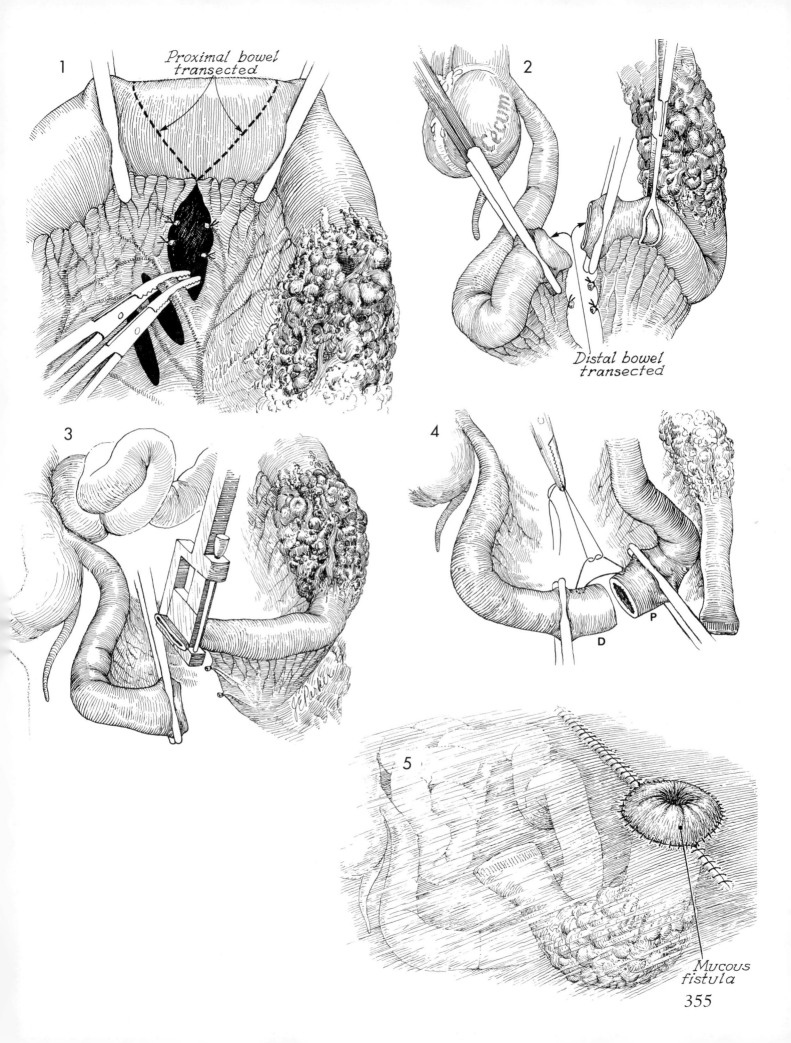

**1** Proximal bowel transected

**2** cecum

Distal bowel transected

**3**

**4** D     P

**5** Mucous fistula

# Small Bowel Bypass With Ileotransverse Colostomy and Mucous Fistula

Ileotransverse colostomy with mucous fistula is utilized when the disease process involves the major portion of the terminal ileum plus the ascending colon. The transverse colon may be the ideal site for a small bowel bypass, since it has had little if any ionizing irradiation. Anastomosis at this site reduces the length of colon available for the absorption of intestinal contents, however, and the patient must adapt to living with a more liquid fecal stream than if additional colon were usable. The technique for performing the operation is similar to the other small bowel bypasses with end-to-side anastomosis of the ileum into the colon.

The purpose of the operation is to reestablish intestinal continuity and bypass the diseased segment of small intestine.

**Physiologic Changes.** Once the anastomoses are begun between the small bowel and the transverse colon, the length of colon available for absorption of intestinal contents is reduced. This is particularly true if the disease process is such that a diverting cutaneous colostomy is needed. The patient can "run out" of colon. Care must be taken to ensure that at least 20–25 cm of colon are available for anastomosis. There will be a marked difference in the quality of life for the patient if sufficient colon is available to absorb fluid from the fecal stream and produce a firm stool rather than a continuous flow of liquid.

**Points of Caution.** The points of caution are the same as for other small bowel bypasses. Care must be taken to avoid spillage of raw stool into the peritoneal cavity. Preoperative antibiotics should be used. The peritoneal cavity should be thoroughly lavaged after the procedure. A closed suction drain should be placed adjacent to the anastomosis.

---

## Technique

The technique for ileotransverse colostomy with mucous fistula is similar to that for the ileoascending colostomy with mucous fistula.

**1** The bowel proximal to the diseased segment is identified and elevated, its mesentery is opened, and the vessels are clamped and tied. The bowel is transected in an oblique fashion.

**2** The proximal bowel is brought to a convenient site on the transverse colon. The site should be selected as far proximal on the large bowel as possible. This will supply a greater length of colon for absorption of fluid from the fecal stream.

The colon is cross-clamped with linen-shod intestinal clamps. The cross-clamped piece of proximal small bowel is brought adjacent to the opening made over the teniae coli on the antimesenteric surface of the colon.

The technique for anastomosis of the small bowel to the colon in an end-to-side fashion is the same as that shown on page 351, demonstrating the Gambee anastomosis technique with an ileoileostomy and mucous fistula.

**3** The distal small bowel has been exteriorized through the anterior abdominal wall via the lower midline incision, and a stoma has been created. The completed anastomosis from the small bowel to the transverse colon is shown. The abdomen has been closed.

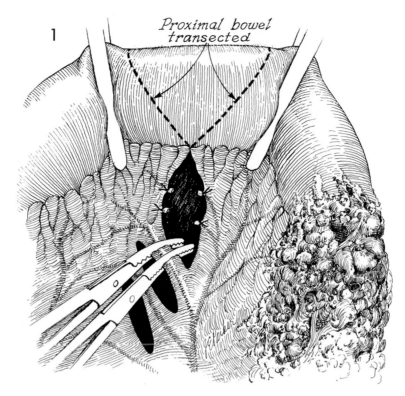

1 — Proximal bowel transected

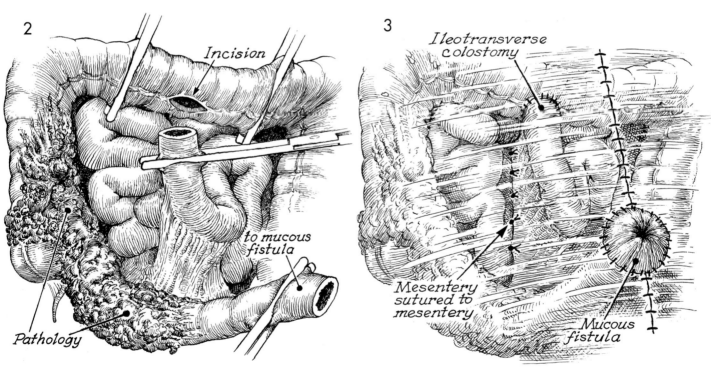

2 — Incision — Pathology — to mucous fistula

3 — Ileotransverse colostomy — Mesentery sutured to mesentery — Mucous fistula

357

# Terminal Ileectomy With Right Colectomy and Ileotransverse Colostomy

The presence of a tumor or severe irradiation damage to the terminal ileum and the right colon, with or without obstruction, may require resection of the affected area.

**Physiologic Changes.** Resection of a portion of the terminal ileum is associated with a loss of absorption of the fat-soluble vitamins A, D, C, and K. Vitamin $B_{12}$ is normally absorbed in the terminal ileum; thus when the terminal ileum is absent, $B_{12}$ must be given systemically.

Loss of the terminal ileum creates changes in cholesterol metabolism and bowel salt reabsorption. If undigested fats are dumped directly into the transverse colon, the osmotic pressure of the colon is elevated, and diarrhea results.

**Points of Caution.** After the abdomen has been opened through a midline incision extended to the xiphoid, care should be taken to identify the blood supply to the right colon and terminal ileum. If at all possible, the colon should be transected distal to the middle colic artery. The ileocolic artery frequently has to be clamped and tied.

## Technique

**1** The line of transection from the transverse colon to the ileum is shown. These transections are frequently made with the gastrointestinal anastomosis (GIA) stapler to minimize spill from the intestine. The ileocolic and the right colic artery should be identified, transected, and tied. The line of Toldt lateral to the right colon should be excised with scissors or cautery. The hepatocolic ligament should be incised with a cautery or clamped and tied.

**2** The resected terminal ileum and right colon can be seen. Care should be taken to fully identify the right ureter prior to resection. A indicates aorta; and *IVC*, inferior vena cava.

**3** The GIA stapler connects a side-to-side anastomosis of the ileum and colon.

**4** A TA-55 stapler has closed the defect in the bowel. A large anastomosis has been made between the terminal ileum and the transverse colon. The mesentery between these two pieces of bowel is closed with interrupted suture to prevent internal hernia.

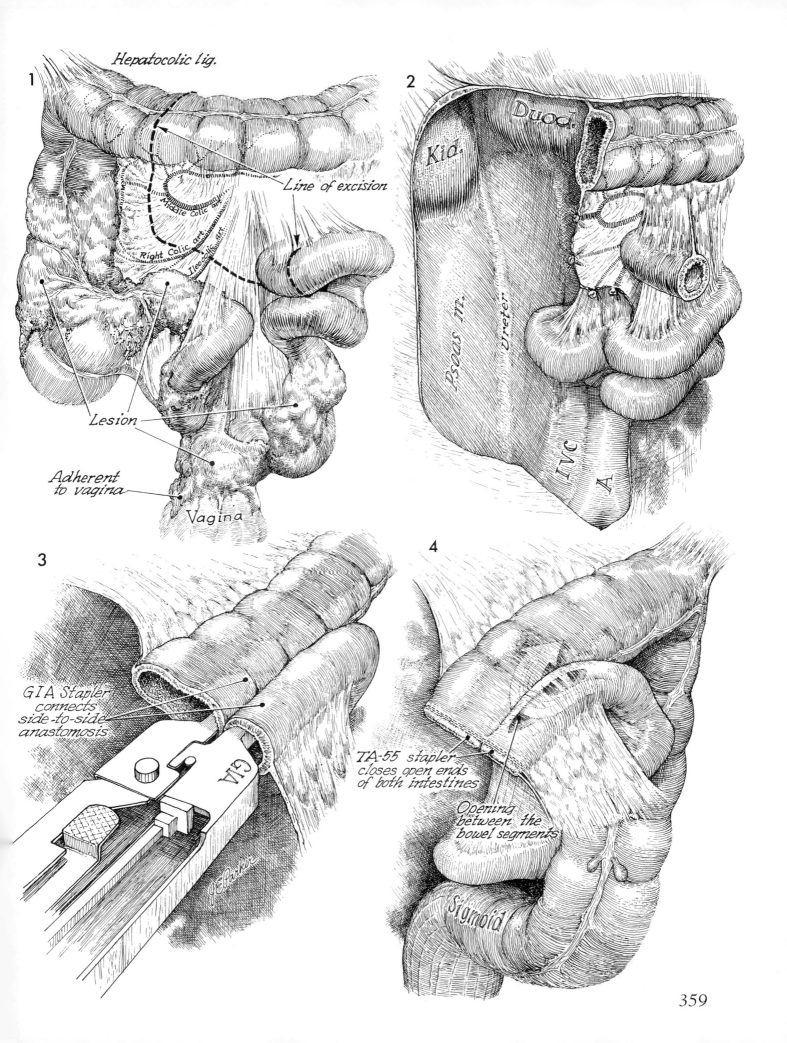

**1**

Hepatocolic lig.

Line of excision

Middle Colic art.

Right Colic art.

Ileocolic art.

Lesion

Adherent to vagina

Vagina

**2**

Kid.

Duod.

Psoas m.

Ureter

IVC

A.

**3**

GIA Stapler connects side-to-side anastomosis

GIA

J. Parker

**4**

TA-55 stapler closes open ends of both intestines

Opening between the bowel segments

Sigmoid

359

# 9
## Abdominal Wall

# Pfannenstiel Incision

The Pfannenstiel incision has become popular in the past decade for cosmetic reasons. This is particularly true in younger women having surgery for benign gynecologic and pelvic problems. If properly placed, it is generally concealed by regrowth of the pubic hair.

The purpose of the technique is to provide a cosmetic incision for pelvic surgery.

**Physiologic Changes.** The Pfannenstiel incision transects neurovascular pathways in the skin of the abdominal wall and frequently requires partial or complete transection of the rectus abdominis muscle. It is rarely associated with incisional hernia, has a low incidence of wound dehiscence, and heals without significant scarring. The latter fact may be due to the copious blood supply in the mons pubis.

**Points of Caution.** A Pfannenstiel incision should never be used in oncologic surgery. It does not give exposure to the upper abdomen and provides only limited exposure to aortic and lymph nodes for their analysis and dissection. Care must be taken to avoid incidental laceration of the inferior epigastric artery and vein on the lateral margin of the rectus muscles. If the muscles are to be transected, the epigastric artery and vein should be identified, clamped, and ligated prior to transection of the muscle. In addition, care should be taken with regard to the point of entry into the peritoneum. If the incision is made too low, the bladder can be entered.

Hemostasis is particularly important during this incision. The vascularity of the mons pubis increases the risk of hemorrhage, formation of hematoma, and infection. The surgeon should ensure that the incision is dry before closure of the wound. If there is any question, a small suction drain should be left in the incision for 24–48 hours.

## Technique

**1** The patient's position for this operation can be lithotomy, supine, or modified dorsal supine lithotomy. The latter is shown here.

**2** The Pfannenstiel incision is semicircular and is made slightly above the mons pubis for a length of about 12 cm. Care must be taken to ensure that hemostasis is complete prior to entering the peritoneal cavity. The rectus fascia is opened transversely.

**3** After the rectus fascia is opened, the rectus muscles are separated and dissected off the peritoneum. If the rectus muscles cannot be separated sufficiently by lateral retraction, they should be transected. In general, the muscles are easier to separate in patients who have had a previous term pregnancy. In some patients with strong, tight rectus muscles, adequate exposure may not be achieved without transection of the muscle. If the muscle is to be transected, the inferior epigastric artery and vein on the lateral border of the muscle must be clamped, incised, and ligated prior to cutting the muscle.

**4** The peritoneum is picked up between tissue forceps and opened with either a longitudinal or a transverse incision.

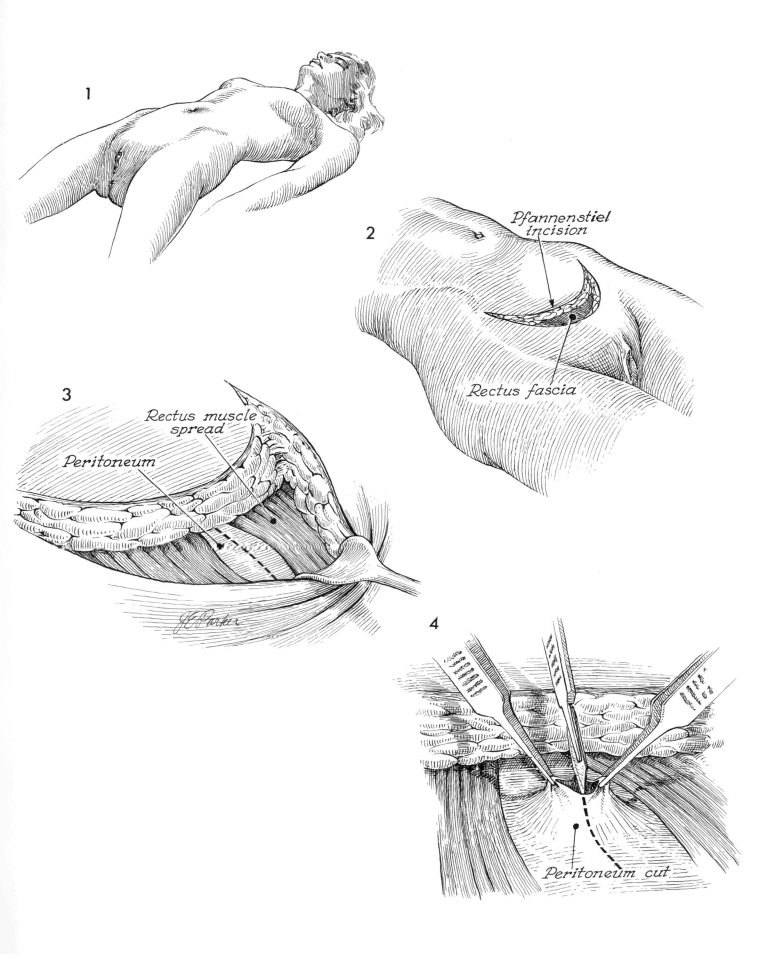

**1**

**2**

*Pfannenstiel incision*

*Rectus fascia*

**3**

*Rectus muscle spread*

*Peritoneum*

*J C Parker*

**4**

*Peritoneum cut*

# Maylard Incision

The Maylard incision is an abdominal incision that can afford extensive exposure to the pelvic organs when this is needed. Although it can be used for most gynecologic procedures, it is not particularly useful in such upper abdominal surgeries as ovarian cancer that may be associated with tumor in and around the liver or spleen.

Its main disadvantage is that it is a more painful incision for the patient during the first postoperative week. This may be weighed against its reduced rate of incisional hernia and the fact that it is cosmetically advantageous, since it does not scar the midabdomen.

**Physiologic Changes.** None.

**Points of Caution.** Care must be taken to ensure the integrity of the ligature on the inferior epigastric artery lateral to the rectus fascia. We prefer a sloping U-shaped incision from the anterior superior iliac spine down slightly superior to the mons pubis to the superior iliac spine on the opposite side. This course should definitely be marked on the patient with brilliant green solution prior to making the incision.

## Technique

**1** With the patient in the dorsal supine position, the proposed incision is marked on the abdomen with brilliant green solution.

**2** The incision is made down to the rectus fascia.

**3** The rectus fascia and rectus muscles are transected by using the electrosurgery technique. Care must be exercised at the lateral margin of the rectus muscle to ensure the integrity of the inferior epigastric artery and vein. The muscle is totally transected.

**4** A small area of the peritoneal cavity is opened. A finger is placed in this opening, and the remaining portion of the peritoneum is opened with electrocautery.

Closure of a Maylard incision does not require suturing the rectal muscle stumps together. We have been impressed with the simple running suture for closing this incision. The skin and subcutaneous tissue can be closed with the automatic surgical stapler or a subcuticular suture.

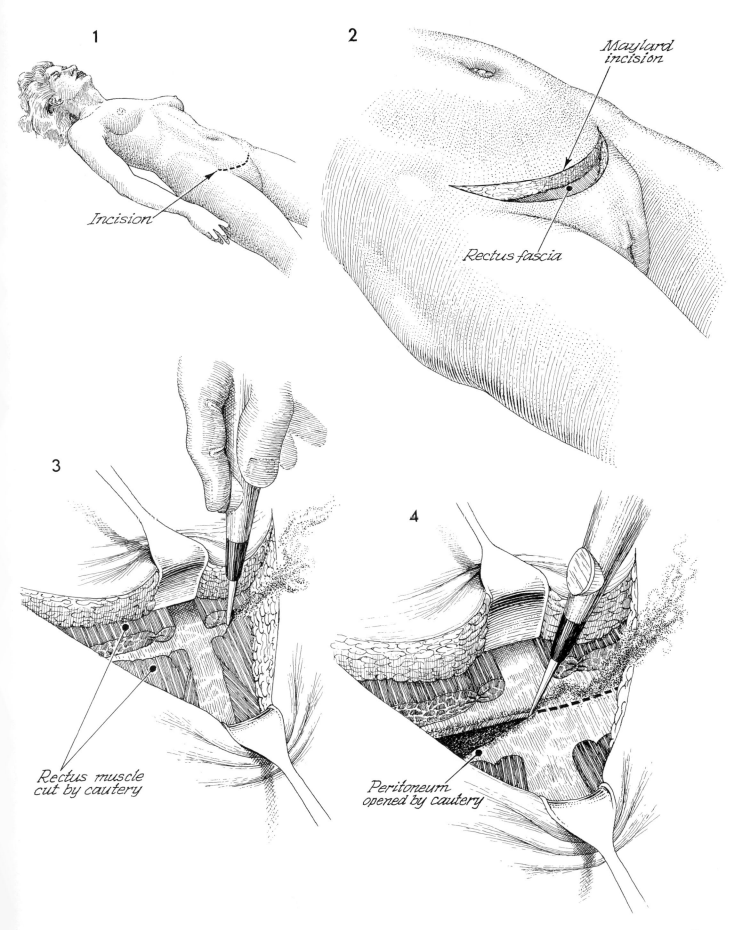

**1**

Incision

**2**

Maylard
incision

Rectus fascia

**3**

Rectus muscle
cut by cautery

**4**

Peritoneum
opened by cautery

365

# Panniculectomy

A large abdominal panniculus after weight reduction in a patient who has had excessive obesity can be associated with excoriation and breakdown of the underside of the panniculus. In these cases, panniculectomy is indicated.

The purpose of panniculectomy is to remove the large abdominal panniculus.

**Physiologic Changes.** Large panniculi will frequently contain 500–700 mL of blood within the mass of tissue. Therefore, this procedure can be associated with excessive blood loss. Postoperative hypovolemia and its clinical sequelae may result.

**Points of Caution.** The patient should be evaluated in both the standing and the supine position prior to the operation to design an incision that will prevent the "dog ears" that frequently occur after a panniculectomy in the area of the anterior iliac spine.

One assistant must be constantly available to keep traction on the panniculus.

Meticulous attention to hemostasis is essential. The wound should be drained with suction catheters.

---

## Technique

**1** The patient is placed in the dorsal supine position. Brilliant green surgical dye is used to design and mark off the lines of incision.

**2** Large fishhooks are inserted into the panniculus and connected to an orthopedic frame erected over the operating table to elevate the panniculus. The inferior margin of the panniculus can be marked. A V-shaped incision over the mons pubis and a Z-shaped incision at the lateral margins are made to prevent overlapping of the abdominal flaps and the "dog ear" protrusion of tissue at the iliac spines.

**3** While the flap is held on traction with the fishhooks, the incisions are carried down to the rectus fascia.

**4** Unless meticulous hemostasis is maintained throughout the operation, blood loss will become excessive. The V-shaped incision in the mons pubis should be closed with interrupted 2-0 synthetic absorbable sutures.

**5** The reconstruction of the mons pubis has been completed with placement of the subcutaneous row of interrupted 3-0 synthetic absorbable sutures.

**6** Suction drains are placed in the wound and may be anchored to the rectus fascia with a 5-0 synthetic absorbable suture to prevent displacement. The skin stapler is used to close the edges of the wound.

**7** The cephalad margin of the abdominal flap should be mobilized up to the umbilicus. If a great deal of mobilization is required, an elliptical incision can be made around the umbilicus, and a matching elliptical defect can be created cephalad to the umbilicus. Then, when the abdominal wall is completely mobilized and moved caudad to match the inferior margin of the incision, the elliptical umbilical incision can be closed, and the umbilicus can be sutured to the edges of the newly created abdominal defect. The abdominal incision should be closed with interrupted 2-0 synthetic absorbable sutures.

**8** A second layer of subcutaneous sutures is placed with 3-0 synthetic absorbable sutures.

**9** The remaining portions of the skin are approximated with stainless steel skin clips. The suction drains are connected to continuous suction. They are removed when they are no longer productive.

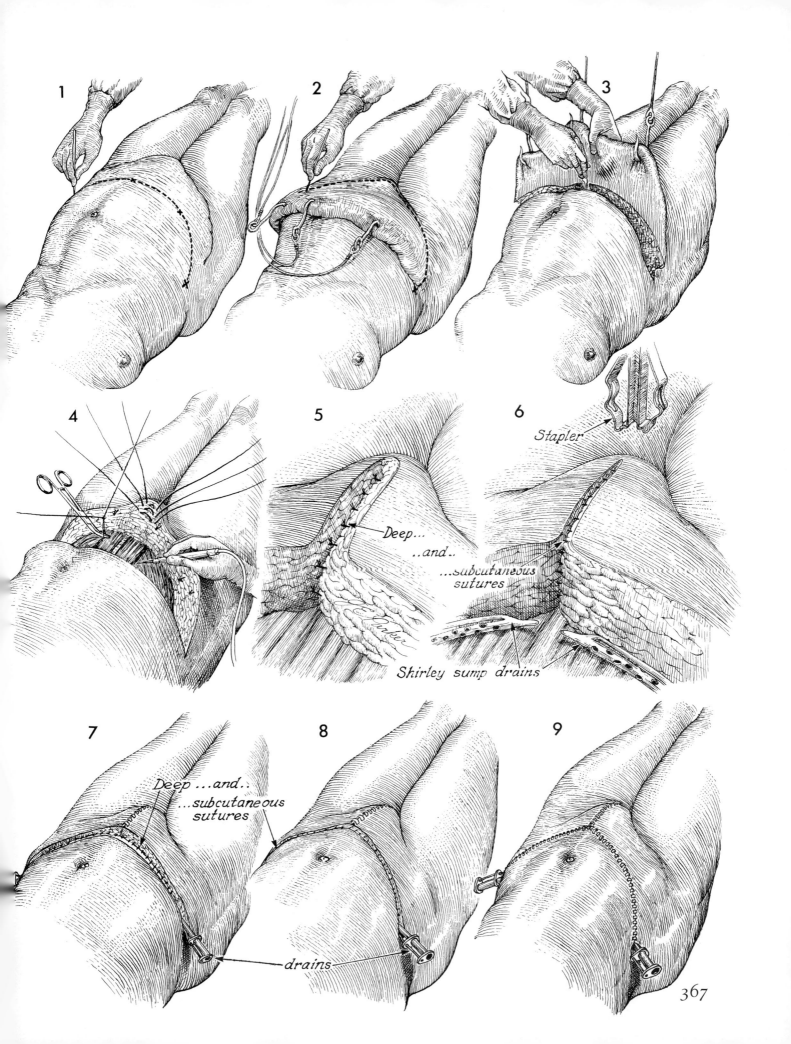

**1**

**2**

**3**

**4**

**5**

Deep...

..and..

...subcutaneous sutures

*Clarke*

**6**

Stapler

Deep...

..and..

...subcutaneous sutures

Shirley sump drains

**7**

Deep ...and..

...subcutaneous sutures

drains

**8**

drains

**9**

367

# Incisional Hernia Repair

Although improved suture materials (stainless steel wire, monofilament nylon, Prolene, etc.), in addition to improved techniques in closing the rectus fascia, have significantly reduced the incidence of incisional hernia, such hernias do occasionally occur.

They are, interestingly, rarely seen with the lower transverse Pfannenstiel-type incision. The etiology of incisional hernia can range from wound infection and subfascial hematoma to a disruption of the suture line secondary to coughing during the immediate postoperative period.

The purpose of the operation is to close the hernia and reinforce the fascia to reduce recurrence.

**Physiologic Changes.** The overall comfort of a patient is increased by eliminating the incisional hernia. Although the incidence of bowel obstruction is small, it can occur. The traditional physiologic principles of hernia repair apply equally to incisional hernias and inguinal hernias (i.e., high ligation and excision of the hernial sac and double reinforcement of the rectus fascia).

**Points of Caution.** Care must be exercised in making the initial incision to avoid lacerating a loop of bowel adherent in the hernial sac.

Adequate mobilization of both fascia and subcutaneous tissue should be made to allow both tissues to come together without tension.

---

## Technique

**1** The patient is placed on the operating table in a supine position. Palpation of the abdomen reveals the hernia. No attempt is made to excise the cutaneous portion of the hernial sac. A midline incision is made over the hernial area, excising the previous scar.

**2** The incision is carried down to the hernial sac, which generally represents the peritoneum or attenuated rectus fascia. The hernial sac is located, a small hole is made, the sac is completely explored with the finger, the peritoneal incision is extended, and all contents are removed from the sac. The margins of the sac itself are identified and excised with scissors. The margins of the rectus fascia are then identified, and the skin and subcutaneous fat overlying the rectus fascia are sufficiently mobilized to allow the rectus fascia to be developed as two overlying flaps similar to a double-breasted coat. This is initiated by placing a retractor under the skin margin, applying two Kocher clamps to the margin of the rectus fascia, and dissecting the skin and subcutaneous tissue from the rectus fascia with sharp dissection. The same procedure is carried out on the opposite side. The peritoneum is closed with a running 0 synthetic absorbable suture.

**3** A row of 28-gauge stainless steel wire or 0 nylon sutures is placed in the base of one flap and through the margin of the opposite flap as interrupted mattress sutures. These are tied in progression. The margin of the overlying flap is elevated by traction with small hemostats.

**4** The line of sutures from the inner flap is completed. The outer layer of rectus fascia is pulled over the inner layer and sutured with interrupted 28-gauge wire or 0 nylon mattress sutures.

**5** Any existing scar tissue in the skin and subcutaneous incision is surgically excised.

**6** The subcutaneous tissue is closed with interrupted 2-0 synthetic absorbable suture, and the skin is closed with a subcutaneous 3-0 Dexon suture.

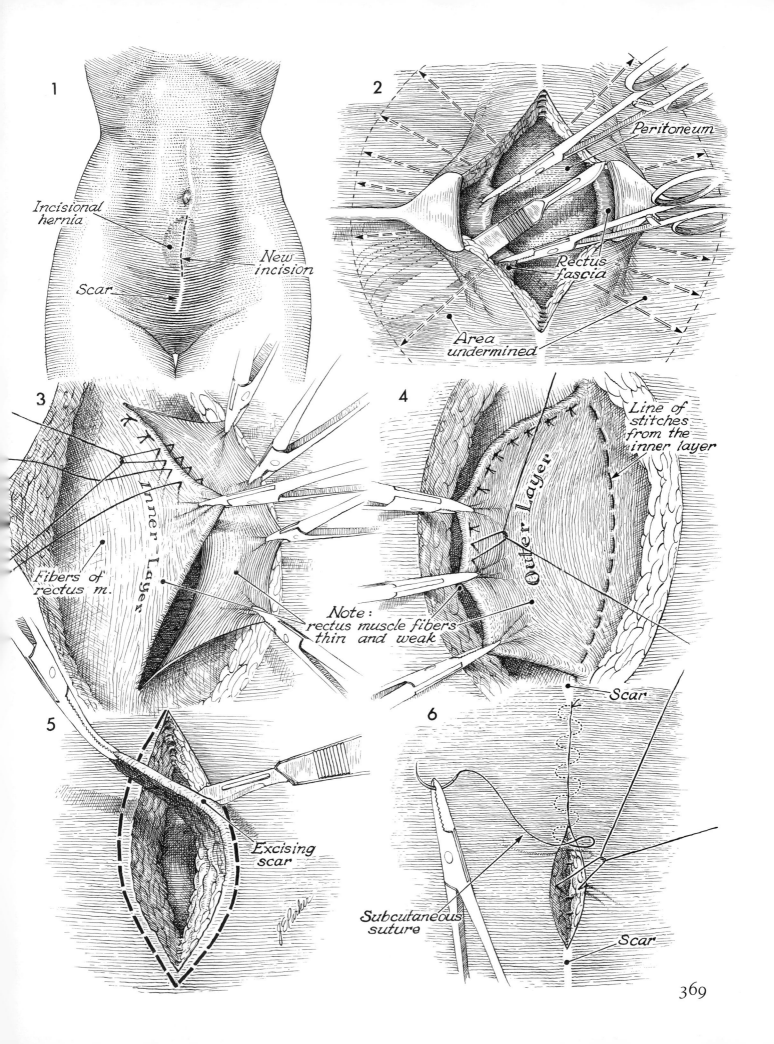

**1**

Incisional hernia

Scar

New incision

**2**

Peritoneum

Rectus fascia

Area undermined

**3**

Inner Layer

Fibers of rectus m.

Note: rectus muscle fibers thin and weak

**4**

Outer Layer

Line of stitches from the inner layer

Scar

**5**

Excising scar

J. C. Parker

**6**

Subcutaneous suture

Scar

369

# Abdominal Wound Dehiscence and Evisceration

The seepage of serosanguineous fluid through a closed abdominal wound is an early sign of abdominal wound dehiscence with possible evisceration. When this occurs, the surgeon should remove one or two sutures in the skin and explore the wound manually, using a sterile glove. If there is separation of the rectus fascia, the patient should be taken to the operating room for primary closure. Wound dehiscence may or may not be associated with intestinal evisceration. When the latter complication is present, the mortality rate is dramatically increased and may reach 30%.

The basic principles of management of abdominal wall dehiscence and evisceration are early diagnosis and surgical closure. The latter is accomplished by mass closure with wide sutures of heavy delayed synthetic absorbable suture.

The purpose of the operation is to close the abdominal wall.

**Physiologic Changes.** Dehiscence may stem from wound hematomas or from excessive intra-abdominal pressure secondary to abdominal coughing or vomiting that has disrupted the sutures. It is most commonly seen in patients with properties of poor wound healing, such as patients with diabetes, oncology patients, and patients taking steroid medications.

**Points of Caution.** All attempts should be made to diagnose and manage this problem promptly to minimize the risk of intestinal evisceration.

All sutures should be placed prior to tying any one suture.

---

## Technique

**1** The patient showing abdominal wall dehiscence with evisceration of the small intestine is placed in the supine position under general anesthesia.

**2** The contaminated edges of the wound including a combination of the peritoneum and rectus fascia are excised.

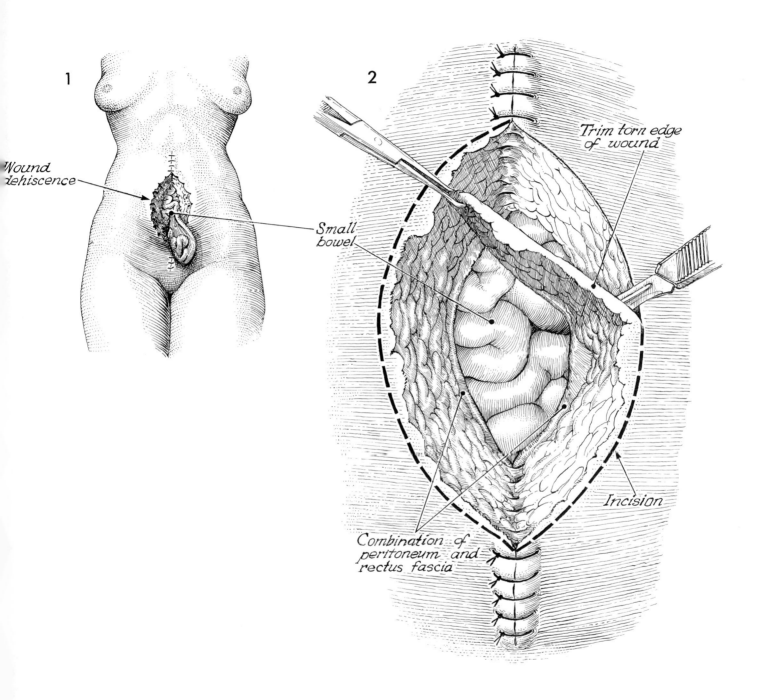

1

*Wound dehiscence*

2

*Trim torn edge of wound*

*Small bowel*

*Incision*

*Combination of peritoneum and rectus fascia*

371

# Abdominal Wound Dehiscence and Evisceration

## (Continued)

**3** At the xiphoid end of the incision, the needle is placed through *point a* to *point a'* through all layers of the rectus fascia muscle and peritoneum. When the needle is brought out of *point a'*, it is passed through the loop end of the suture.

**4** The needle is brought through *point b* to *point b'*, 2½ cm from *point a* and *point a'*, respectively.

**5** The sutures are not pulled taut for the remainder of the sutures *c* through *n*, *m*, etc. By leaving the sutures loose, the surgeon has the best opportunity to place the sutures precisely. When the sutures have been completely placed, they can be cinched up taut. Here one sees the technique of placing the final sutures from *m'* to *n*. One strand of the double suture is cut, while the uncut strand is passed through the wound opening beneath the abdominal wall and out of *point n* from inside to out.

**6** The sutures are cinched up snugly but are not tight. The two single-suture strands are tied after all loops have been tightened. Multiple throughs, more than five, are placed in this knot.

**7** The suture has been tied. To date, there has been no item of data to show that this closure has any less or any greater strength than the more time-consuming Smead-Jones closure with running far-to-near–near-far suture.

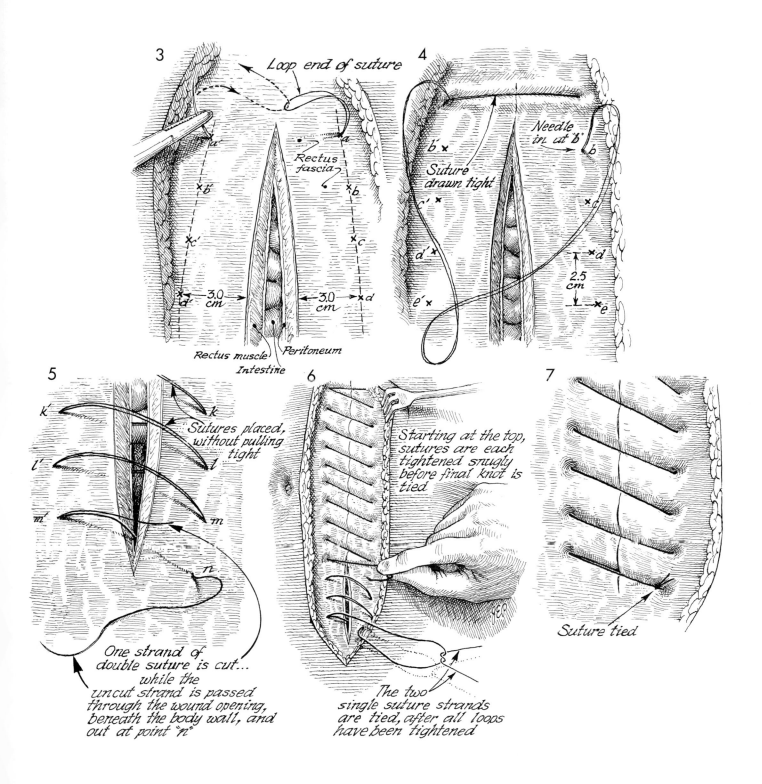

**3**

Loop end of suture

Rectus fascia

a′ ×

×b′

×c′

×d′ — 3.0 cm

a

×b

×c

×d — 3.0 cm

Rectus muscle    Peritoneum
Intestine

**4**

b′ ×

c′ ×

d′ ×

e′ ×

Suture drawn tight

Needle in at "b"

b

× c

× d    2.5 cm

× e

**5**

k′

l′

m′

Sutures placed, without pulling tight

k

l

m

n

One strand of double suture is cut...
while the uncut strand is passed
through the wound opening,
beneath the body wall, and
out at point "n"

**6**

Starting at the top,
sutures are each
tightened snugly
before final knot is
tied

The two
single suture strands
are tied, after all loops
have been tightened

**7**

Suture tied

373

# Massive Closure of the Abdominal Wall With a One-Knot Loop Suture

Techniques for closure of the midline abdominal incision have varied over time with better understanding of the physiology and engineering of closure of the abdominal wall and changes in materials in surgical suture. Closure of the midline through multiple layers including (1) the peritoneum and (2) the edges of the rectus fascia has evolved from braided products such as silk and cotton to synthetic braided products such as Teflon and braided nylon.

Contemporary surgical data show that closure of the peritoneum in a single layer in the pelvis or on the abdominal wall is unnecessary. Engineering sciences applied to wound healing have shown that the interrupted sutures have a weaker suture line than do running sutures. The weakest point in any suture line is the knot. Therefore more knots equal a weaker suture line, and less knots equal a stronger suture line. With the advent of delayed synthetic absorbable sutures, especially monofilament sutures, an entire abdominal midline incision from xiphoid to symphysis can be closed with the mass closure technique utilizing one knot.

**Physiologic Changes.** The physiology and engineering of this suture rely on the give and take of a suture line or cable line in any situation where total fixation of a suture through tissue with movement results in a "giggly saw" technique of tearing the tissue. Mass closure with the one-knot loop suture technique allows give of the suture with coughing, respiration, and movement. It basically holds the wound together and allows the properties of wound healing, the strongest of all wound-healing techniques, to take place without necrosis and closure by second intention.

**Points of Caution.** Monofilament suture should be used. Most wounds can be completely closed with delayed monofilament synthetic suture. There may be a place for monofilament synthetic permanent suture such as nylon or Prolene. The loop suture eliminates all the knots except one. Care must be taken to allow a 3-cm margin, wider than a man's finger, and to place the sutures 2½–3 cm apart. These characteristics of the length and width of the mass closure are necessary to conform to engineering principles.

## Technique

**1** An incision has been made from the xiphoid to the abdomen.

**2** At the xiphoid end of the incision, the needle is placed through *point a* to *point a'* through all layers of the rectus fascia muscle and peritoneum. When the needle is brought out of *point a'*, it is passed through the loop end of the suture.

**3** The needle is brought through *point b* to *point b'*, 2½ cm from *point a* to *point a'*.

**4** The sutures are not pulled taut for the remainder of the sutures from *c* through *n*, *m*, etc. By leaving the sutures loose, the surgeon has the best opportunity to place the sutures precisely. When the sutures have been completely placed, they can be cinched up taut. Here one sees the technique of placing the final sutures from *m'* to *n*. One strand of the double suture is cut, while the uncut strand is passed through the wound opening beneath the abdominal wall and out of *point n* from inside to out.

**5** The sutures are cinched up snugly but are not tight. The two single-suture strands are tied after all loops have been tightened. Multiple throughs, more than five, are placed in this knot.

**6** The suture has been tied. To date, there has been no item of data to show that this closure has any less or any greater strength than the more time-consuming Smead-Jones closure using a running far-to-near–near-far suture.

374

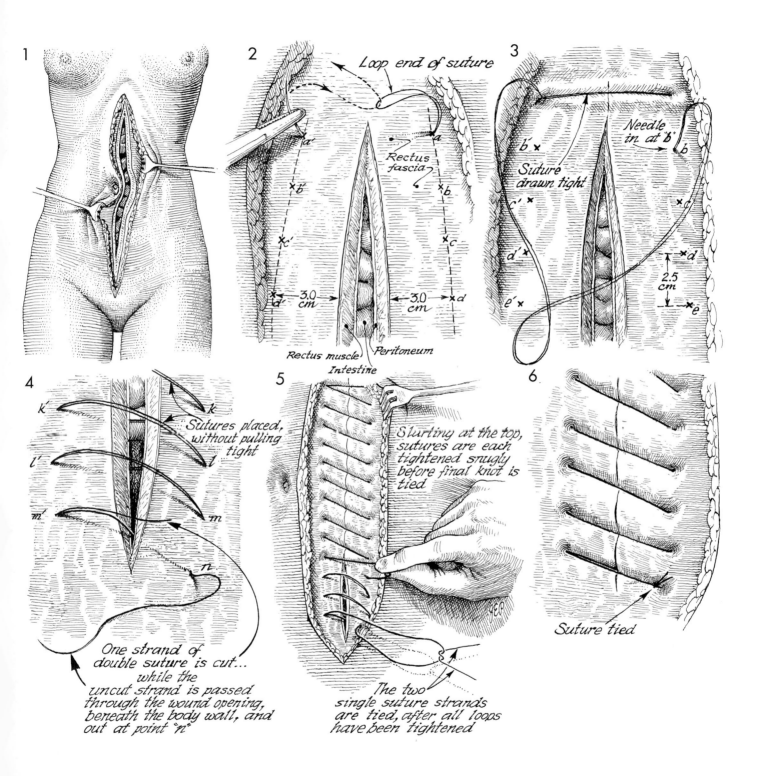

**1**

**2**

Loop end of suture

Rectus
fascia

a'    a

b'    b

c'    c

←3.0 cm    ←3.0 cm

d'    d

Rectus muscle
Intestine
Peritoneum

**3**

Needle
in at "b"

b'    b

Suture
drawn tight

c'    c

d'    d

2.5
cm

e'    e

**4**

k'    k

Sutures placed,
without pulling
tight

l'    l

m'    m

n

One strand of
double suture is cut...
while the
uncut strand is passed
through the wound opening,
beneath the body wall, and
out at point "n"

**5**

Starting at the top,
sutures are each
tightened snugly
before final knot is
tied

The two
single suture strands
are tied, after all loops
have been tightened

**6**

Suture tied

375

# Hemorrhage Control Following Laceration of Inferior Upper Epigastric Vessels

With the use of multiple trocar insertions through the abdominal wall, especially the left and right lower quadrants of the abdomen, there is a significant chance of the trocar injuring the inferior epigastric vessels located on the lateral aspects of the rectus abdominis muscle. Laceration of these vessels creates a significant abdominal wall hematoma. If the tears in the subfascia and peritoneum are significant, uncontrolled bleeding from the inferior epigastric vessels may enter the peritoneal cavity, and the patient could progress into hypovolemic shock without the appearance of an abdominal wall hematoma.

Before resorting to a laparotomy to control the bleeding, the surgeon is advised to first attempt hemorrhage control with a simple procedure using equipment available in any hospital, i.e., a Foley catheter and Kelly clamp.

**Physiologic Changes.** The changes are those of blood loss.

**Points of Caution.** Care must be utilized to select a Foley catheter that will easily fit the trocar sheath. After the hemorrhage has been controlled, the patient must be admitted to the hospital for close observation to ensure that the inferior epigastric vessels are adequately entrapped between the balloon of the Foley catheter and the Kelly clamp placed adjacent to the skin.

## Technique

1 The frontal view shows the relationship between the rectus muscle, the inferior epigastric vessels, and the insertion of a laparoscopic trocar in the lower quadrant of the abdomen. The cross-sectional view shows the relationship between the skin, rectus fascia, rectus muscle, inferior epigastric vessels, and the trocar that has perforated these vessels.

2 The trocar is withdrawn from the trocar sleeve. A Foley catheter is inserted down the trocar sleeve, and the balloon is inflated.

3 The trocar sleeve is advanced up the shaft of the Foley catheter, and traction is placed ventrally on the Foley catheter against the abdominal wall from within the abdominal cavity outward. The balloon is tightly lodged against the bleeding vessels to control hemorrhage.

4 To maintain the traction and thus the pressure on the bleeding vessels, a Kelly clamp is applied to the catheter adjacent to the abdominal wall skin.

The catheter balloon remains in place for 24–36 hours, after which the Kelly clamp is released, the balloon on the Foley is deflated, and the catheter is withdrawn from the wound. Additional observation is required to ensure that the bleeding is controlled. In most cases, this technique will control the bleeding without laparotomy.

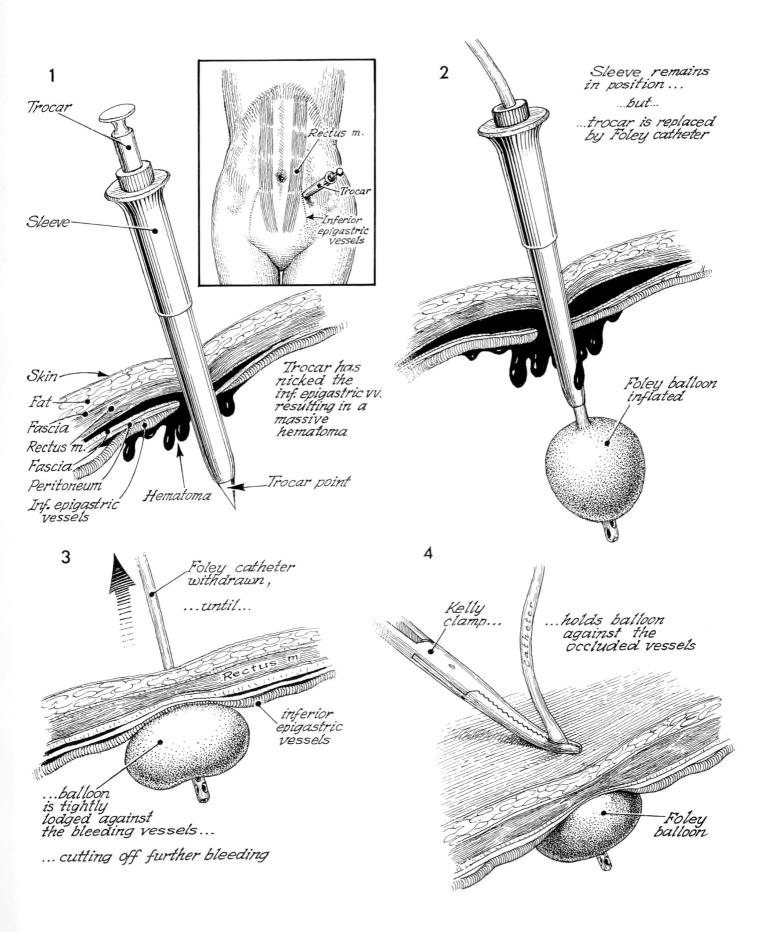

**1**

Trocar

Sleeve

Skin
Fat
Fascia
Rectus m.
Fascia
Peritoneum
Inf. epigastric
vessels

Hematoma

Trocar point

Rectus m.

Trocar

Inferior
epigastric
vessels

*Trocar has
nicked the
inf. epigastric vv.
resulting in a
massive
hematoma*

**2**

*Sleeve remains
in position...
...but...
...trocar is replaced
by Foley catheter*

Foley balloon
inflated

**3**

*Foley catheter
withdrawn,
...until...*

Rectus m.

inferior
epigastric
vessels

*...balloon
is tightly
lodged against
the bleeding vessels...*

*...cutting off further bleeding*

**4**

*Kelly
clamp...*

Catheter

*...holds balloon
against the
occluded vessels*

Foley
balloon

# 10

## Malignant Disease: Special Procedures

# Staging of Gynecologic Oncology Patients With Exploratory Laparotomy

Modern gynecologic oncology demands accurate staging of cancer patients in order to determine the most effective method of treatment. The noninvasive techniques formerly required for staging are being expanded to include extensive exploratory laparotomy. A significant percentage of patients may have more advanced disease than was noted with noninvasive clinical staging procedures.

Surgical staging as described in this section is of particular value in ovarian and endometrial carcinoma. Its role in epidermoid carcinoma of the cervix remains debatable at this time. The debate is not whether additional information can be gained; it can. The question is whether the overall end results warrant the additional morbidity associated with total pelvic and aortic irradiation following this type of surgical staging. Since it is particularly important for the surgeon to search under the diaphragm and to explore the aorta up to the level of the renal vessels, the Pfannenstiel incision is not advised.

The purpose of the operation is to gain detailed knowledge of the extent of metastasis of the pelvic malignancy.

**Physiologic Changes.** The most significant physiologic change is adhesion formation secondary to the procedure. This has an adverse effect if one contemplates total pelvic and aortic irradiation or intraperitoneal therapy. The adhesions fix the intra-abdominal structures, such as the bowel, thereby giving them maximum irradiation. Adhesions form pockets and block diffusion of intraperitoneal drugs to their targets.

**Points of Caution.** It is difficult to perform this procedure through a lower transverse incision because adequate exposure to the upper abdomen is compromised.

To adequately expose the renal vessels, the ligament of Treitz and the third portion of the duodenum frequently require mobilization.

## Technique

**1** The patient is placed in the supine position or the dorsal modified lithotomy position with the hips slightly abducted, the thighs parallel to the floor, and the knees flexed in obstetric stirrups. The incision should extend from the symphysis pubis to well above the umbilicus and, in many cases, up to the xiphoid.

**2 & 3** The initial exploration should start under the diaphragm. This area should be visualized directly or with the aid of a laparoscope. If studding is found under either the left or the right diaphragm, biopsy of the small lesions should be done.

**4** Washings should be obtained from five separate areas in the abdominal cavity under each diaphragm, in each lateral colonic gutter, and in the pelvis. These should be sent to the laboratory for cytopathologic studies.

**5** The exploration of the retroperitoneal space is begun by excising the peritoneum in the area of the cecum and terminal ileum.

**6** The peritoneum is incised parallel to the right common iliac artery. The incision is then advanced up the aorta until the third portion of the duodenum is encountered.

**7** At the third portion of the duodenum, the ligament of Treitz is noted and mobilized along with the duodenum to allow adequate exposure to the renal vessels.

**8** Lymph node excision is begun at the level of the left renal artery and vein, the origin of the right and left ovarian vessels. Adequate lymph sampling is performed along the aorta. VC indicates vena cava.

**9** The peritoneum overlying the aorta is closed with 3-0 synthetic absorbable sutures.

At this point, the oncologic procedure, whether it be a Wertheim hysterectomy for cervical carcinoma, tumor debulking for ovarian carcinoma, or extra fascia hysterectomy for uterine carcinoma, can begin.

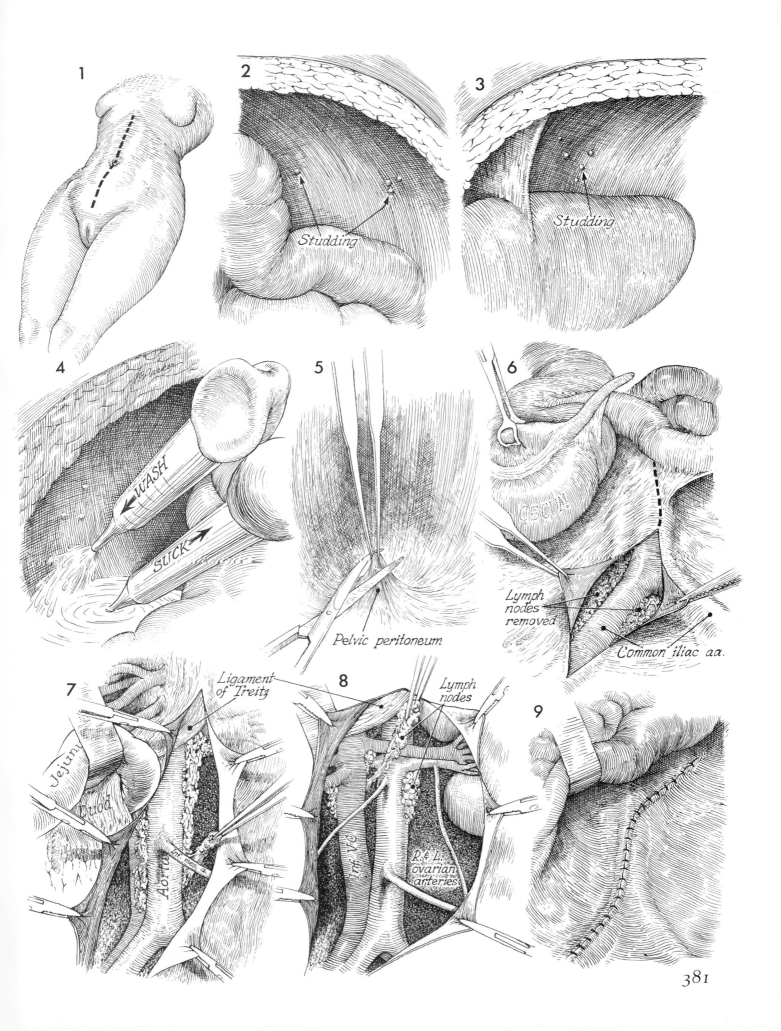

**1**

**2**

Studding

**3**

Studding

**4**

WASH

SUCK

**5**

Pelvic peritoneum

**6**

CECUM

Lymph
nodes
removed

Common iliac aa.

**7**

Jejunum

Duod.

Aorta

Ligament
of Treitz

**8**

Lymph nodes

Inf. V.C.

R. & L.
ovarian
arteries

**9**

# Subclavian Port-A-Cath

Oncology patients frequently require central venous access by catheter for chemotherapy, parenteral nutrition, and blood withdrawal. In some patients, after multiple surgical procedures and/or chemotherapy, venous access to the arms rapidly becomes unavailable. The same technique for Port-A-Cath can be used for Hickman and Gresbourg catheters required for total parenteral nutrition.

**Physiologic Changes.** Because there is greater blood flow through the central veins than through the peripheral veins, parenteral nutrition and chemotherapy can be administered through the central lines with less risk of causing chemical phlebitis.

**Points of Caution.** The patient must be placed in the Trendelenburg position. This increases the central venous pressure and avoids the possibility of an air embolism rising in the central venous system.

The guidewire or catheter should not be left in the atrium because its presence may cause arrhythmia.

The Silastic catheter should never be pulled back through the shaft of a needle. The tip of the needle can lacerate the catheter and release it as a foreign body within the venous system.

To prevent the development of a gas embolus, all syringes or catheters that are placed in the central venous system should be filled with a heparinized saline solution.

# Subclavian Port-A-Cath

## (Continued)

## Technique

**1** The patient is placed in a 15° Trendelenburg position to increase central venous pressure and thereby reduce the chances of air embolism. The subclavian vein has greater exposure if the shoulders are hyperextended over a rolled towel placed longitudinally between the scapula under the thoracic spine. The head should be turned to the opposite side. Under these conditions, the subclavian vein becomes more accessible. The skin over the neck and upper thorax is prepped in a routine fashion. Aseptic technique should be followed. A 2-inch, 14-gauge needle attached to a 10-mL syringe with 2–3 mL of heparinized saline solution in the syringe should be inserted through the skin with the bevel of the needle pointing down. The ideal site for the puncture is at the inferior border of the middle of the clavicle directed toward a fingertip pressed firmly into the suprasternal notch. The needle should be passed beneath the inferior margin of the clavicle in a horizontal plane and directed toward the anterior margin of the trachea at the level of the suprasternal notch. The needle and syringe are kept parallel to the surface of the patient's bed and adjacent to the anterior wall of the subclavian vein in the direction of its long axis. The accuracy of the placement into the subclavian vein can be demonstrated by a copious flow of blood into the barrel of the syringe with slight negative pressure. The syringe is removed from the hub of the needle, and the thumb is immediately placed over the hub.

**2** A flexible guidewire is inserted through the hub of the needle and passes into the superior vena cava (SVC).
When the guidewire is securely in the superior vena cava, the needle is withdrawn over the guidewire and removed.

**3** The guidewire is shown as it enters the skin under the clavicle. The ideal site for the Port-A-Cath chamber is selected; it is between two ribs, approximately 8 cm from the point where the guidewire enters the skin. A 4-cm incision is made in this area, and a pocket is created under the subcutaneous fat on top of the pectoralis fascia. Hemostasis in this pocket is essential.

**4** The subcutaneous pocket is demonstrated by placing the Port-A-Cath, with the catheter attached, into the pocket. At this point, the eyes on the Port-A-Cath flange are sutured to the fascia of the pectoralis muscle with 3-0 nylon sutures.
The Port-A-Cath and the catheter are filled with heparinized saline solution. This is achieved by inserting a Huber needle attached to a syringe of heparinized saline. The entire Port-A-Cath and catheter are filled with saline solution before any attempt is made to insert the catheter into the venous system.

**5** A 1-cm incision is made adjacent to the guidewire underneath the clavicle. An alligator-mouth grasping forceps is tunneled through the small incision down to the larger subcutaneous pocket. The alligator-mouth jaws grasp the catheter and pull it through the subcutaneous pocket, out through the incision next to the guidewire in the subclavian vein.

**6** The Port-A-Cath chamber is shown at the lower right. The skin incision over the Port-A-Cath is closed with fine suture or the skin stapler. At this point, a vein dilator sheath is inserted over the guidewire through the 1-cm skin incision under the clavicle and down into the subclavian vein. Note that the catheter exits the skin adjacent to the vein dilator sheath.

**7** The guidewire is withdrawn through the vein dilator sheath and removed. A finger is inserted over the vein dilator to prevent air from entering the subclavian vein. The Port-A-Cath catheter is measured from the subcutaneous pocket up to the subclavian vein and down an estimated distance in the superior vena cava. The excess catheter is cut away with sharp scissors.
The catheter is threaded through the vein dilator sheath into the subclavian vein and, ultimately, into the superior vena cava.

**8 & 9** The vein dilator sheath is constructed so that it will tear away as it is pulled out of the subclavian vein. This is achieved by placing the finger on each flange of the vein dilator sheath. An assistant threads the catheter farther into the superior vena cava. The sheath is withdrawn as it is split apart. The vein dilator sheath is removed entirely.
At this time an x-ray picture is taken (either by fluoroscopy or from the flat plate of the chest) to ascertain the position of the catheter. If it is in the right atrium, it is withdrawn 4–5 cm through the skin incision. When the catheter is in the appropriate position, the skin incision is closed with fine suture or skin staples. A heparinized saline solution in a 10-mL syringe with a Huber needle is placed through the skin into the Silastic diaphragm Port-A-Cath, and the entire system is flushed with 10 mL of heparinized saline solution.

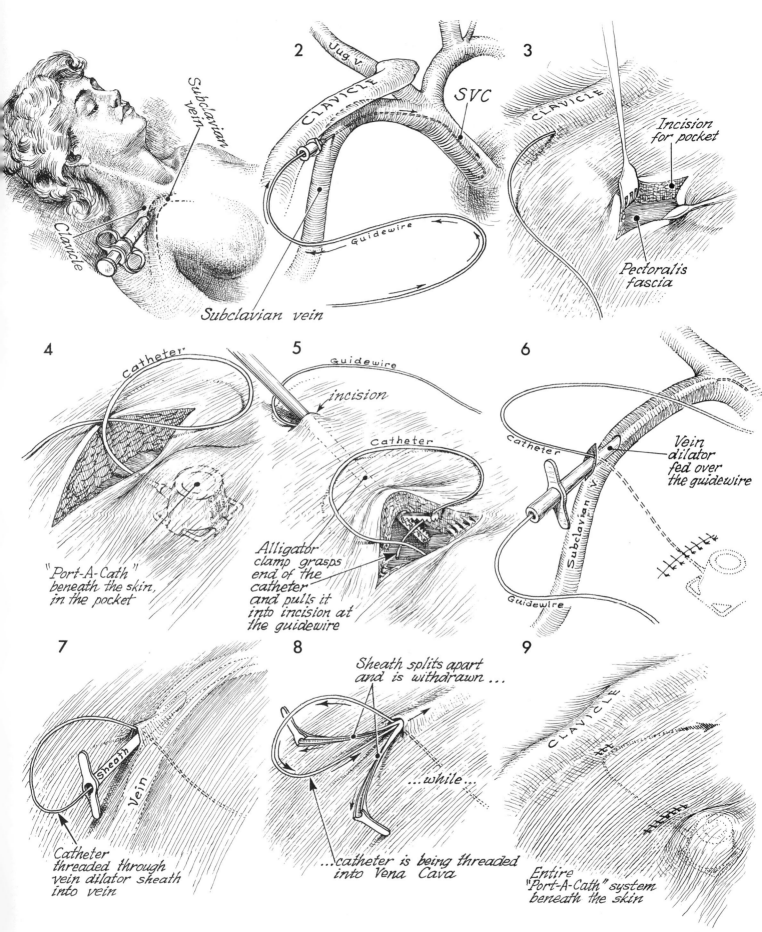

**2**

Jug. V.

CLAVICLE

SVC

Subclavian vein

Guidewire

**3**

CLAVICLE

Incision for pocket

Pectoralis fascia

Subclavian vein

Clavicle

**4**

Catheter

"Port-A-Cath" beneath the skin, in the pocket

**5**

Guidewire

incision

Catheter

Alligator clamp grasps end of the catheter and pulls it into incision at the guidewire

**6**

Catheter

Vein dilator fed over the guidewire

Subclavian V.

Guidewire

**7**

Sheath

Vein

Catheter threaded through vein dilator sheath into vein

**8**

Sheath splits apart and is withdrawn ...

...while...

...catheter is being threaded into Vena Cava

**9**

CLAVICLE

Entire "Port-A-Cath" system beneath the skin

385

# Peritoneal Port-A-Cath

Recent data indicate that some forms of intraperitoneal chemotherapy for ovarian malignancies with small volume disease may be more efficacious than intravenous chemotherapy.

**Physiologic Changes.** Intraperitoneal chemotherapy allows a greater dose of drug to come into direct contact with tumor cells and, at the same time, secondary to the large molecular weight of the chemical, facilitates a delayed absorption across the peritoneum into the vascular space. Therefore, a smaller dose of the drug arrives at sensitive target organs, such as kidney, nerve, and heart, per unit of time.

The length of time the cancer cells spend under the curve of the ultimate dose of chemotherapy is important. After an appropriate time under the "curve," the adjacent normal cells receive no further damage from the drug because the chemotherapy can then be withdrawn. Withdrawal reduces the time that the drug is administered to the systemic circulation. This reduces the toxicity associated with chemotherapy.

**Points of Caution.** A Port-A-Cath intraperitoneal chemotherapy device should not be inserted if there is bacterial contamination of the peritoneal cavity.

The Port-A-Cath system should be flushed frequently with heparinized saline solution. Ideally, it should be flushed once a week to prevent clogging of the system with peritoneal fluid. It should always be flushed thoroughly after any infusion of chemotherapy.

## Technique

**1** The patient is placed in the supine position. The surgeon selects a site for the Port-A-Cath by penetrating the abdominal wall with a 17-gauge Tuohy needle. A saline syringe is attached to the needle, and assessment is made for easy flow into the peritoneal cavity to ascertain when the point of the needle is free in the peritoneal cavity and when it is in an intraperitoneal organ or trapped between adhesions.

Another technique used to locate a site for the Port-A-Cath is to attach the hub of the needle to a pneumoperitoneum device, such as the laparoscopy carbon dioxide gas machine. If the needle is free in the peritoneal space, the flow pressure will be no higher than 10 mm Hg.

Several attempts are often required for placement of the needle several weeks after radical cytoreductive surgery.

When the appropriate spot has been located, a 6-cm "minilaparotomy" longitudinal incision is made in that area.

**2** The incision is carried down to the peritoneum, and the peritoneal cavity is entered. Dissection of bowel and adhesions may be required to achieve complete flow into the intraperitoneal space.

**3** A subcutaneous pocket of 6–7 cm is created on top of the rectus fascia. The Port-A-Cath is placed on top of the rectus fascia and secured with interrupted 3-0 nylon suture. At this point, the Port-A-Cath and its catheter are filled with heparinized saline solution.

**4** The incision in the rectus fascia peritoneum remains open, and the catheter from the Port-A-Cath is brought near that incision. A clamp is inserted through the fascia and peritoneum, and a small cutdown is made onto the tip of this clamp, approximately 3–4 cm lateral to the fascia and the peritoneal incision. The catheter is brought through this stab wound into the peritoneal cavity.

The Port-A-Cath catheter is arranged in a manner that will allow it to traverse the entire peritoneal cavity. The Port-A-Cath can be sutured to various points in the peritoneal cavity to allow maximum distribution of infused drug without creating the potential of a "clothesline" effect of the catheter whereby a knuckle of bowel can become involved in an internal hernia.

The incision in the peritoneum and rectus fascias are closed in layers with delayed absorbable sutures.

**5** The Port-A-Cath is in its pocket under the skin. The catheter travels through the peritoneal cavity to deliver the drug to the pelvis and upper abdomen.

The surgeon can adjust the placement of the catheter to meet individual needs. It can be placed adjacent to the liver, diaphragm, or wherever the maximum tumor burden lies.

The Port-A-Cath is flushed at the end of the procedure with heparinized saline solution.

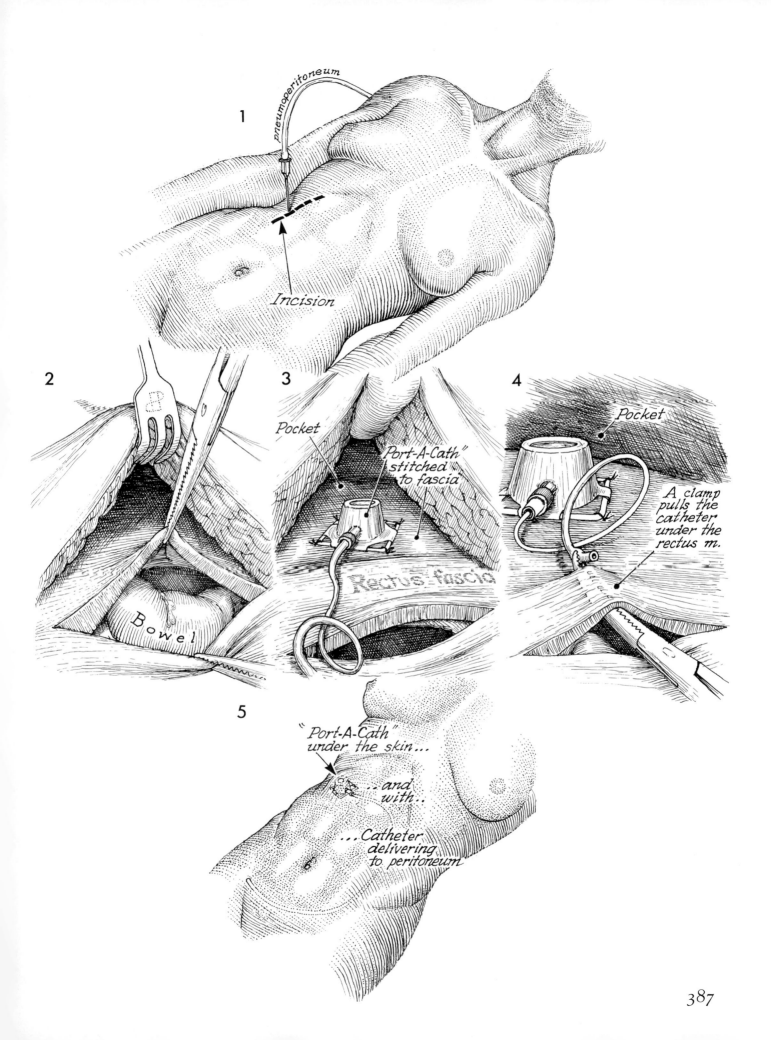

1

*pneumoperitoneum*

*Incision*

2

*Bowel*

3

*Pocket*

*Port-A-Cath" stitched to fascia*

*Rectus fascia*

4

*Pocket*

*A clamp pulls the catheter under the rectus m.*

5

*"Port-A-Cath" under the skin...*

*...and with...*

*...Catheter delivering to peritoneum*

# Application of Vaginal Cylinders for Intracavitary Radiation Therapy

Vaginal intracavitary radiation therapy is applied for two reasons: (1) to treat carcinoma directly in the vagina, the subvaginal mucosa and, in adenocarcinoma of the endometrium, the lymphatic and (2) to add radiation to *point* A in the isodose curve.

The largest cylinder that can comfortably fit the vagina should be used to achieve the most favorable isodose curve with the lowest surface dose. An intrauterine tandem can be inserted through the vaginal cylinder and can be loaded as the length of the uterus dictates. If the uterus is absent, the cylinders can be used alone to apply radiation therapy to the vagina.

The purpose of applying intracavitary therapy to the vagina is to irradiate the vaginal canal with ionizing radiation. In general, attempts are made to deliver 4000 cGy of radiation to the depth dose of 1.5 cm.

**Physiologic Changes.** The physiologic changes in this procedure are the same as for all procedures in which ionizing radiation is passed through normal and malignant tissue.

**Points of Caution.** The vaginal cylinders should be constructed so that they will fill the entire vaginal canal up to, but not beyond, the introitus. Care should be taken that no radium source extends beyond the vaginal introitus for fear that ulceration of the labia minora and majora will occur.

Fixation of the device should be made to ensure that the cylinder will not slip toward the introitus. This usually can be performed by suturing the labia together in the midline.

## Technique

**1** Cylinders of varying diameter can be easily constructed out of Silastic. The cylinders can be fashioned so that they can be added to each other in tandem to accommodate different vaginal lengths.

**2** If a Fletcher uterine tandem is to be used, it should be inserted into the entire length of the endometrial canal. The vaginal cylinders can then be loaded on the tandem. The radium sources can be inserted through the center of the tandem in a manner that will deliver the desired isodose curve for the uterus, cervix, and vagina.

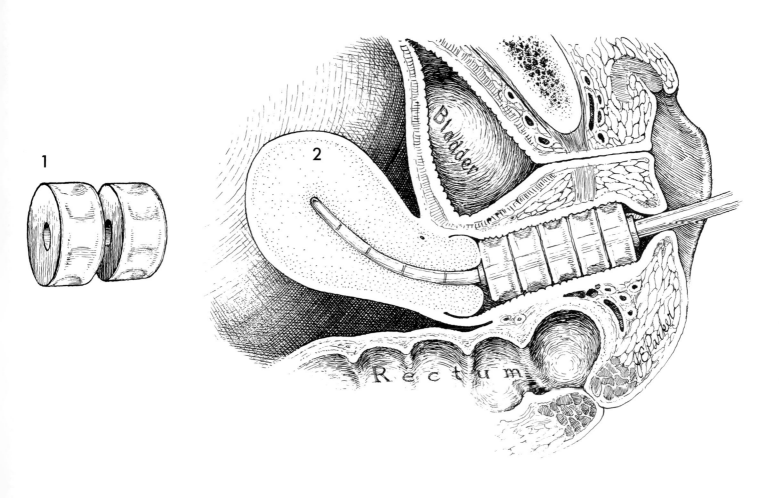

1

2

Bladder

Rectum

# Application of Uterine Afterloading Applicators for Intracavitary Radiation Therapy

Therapy for carcinoma of the cervix can be achieved with pelvic irradiation. It is difficult to deliver appropriate doses of ionizing irradiation to the cervix with external beam therapy alone. Therefore, the proper application of intracavitary radiation therapy to the cervix in a manner that produces an isodose curve that will deliver maximum irradiation to the cervix, lower uterine segment, parametrium, and upper vagina is vital.

It is not the purpose of intracavitary therapy to irradiate the pelvic wall. This must be done by external beam therapy. To date, a combination of properly applied paracervical and intrauterine irradiation along with external beam therapy has given the best results for cure of carcinoma of the cervix in advanced stages.

The purpose of this operation is to apply a uterine tandem with symmetrically placed paracervical ovoids in a manner that will deliver maximum irradiation to the cervix without excessive irradiation to the base of the bladder or rectum.

**Physiologic Changes.** Physiologic changes in this operation are those of ionizing irradiation passing through malignant tissue.

**Points of Caution.** It is vital that the cervical os be identified and the endocervical canal and endometrial cavity be sounded prior to insertion of the intracavitary therapy applicators. This can be one of the most difficult parts of this procedure. The cervical os is generally more posterior than it would seem because the malignant tissue expands from the anterior lip and distorts the configuration of the cervix.

The uterine tandem should be inserted into the entire length of the endometrial canal.

The ovoids should be positioned so that they are in the vaginal fornices and there is approximately 3.0 cm between the surfaces of the two ovoids. The upper vagina should not be stretched.

Gauze packing should be applied in a manner that gives maximum distance between the sources and the base of the bladder and rectum.

## Technique

**1** A weighted posterior retractor is placed in the vagina. The anterior lip of the cervix is grasped with a wide-mouth tenaculum, such as a Jacobs tenaculum. Single-toothed tenacula should be avoided to prevent tearing of tumor tissue. The cervical os is identified, and the uterus is sounded for depth and direction. A tapered cervical dilator, such as a K-Pratt dilator, is used to dilate the cervical canal to 6 mm.

**2** The Fletcher tandem is inserted up to the uterine fundus, and the flange on the tandem is locked into position. If perforation occurs and the position of the tandem is in doubt, diagnostic laparoscopy may aid the surgeon in repositioning the tandem within the uterus.

**3** The largest Fletcher ovoid is fitted for size. The largest ovoids that will symmetrically fit into the vaginal fornices are selected and placed. The upper vagina should not be stretched. The fulcrum of the ovoid applicator is locked.

**4** The tandem and ovoid applicator are packed into the vagina, leaving the maximum distance between the bladder and radium sources.

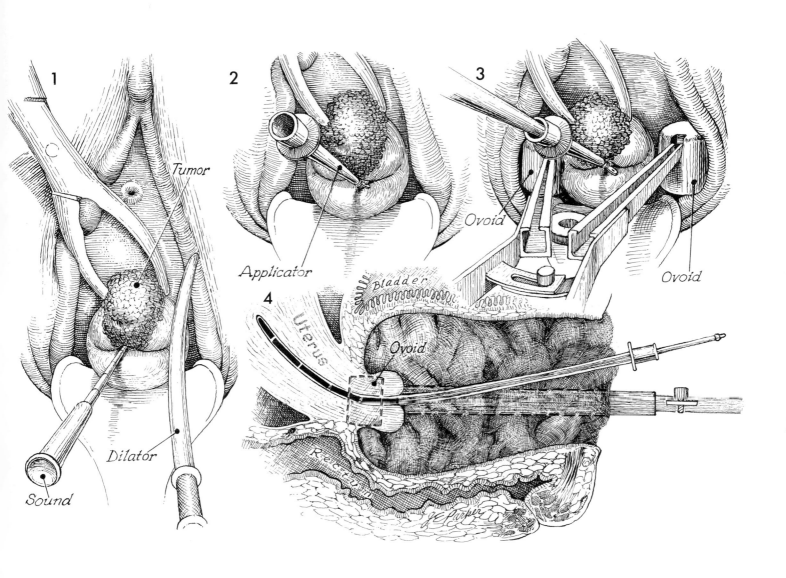

**1**

Tumor

Dilator

Sound

**2**

Applicator

**3**

Ovoid

Ovoid

**4**

Bladder

Uterus

Ovoid

Rectum

391

# Pelvic High-Dose Afterloader

If, at the time of total pelvic exenteration, tumor margins are close to the pelvic wall or if microscopic tumor remains on the pelvic wall in the area of radical excision of the pelvic wall, it is recommended that the tumor bed be irradiated even if the patient has already received total pelvic irradiation and intracavitary radiation therapy.

**Physiologic Changes.** After total pelvic irradiation to 5000 cGy plus intracavitary radiation sources, either intracavitary radiation therapy with tandem and ovoid or high-dose afterloader techniques, the tumor on the pelvic wall frequently has not received enough irradiation to destroy it. In fact, the pelvic wall frequently receives no more than 5600 cGy in most techniques. Thus after total pelvic exenteration, there may be additional microscopic tumor present. It would be extremely difficult and dangerous to give more external beam therapy to the pelvic wall, and because of the inverse square law, there would be no method of giving standard tandem and ovoid therapy in the vagina that would significantly reach the pelvic wall.

Therefore, if, following total pelvic exenteration, microscopic tumor remained on the pelvic wall, the high-dose afterloader technique could be used through a standard support frame device to give an additional cytoreductive dose of radiation to the tumor.

**Points of Caution.** The destructive effect of radiation on the external iliac artery and vein and the possibility of radiation osteomyelitis to the ischial bones of the pelvis must be considered. In addition, the radiation should be covered by omental flaps or a rectus abdominal flap to give greater distance from the high-dose afterloader tubes in order not to damage adjacent intestine and allow neoangiogenesis to revascularize the pelvic wall.

---

## Technique

**1** A total pelvic exenteration has been performed. Microscopic tumor remains on the pelvic side wall. One notes the stump of the rectum, the vagina, and the urethral meatus. The ureters have been cut at the pelvic brim.

**2** The high-dose afterloader tubes for delivery of the radioactive material are seen placed into the slots of the frames that have been designed to deliver an even isodose curve of irradiation to the tumor. The high-dose afterloader frames manufactured out of a modified polygalactide L-lactide material that will undergo hydrolysis when left in the pelvis do not require removal.

**3** The omental flap plus a rectus abdominis muscle flap ("VARM" flap) is moved over the frames and the radiation tubes to protect the adjacent intestine by at least 4 cm and allow neoangiogenesis to revascularize the pelvic wall.

**4** The radiation tubes are exteriorized through the right flank or right lower quadrant and attached to the high-dose afterloader device. At the completion of the radiation treatment, the tubes can be surgically removed. The frames, made of polygalactide L-lactide, will dissolve.

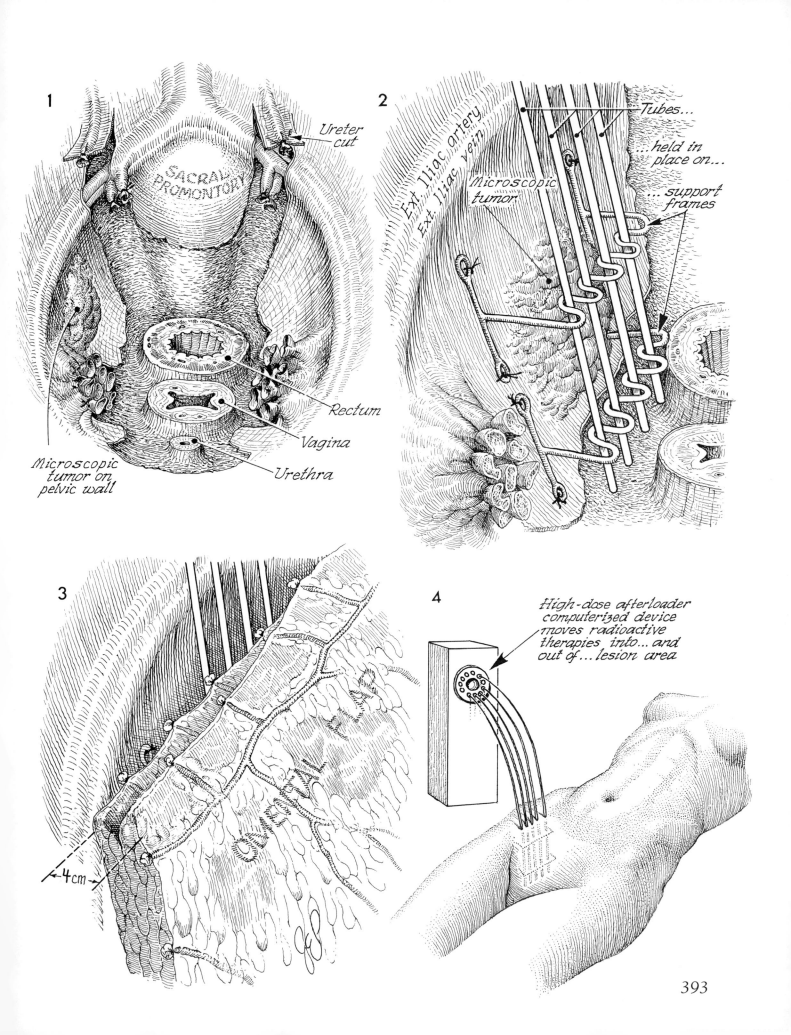

**1**

Ureter cut

SACRAL PROMONTORY

Rectum

Vagina

Urethra

Microscopic tumor on pelvic wall

**2**

Ext. Iliac Artery
Ext. Iliac vein

Microscopic tumor

Tubes...

...held in place on...

...support frames

**3**

4cm

**4**

High-dose afterloader computerized device moves radioactive therapies into...and out of...lesion area

393

# Abdominal Injection of Chromic Phosphate ($^{32}$P)

$^{32}$P is indicated in those cases of ovarian carcinoma where all bulk disease has been removed, and it is necessary to destroy tumor cells or micronodules of tumor less than 4 mm in diameter.

Although a Silastic catheter can be inserted at the time of laparotomy, it should not be exteriorized but left in a subcutaneous pocket, because if it is exteriorized, by the seventh or eighth postoperative day it will be grossly contaminated and the patient will be at risk for peritonitis. Care should be taken to ensure that there is no drainage of fluid from old closed suction drain sites prior to injecting the radionucleotide.

The purpose of the operation is to inject $^{32}$P into the peritoneal cavity in a manner that will allow free flow of the fluid throughout the peritoneal cavity. It should deliver 6000 rads to a depth of 3 mm on the peritoneal surfaces.

**Physiologic Changes.** $^{32}$P is an emitter of a beta particle. The penetration power of a beta particle is 4 mm. It has its effect on cells and micronodules of tumor. It is not effective against bulk tumor.

**Points of Caution.** It is imperative that the paracentesis needle be properly placed in the peritoneal cavity and not in an organ or a pouch formed from postoperative adhesions.

## Technique

**1 & 2** The patient is placed in the supine position on the radiology fluoroscopy table. A 16-gauge needle is used to perforate the anterior abdominal wall under local anesthesia. A Silastic catheter is threaded through the needle into the peritoneal cavity, and a test dose of radiopaque dye and saline solution is injected under fluoroscopic control. If the dye diffuses throughout the abdomen and there is no pooling, the position of the catheter is accepted.

**3** $^{32}$P is drawn up in a syringe, attached to a three-way stopcock, and injected in one push. A container of intravenous saline solution is then attached to the other arm of the three-way stopcock, and 1000 mL are allowed to flow into the peritoneal cavity, diluting the $^{32}$P and promoting a flow of the radionucleotide throughout the abdomen.

**4** The patient is rotated from side to side and from the Trendelenburg to reverse Trendelenburg position to facilitate the spread of the radionucleotide over the liver, under the diaphragm, and throughout the peritoneal cavity.

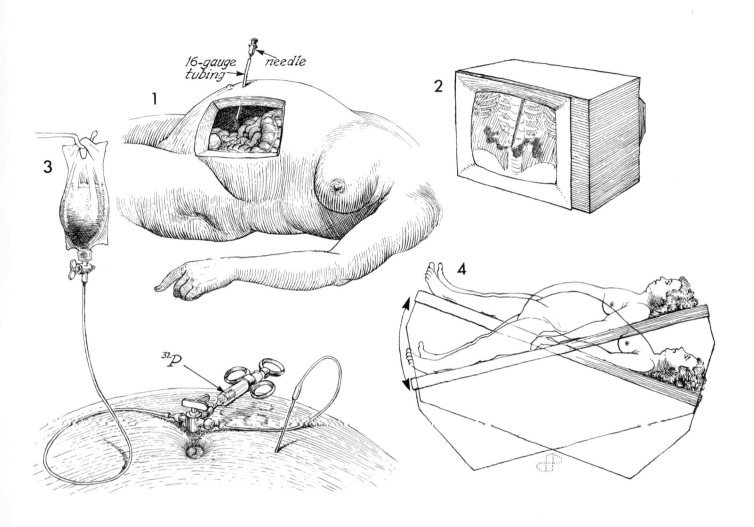

1

16-gauge tubing     needle

2

3

$^{32}P$

4

395

# Supracolic Total Omentectomy

Supracolic total omentectomy is performed in conjunction with surgery for ovarian carcinoma. It is important that patients with ovarian carcinoma be operated on through an extended midline incision, generally one from the xiphoid to the symphysis. It is difficult to perform an adequate omentectomy through a transverse or Pfannenstiel incision, and all too often such omentectomies result in incomplete excision of the tumor-bearing omentum, leaving tumor in the remaining portion of the omentum. It is instructive to discover on pathology the degree of micrometastasis in the omentum associated with ovarian carcinoma when clinically the omentum appears to be tumor free.

The purpose of the operation is to remove the total omentum and all gross and microscopic metastases therein.

**Physiologic Changes.** None

**Points of Caution.** The omentum should be removed from the greater curvature of the stomach and transverse colon. Care must be taken to secure the small omental branches of the right gastric artery. Meticulous hemostasis should be achieved.

---

## Technique

**1** The incision for total omentectomy must allow exposure to the upper abdomen. This is very difficult with a Maylard-type incision or any type of lower transverse abdominal incision.

**2** There is possible pathology in the omentum. The *dotted line* represents the line of excision for a supracolic omentectomy. Key anatomical features are the hepatic flexure of the colon, the spleen and its vascular supply, the splenic flexure of the colon, the cecum, and the rectum.

**3** After removing the omentum from the hepatic flexure of the transverse colon, the right gastroepiploic artery and its short gastric branches are identified. Small defects are made between each of the short gastric branches.

**4** The LDS (linear dissecting) stapler (United States Surgical Corp.) is applied to each of the short gastric branches by manipulating the stapler into the defects created in the omentum.

**5** The omentum is completely removed from the stomach.

**6** The left gastroepiploic artery has been stapled. The remaining omentum is removed from the transverse colon.

**7** The stomach and short gastric arteries are noted. The transverse colon has been cleaned, and the omentum totally removed.

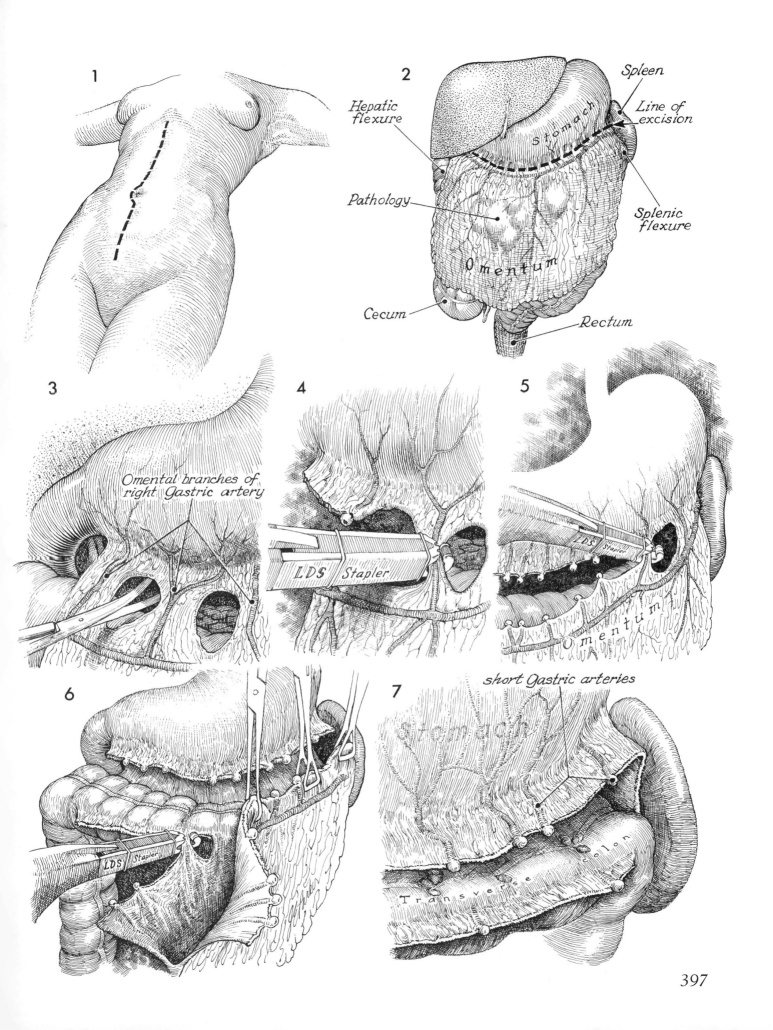

1

2

Hepatic
flexure

Spleen

Line of
excision

Pathology

*Stomach*

Splenic
flexure

Cecum

*Omentum*

Rectum

3

Omental branches of
right Gastric artery

4

LDS   Stapler

5

LDS   Stapler

*Omentum*

6

LDS   Stapler

7

short Gastric arteries

*Stomach*

*Transverse   colon*

397

# Omental Pedicle "J" Flap

An omental "J" flap provides (1) a nonirradiated vascular pedicle flap to cover intestinal anastomoses and (2) vesicovaginal-rectovaginal fistula repairs to form a lid on the inlet of the true pelvis after exenteration and to form a cylinder for a neovagina.

The purpose of this operation is to create a flap from the omentum by transecting the omentum from its attachments to the stomach, leaving enough branches of the left gastroepiploic vessels to provide an adequate blood supply for the flap.

**Physiologic Changes.** Irradiation produces obliterative endarteritis, ischemia, and fibrosis, all of which retard healing. By applying a vascular pedicle that has not been irradiated, the surgeon attempts to reverse some of the ischemia present in the irradiated tissue by promoting capillary and arterial ingrowth from the pedicle flap's blood supply. In addition, when the inlet to the true pelvis has been blocked by an omental lid, the small bowel is prevented from dropping into the denuded true pelvis after an extensive operation. Therefore, the possibility of intestinal obstruction and fistula formation is reduced. The omentum has a copious blood supply. Therefore, it is an excellent recipient of a skin graft for a neovagina.

**Points of Caution.** The short gastric vascular arcades to the omentum must be identified on the greater curvature of the stomach prior to initiating the procedure to ensure an adequate blood supply from the gastroepiploic artery remains for the proposed omental flap. The flap should be designed so the stomach is not pulled into the lower abdomen. The flap should not be placed on tension.

---

## Technique

**1** This operation is performed in conjunction with other radical pelvic surgery. Therefore, the appropriate incision for the initial procedure is adequate for the omental "J" flap. It is extremely difficult to perform the omental J flap through a transverse or Pfannenstiel incision, however, so a midline incision extended around the umbilicus is preferred.

**2** The design of the flap prior to transecting the omentum is essential. A centimeter ruler and unfolded sponge are helpful in determining the appropriate length needed for the flap to reach the pelvis without tension. A check of the vascular arcades should be made to ensure that an ample blood supply is entering the base of the flap. Generally, the transection of the omentum is started at the hepatic flexure of the colon and proceeds from the patient's right to her left.

**3** The omentum is opened in avascular areas with a small Kelly clamp or Metzenbaum scissors. The vascular bridges between these openings can be doubly clamped with Kelly clamps, incised, and tied with 2-0 suture.

**4** An alternative to Kelly clamps is the automatic LDS (linear dissecting) stapler (United States Surgical Corp.). This device clamps the vascular bridges between the openings in the omentum with the jaws of the stapler, applies two stainless steel clips, and activates a scalpel within the stapler to cut between the steel clips. It is a valuable, time-saving device.

**5** The omental flap is completed. It can be moved into the pelvis as a cover for a suture line or a pelvic lid.

1

2

* *Location of holes to be made in avascular areas*

*Line of incision*

3

4

stapler

LDS

5

OMENTAL FLAP

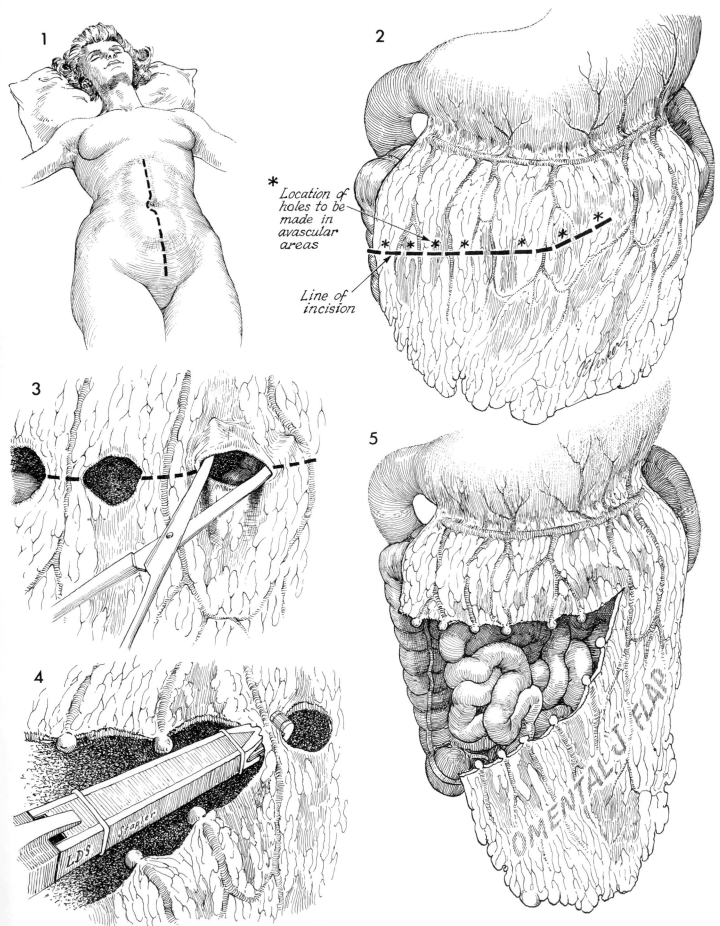

399

# Tube Gastrostomy

A tube gastrostomy can be used following extensive gastrointestinal surgery to decompress the intestines and, when indicated, to supply enteral nutrition.

**Physiologic Changes.** The gastrostomy tube decompresses the stomach and, while the adynamic process is in place, prevents air from passing into the small bowel. Hydrochloric acid is removed from the stomach. The volume of secretions removed from the stomach should be replaced intravenously with sodium chloride. The alternative to tube gastrostomy is a nasogastric tube. This is a space-occupying mass in the mediastinum. The tube gastrostomy eliminates the need for a nasogastric tube, thereby reducing dead space and improving respiratory function.

**Points of Caution.** Care must be taken to see that the gastrostomy tube is within the lumen of the stomach and has not been pulled back into the peritoneal cavity. This is accomplished by suturing the parietal peritoneum to the visceral peritoneum surrounding the gastrostomy and placing skin sutures to the gastrostomy tube.

## Technique

**1** This automatic pursestring suture device (United States Surgical Corp.) speeds the placement of the feeding gastrostomy.

**2** The stomach wall is picked up with a Babcock clamp. The automatic pursestring instrument is applied to a zone of the stomach.

**3** An incision is made within the circle of staples placed with the automatic pursestring suture device.

**4** An incision is made on the anterior abdominal wall at a convenient point adjacent to where the stomach would come up to the anterior abdominal wall.

**5** A Kelly clamp is inserted through that incision, and a Malecot catheter is grasped in the Kelly clamp.

**6** An incision is made through the middle of the pursestring sutures into the stomach wall. The Malecot catheter is seen piercing the abdominal wall into the peritoneal cavity.

**7** The tip of the Malecot catheter is pushed through the defect in the stomach. The pursestring suture is tied. Additional sutures are placed between the parietal and visceral peritoneum to seal off the stomach, where the catheter goes through both structures.

**8** The Malecot catheter is seen piercing the abdominal wall, piercing the stomach, and resting within the stomach.

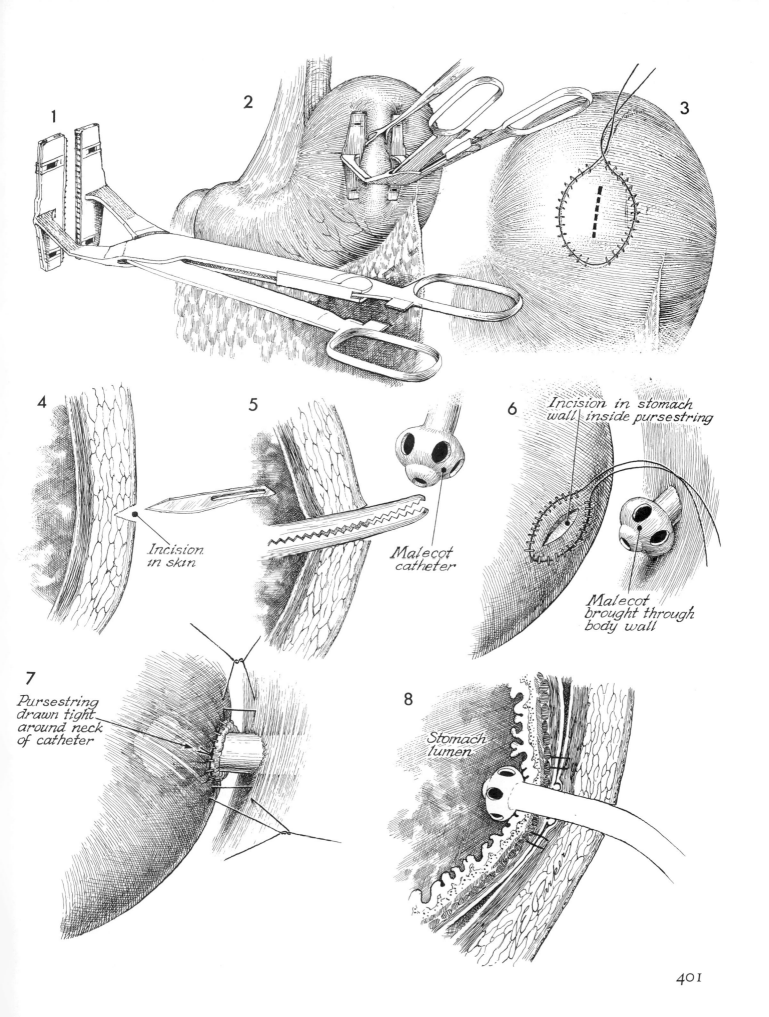

**1**

**2**

**3**

**4**

*Incision in skin*

**5**

*Malecot catheter*

**6**

*Incision in stomach wall inside pursestring*

*Malecot brought through body wall*

**7**

*Pursestring drawn tight around neck of catheter*

**8**

*Stomach lumen*

# Total Vaginectomy

Total vaginectomy is indicated for malignant disease of the vagina. It is frequently required in combination with total abdominal hysterectomy or radical Wertheim hysterectomy. It is the only alternative after total pelvic irradiation for recurrent microinvasive carcinoma of the vagina. The planes of dissection after irradiation are difficult, and there is a high risk of vesicovaginal and rectovaginal fistula. Preoperatively, the surgeon should advise the patient with regard to replacement of the vagina with a skin graft, and a preoperative plan should be made as the patient's sexual status indicates. Although the vagina is occasionally removed abdominally, the procedure is best initiated from the vaginal route. Frequently, an abdominoperitoneal approach is used because the operation is combined with either a radical hysterectomy or simple hysterectomy.

The purpose of the operation is to remove the vagina.

**Physiologic Changes.** If only the vagina is removed and no opening is made into the bladder or rectum, there is little physiologic change.

**Points of Caution.** The major complication of this operation, particularly after pelvic irradiation, is inadvertent vesicovaginal or rectovaginal fistula formation. Therefore, the dissection should be carried out in the most meticulous manner possible. If the surgeon can dissect within a plane outside the pubovesical cervical fascia, fistula formation will be reduced.

Meticulous hemostasis should be performed prior to introducing the split-thickness skin graft.

## Technique

**1** The patient is placed in the dorsal lithotomy position with her buttocks off the end of the table by approximately 8 cm. Adequate vaginal and pelvic examinations are performed, and appropriate biopsies are taken. The bladder is emptied by catheter drainage.

**2** An incision is made around the circumference of the vaginal vault down to the pubocervical fascia underneath the urethra and the perirectal fascia overlying the rectum.

**3** Since the blood supply to the vagina comes predominantly from the lateral side, dissection is begun there first. The vaginal epithelium is deviated to the midline, and Metzenbaum scissors are used to dissect the vaginal mucosa from its lateral wall.

**4** Care is taken to identify the vaginal branches of the pudendal artery, which should be securely clamped and tied.

**5** Dissection underneath the urethra and bladder is generally bloodless as long as it is confined to the plane between the vaginal mucosa and the pubovesical cervical fascia. If the pubovesical cervical fascia becomes involved, the small vessels in the bladder wall make hemostasis difficult.

**6 & 7** The dissection posteriorly should be performed in the plane above the perirectal fascia, or copious bleeding can occur from the hemorrhoidal plexus of vessels. When the dissection has reached the cul-de-sac posteriorly and the vesicouterine peritoneal area anteriorly, the vagina can be removed by itself, but it is generally removed in conjunction with total abdominal hysterectomy. The vaginal canal must then be managed according to the sexual needs of the patient.

If the patient is sexually active, a skin graft can be placed after meticulous hemostasis has been achieved (see Section 2, p. 91, on McIndoe vaginoplasty), or the vaginal canal can be closed by suturing the pubovesical cervical fascia to the rectal fascia posteriorly (see Section 2, p. 78, on the Le Fort operation). If a McIndoe vaginoplasty is to be performed, suction catheters should be left in the pelvic area and brought out through left and right lower quadrant stab wounds; or if closure of the vaginal space is indicated as in the Le Fort operation, they can be brought out through the lateral vaginal vault. A suprapubic Foley catheter is left in the bladder until voiding is established. *B*, bladder.

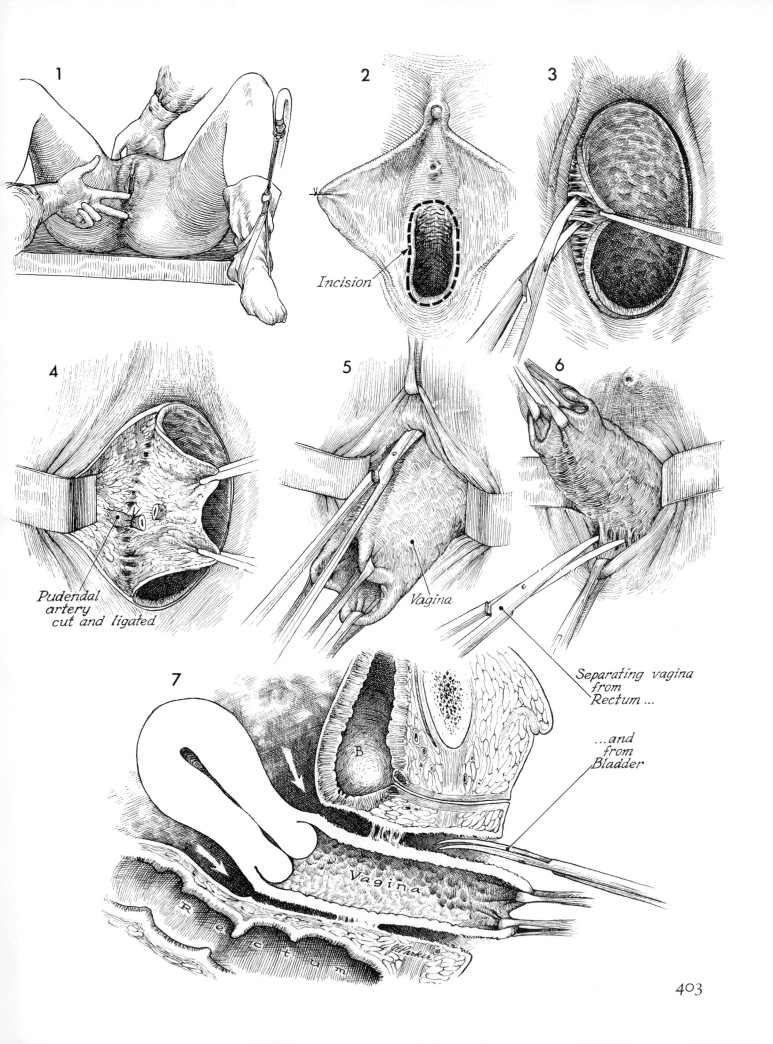

**1**

**2**

*Incision*

**3**

**4**

*Pudendal
artery
cut and ligated*

**5**

*Vagina*

**6**

*Separating vagina
from
Rectum ...*

*...and
from
Bladder*

**7**

*B*

*Vagina*

*Rectum*

403

# Radical Vulvectomy With Bilateral Inguinal Lymph Node Dissection

Radical vulvectomy with bilateral inguinal lymph node dissection is indicated in invasive carcinoma of the vulva. The operation is best performed in a single-stage procedure. Emphasis is placed on removal of the entire lesion with an adequate tumor-free margin.

The purpose of this operation is to remove the vulva, its adjacent structures, a margin of normal tissue, and the inguinal lymph nodes from the anterior superior iliac spine to the abductor canal in the leg.

**Physiologic Changes.** A large surgical wound is created by this operation. If it cannot be closed per primam without tension, it must be sealed with grafting or use of the new Sure-Closure skin stretcher. If it is allowed to granulate slowly, marked physiologic changes similar to those accompanying a burn, i.e., the loss of electrolytes, fluid, and protein and contracture, will occur from contracture.

Trauma to the femoral artery and vein increases the risk of thrombophlebitis and pulmonary embolism.

**Points of Caution.** Care must be taken that all lymph nodes are excised. The Cloquet node should be removed and sent for frozen section analysis. Pathologic analysis of this node determines if a deep pelvic lymph node dissection is indicated.

The surgeon must clearly identify the saphenous vein to avoid its accidental transection.

Before proceeding with dissection below the mons pubis, the surgeon must make an incision around the urethral meatus and vaginal introitus.

Mature surgical judgment is needed to ascertain whether the margins of the wound can be sufficiently undermined and mobilized to be brought together without tension. Radical vulvectomy incisions closed under tension will necrose and open in approximately 1 week. The Sure-Closure skin stretchers are an alternative to undermining skin flaps. Closed suction drainage of the wound has reduced seroma formation and its associated sequelae.

# Radical Vulvectomy With Bilateral Inguinal Lymph Node Dissection

## (Continued)

*Technique*

**1** The patient undergoing radical vulvectomy should be positioned on the operating table in the modified dorsal lithotomy position with the legs extended, giving adequate exposure to the lower abdomen and perineum. The hips should be abducted 30° and extended 5–10° with the knees flexed 90°.

The abdomen and perineum are surgically prepped. A Foley catheter is inserted in the bladder.

Although a variety of incisions can be used for this operation, one shaped roughly like the head of a rabbit is preferred. The proposed incision is marked with brilliant green solution, starting from the anterior superior iliac spine, sloping downward toward the mons pubis, lateral to the inguinal ligament, to a point adjacent to the pubic tubercle. At this point, it proceeds lateral to the labia majora and horizontal with a "W" incision across the perineal body, joining the incision lateral to the labia majora on the opposite side. A second incision, superior and medial to the first, slopes down toward the mons pubis and meets a similar incision from the other side.

This procedure is best carried out with two surgeons, each with an assistant, operating on both sides.

**2** The upper portion of the entire incision is made at one time. The incision is carried from the anterior superior iliac spine down across the mons pubis, up to the opposite anterior superior iliac spine, down lateral to the inguinal ligament to the pubic tubercle. The incision is carried through the skin down to the fascia. Metzenbaum scissors are used to dissect along the fascial surface, removing en bloc the skin and its subcutaneous lymph nodes.

**3** The inguinal ligament and rectus fascia have been cleaned of all nodal tissue. A retractor is used to deflect the skin overlying the sartorius muscle. The right and left fossae ovalis are identified. If identi-

fication of the fossae ovalis proves difficult, the fascia covering the sartorius muscle should be reflected medially to ensure total removal of the lymph nodes without lacerating vascular structures within the fossae ovalis.

**4** Structures within the femoral canal generally follow the code word "navel"; i.e., the most lateral structure is the femoral nerve followed in order by the femoral artery, vein, an empty space, and a lymphatic space. The femoral artery should be identified, and dissection should be carried along the artery until all lymphatic tissue is removed down to the adductor canal. The femoral nerve should be preserved, although occasionally a few of its terminal cutaneous branches must be sacrificed. The femoral vein should be identified along with the saphenous vein. This can be facilitated by noting the anatomic relationship between the circumflex artery, generally 1–2 cm above the junction of the femoral artery, and the saphenous veins.

**5** At this time, the Cloquet node is located, removed, and sent for pathologic analysis. The lymphatic dissection continues along the saphenous vein until it can be sufficiently freed for clamping and ligation.

**6** The saphenous vein is doubly clamped, incised, and tied with a 2-0 suture.

**7** The adductor longus muscle can now be identified and should be cleaned of all fatty nodal tissue by retracting the saphenous vein en bloc with the lymph nodes until the adductor canal is reached.

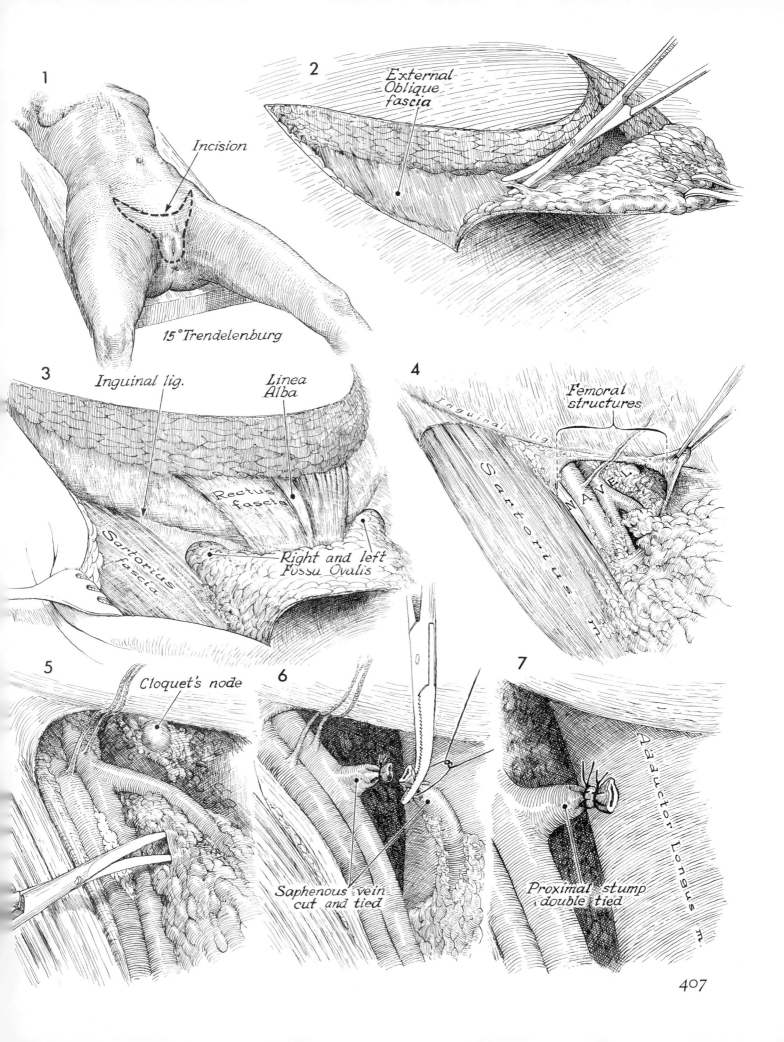

**1**

Incision

15° Trendelenburg

**2**

External
Oblique
fascia

**3**

Inguinal lig.

Linea
Alba

Rectus
fascia

Sartorius
fascia

Right and left
Fossu Ovalis

**4**

Femoral
structures

Inguinal lig.

Sartorius m.

NAVEL

**5**

Cloquet's node

**6**

Saphenous vein
cut and tied

**7**

Proximal stump
double tied

Adductor Longus m.

# Radical Vulvectomy With Bilateral Inguinal Lymph Node Dissection

## (Continued)

**8** The sartorius muscle is identified, mobilized, and transected at its insertion with the electrocautery.

**9** The sartorius muscle is transplanted over the femoral artery and vein.

**10** The sartorius muscle is sutured to the inguinal ligament with interrupted 2-0 suture. To reduce the possibility of hernia, a few 2-0 sutures are placed on the medial border of the sartorius muscle, suturing it to the adductor longus muscle.

**11** The lymph node dissection with the sartorius transplant portion of the operation has now been completed. The saphenous vein adjacent to the adductor canal is identified for the second time. It is clamped and tied with a 2-0 suture.

**12** The surgeon moves from the lateral side of the patient to the perineal area, and the entire surgical specimen is elevated with Allis clamps.

A careful outline of the vaginal introital incision is made with brilliant green solution. The incisions lateral to the labia majora are made down to the fascia.

**13** The pudendal artery and vein are clamped and tied prior to transection. The specimen is retracted medially with multiple Allis clamps. The incision is extended down the lateral border of the labia majora and superficially extended across the perineal body.

**14** The labia minora are retracted laterally with Allis clamps, and an incision is made in the vestibule around the urethral meatus, down around the introitus, across the posterior fourchette, and back up the other side.

**15** The en bloc specimen is retracted downward, and the surgical dissection is made along the fascia until the perineal body is reached.

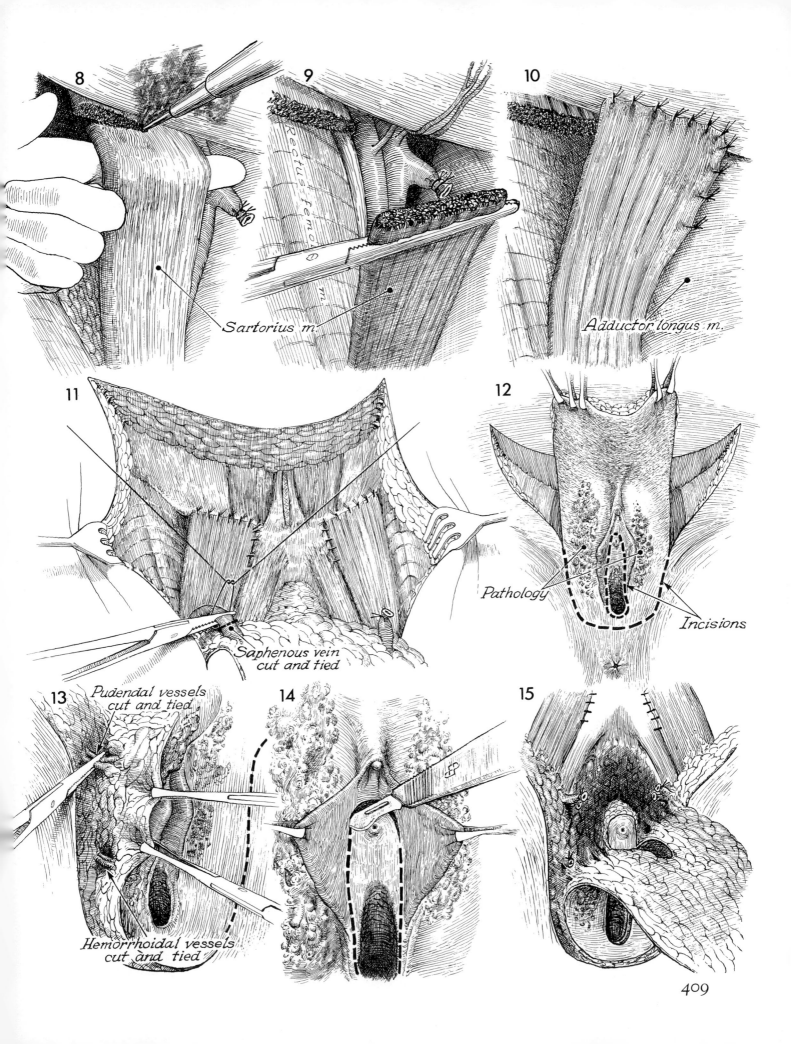

8

9

*Sartorius m.*

10

*Adductor longus m.*

11

*Saphenous vein cut and tied*

12

*Pathology*

*Incisions*

13

*Pudendal vessels cut and tied*

*Hemorrhoidal vessels cut and tied*

14

15

409

# Radical Vulvectomy With Bilateral Inguinal Lymph Node Dissection

## (Continued)

**16** The surgeon elevates the posterior vaginal mucosa with Allis clamps and undermines it for approximately 6–7 cm with curved Mayo scissors, releasing the rectum from the posterior vaginal wall.

**17** A Foley catheter is reinserted into the bladder. The wound is assessed to determine whether it can be closed primarily without tension by mobilizing adjacent tissue, should the Sure-Closure skin stretchers be used, or whether it requires a graft or flap.

Tissue lateral to the margin of the wound is undermined by sharp and blunt dissection. Closed suction drains are placed in the ischial rectal fossa.

**18** Closure of the wound is begun in the perineal body by suturing the subcutaneous tissues for 3 or 4 cm up to the posterior fourchette of the vagina.

The subcutaneous tissue of the thigh is sutured to the paravaginal tissue up to the level of the urethral meatus.

No attempt is made to suspend the urethral meatus to the fascia and periosteum of the pubic symphysis or use it for wound closure. Such a course is apt to produce postoperative urinary incontinence.

The subcutaneous tissue, from both sides of the incision lateral to the labia majora up to the pubic tubercle, is closed to the paravaginal tissue with interrupted 2-0 synthetic absorbable sutures.

Closed suction drains are placed in the ischial rectal fossa and under the closure of the vagina to the skin of the thigh.

**19** The skin of the perineal body is approximated with interrupted 3-0 nylon suture. The vaginal mucosa is sutured to the squamous epithelium around the entire introitus and vestibule with interrupted 3-0 nylon suture. The skin edges above the urethral meatus are sutured together for at least 3–4 cm with interrupted 3-0 nylon sutures.

**20** The skin of the lower abdomen is mobilized up to the umbilicus. There must be no tension on the suture line between the incision overlying the inguinal ligament and the margin of the skin of the lower abdomen.

**21** Suction drains are placed in the area of each sartorius muscle. These are usually sutured to the fascia with 4-0 synthetic absorbable suture to prevent accidental dislodgement. They are, however, easily removed with a gentle tug when they have ceased draining.

The mobilized lower abdomen is pulled down and sutured to the inguinal area in two layers.

**22** The skin margins have been approximated with interrupted mattress sutures of 3-0 nylon. Suction drains have been placed in each inguinal area and through the lower abdomen. A Foley catheter has been placed in the bladder.

Intermittent pneumonic pressure cuffs are applied to the lower legs for thromboembolic prophylaxis. The patient is kept at bed rest for 10 days.

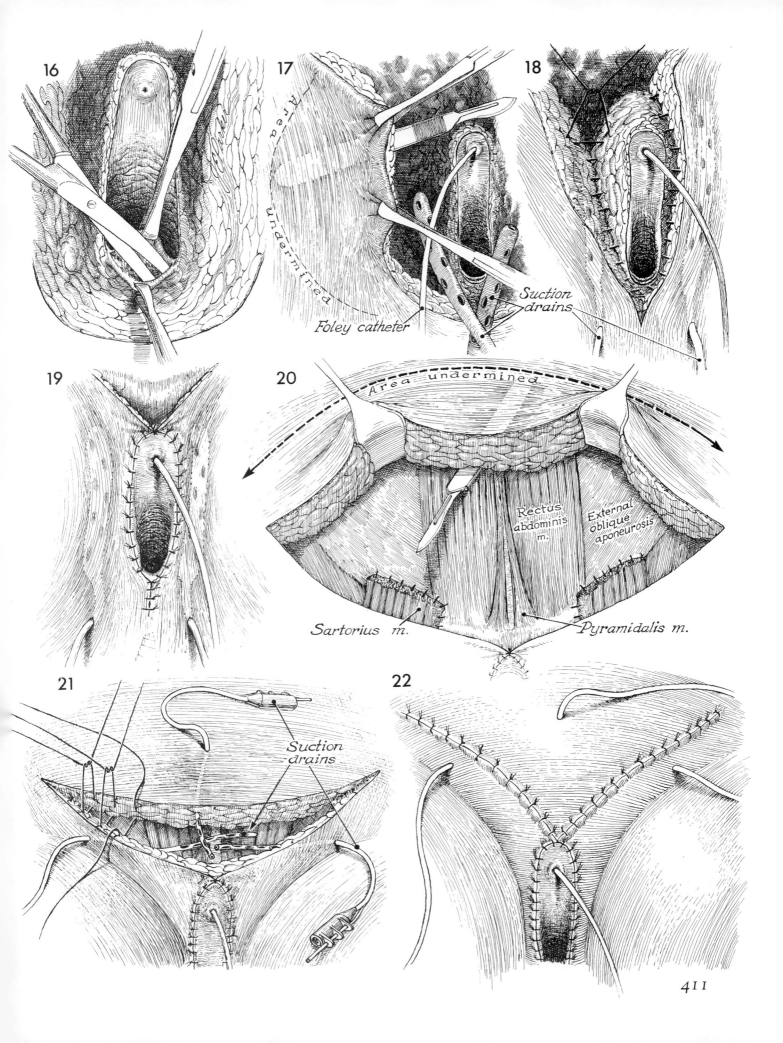

**16**

**17**

Area undermined

Foley catheter

Suction drains

**18**

Suction drains

**19**

**20**

Area undermined.

Rectus
abdominis
m.

External
oblique
aponeurosis

Sartorius m.

Pyramidalis m.

**21**

Suction
drains

**22**

411

# Reconstruction of the Vulva With Gracilis Myocutaneous Flaps

The gracilis myocutaneous flap is useful in those cases of large denuded defects in the perineum following radical vulvectomy or perineal surgery in which primary closure would likely result in postoperative dehiscence of the wound incision. It is not a substitute for the simpler Z-plasty pedicle flap that gives adequate results except when an extended area must be covered.

The principle of a myocutaneous flap is the creation of an island flap that depends on the underlying muscle for its vascular supply. Of course, the blood supply to the muscle underneath the flap must remain intact and viable, or the graft will not survive.

The purpose of the operation is to cover the vulvar defect with a cutaneous structure having its own nonirradiated or traumatized blood supply that can produce a healed wound per primam with a normal functioning vulva.

**Physiologic Changes.** The predominant physiologic change is the production of a vulva that is healed per primam without scarring or contracture.

**Points of Caution.** Care must be taken to accurately identify the gracilis muscle and not mistake it for the sartorius muscle. This is facilitated by extending the knee of the patient while abducting the hip 30°. With the patient in this position, the gracilis muscle is generally palpable.

Care must be taken to determine the size of flap needed prior to making the skin incision over the gracilis muscle. One of the most important points in the operation is to ensure that the neurovascular bundle of the gracilis muscle is preserved.

## Technique

**1** This patient has had a radical vulvectomy necessitating extensive removal of pelvic tissue. The patient is in a modified lithotomy position in which the hips are slightly flexed and the knee is extended but elevated approximately 30° off the operating table. The legs are abducted approximately 30° at the hip joint to give adequate exposure to the perineum and the skin of the inner thigh.

**2** The area of the defect is measured in centimeters to determine the size of graft needed. With the legs in this position, the gracilis muscle stands out. Its origin is on the ischial rami, and its insertion is at the knee.

**3** The anatomy of the inner thigh and vulva is shown, and the important anatomic landmarks are noted. The gracilis muscle is shown with its insertion on the ischial rami, with a cross section of the leg demonstrating the location of the essential neurovascular bundle that enters at the upper third of the gracilis muscle and exits between the adductor longus and adductor magnus muscles. Because of this consistent anatomic arrangement, the gracilis muscle is an ideal structure for the myocutaneous flap.

**4** After the measurements taken in Step 2 are recorded, a line is drawn on the skin down the middle of the gracilis muscle. A skin flap matching the dimensions of the defect is outlined on the inner thigh. The maximum flap that can survive from the neurovascular bundle feeding the gracilis muscle is approximately 24 × 8 cm. Such a large flap, however, is rarely required for gynecologic purposes. As demonstrated in Step 2, the defect in this case measures 19 cm in length and 6 cm in width. Therefore, a flap 21 cm long is drawn, leaving 2 cm for "overage."

**5** An incision is made full thickness through the skin and subcutaneous fat down to the muscular bundles.

**6** The gracilis muscle (G) must be identified after the distal skin incisions are made, prior to extension of the skin incision proximal to the vulvar defect. Otherwise, skin may be included in the flap that is not supplied by the gracilis muscle.

**7** The gracilis muscle (G) is isolated with an umbilical tape. The adductor longus (Al) and adductor magnus (Am) muscles are identified.

**8 & 9** The gracilis muscle is transected.

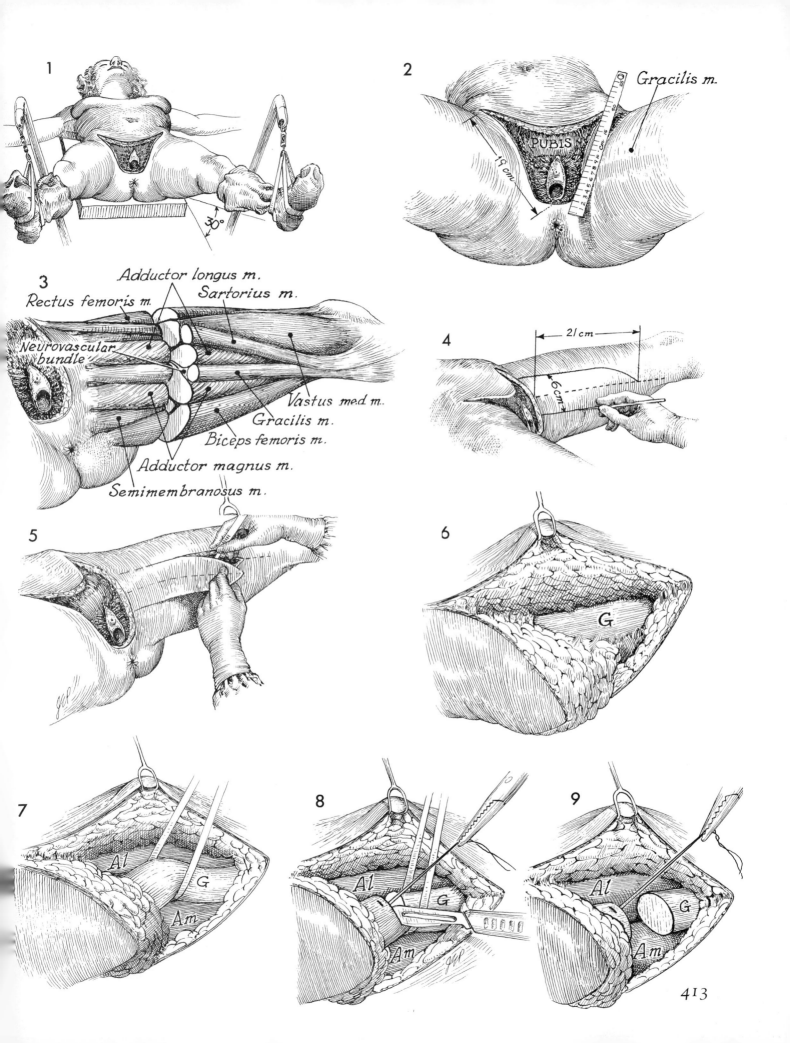

**1**

**2** *Gracilis m.*

PUBIS

19 cm

**3**
*Adductor longus m.*
*Rectus femoris m.*
*Sartorius m.*
*Neurovascular bundle*
*Vastus med. m.*
*Gracilis m.*
*Biceps femoris m.*
*Adductor magnus m.*
*Semimembranosus m.*

**4**
21 cm
6 cm

**5**

**6**
G

**7**
Al
G
Am

**8**
Al
G
Am

**9**
Al
G
Am

413

# Reconstruction of the Vulva With Gracilis Myocutaneous Flaps

## (Continued)

**10** The gracilis muscle is sutured to the overlying subcutaneous flap by interrupted 4-0 synthetic absorbable sutures.

**11** The vulvar defect is seen on the left, and the full-thickness flap is dissected off the underlying muscle with small Metzenbaum scissors. Extreme care is taken as the area of the neurovascular bundle is approached.

**12** Locating the neurovascular bundle of the gracilis muscle is vital to the success of the procedure. Identification is facilitated by incising the fascia over the adductor magnus muscle and dissecting this fascia medially with a blunt instrument.

**13** Assistance can be obtained from a small ultrasound Doppler that can probe each possible pedicle for the exact location of the gracilis artery and vein. The proximal portion of the gracilis muscle is transected from the ischial rami and

sutured to the subcutaneous tissue of the graft. At this point, the gracilis muscle is totally isolated and completely dependent on its vascular supply that enters from the border of the adductor longus and adductor magnus muscles.

**14** After the flap on the opposite thigh has been developed, the patient is given 1 g of fluorescein dye intravenously. After 3–5 minutes, the operating room is darkened, a Wood's lamp is focused on the myocutaneous flap, and the viable area of the flap will fluoresce with a brilliant yellow color. Nonviable areas are rendered as dark purple and should be excised at this time, as shown in Figure 14.

**15** The flap is completely isolated. The neurovascular bundle is identified. A closed suction drain is placed in the space previously occupied by the gracilis muscle and is brought out at the distal end of the leg incision.

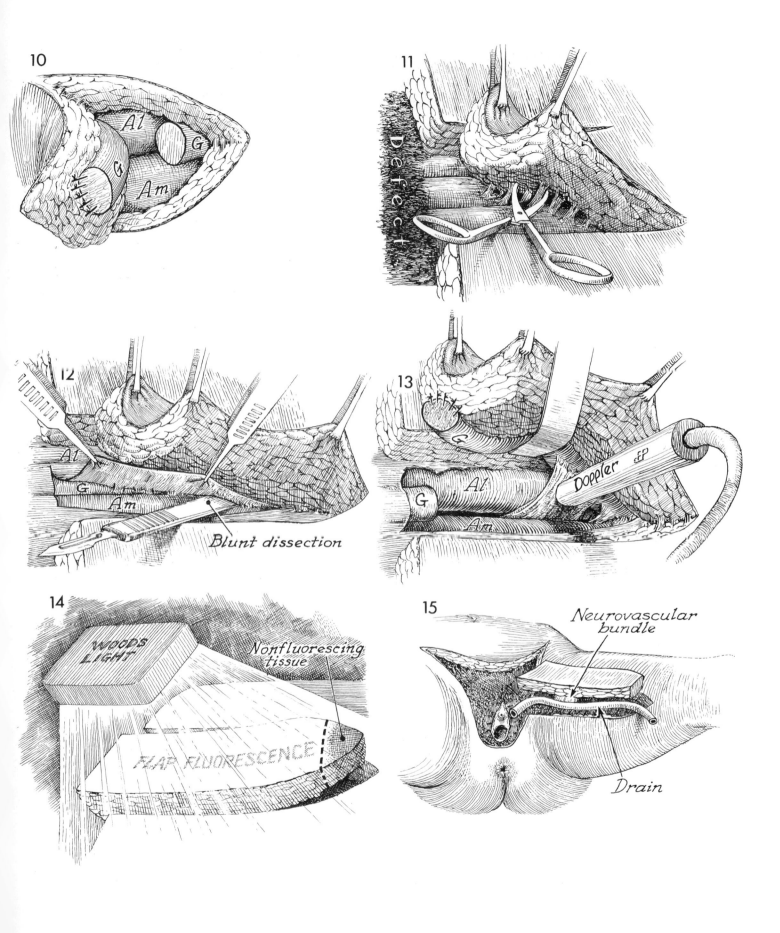

# Reconstruction of the Vulva With Gracilis Myocutaneous Flaps

## (Continued)

**16** The flap may be rotated clockwise or counterclockwise, at the discretion of the surgeon, to provide the best coverage for the vulvar defect.

**17** The flap is rotated into place, and a subcutaneous 3-0 synthetic absorbable suture is placed between the flap and the edge of the defect. Fine skin sutures of 4-0 Prolene are placed between the skin and the vulvar defect. Some surgeons prefer a subcuticular suture of 4-0 Dexon, finding it less compromising to the vasculature of the flap edge.

**18** The defect in the leg is closed in layers with a synthetic absorbable suture. The drain is brought out through the distal end of the incision. The proximal end of the drain is placed under the flap. The medial border of the flap is sutured to the edge of the vagina.

**19** The remaining portion of the inguinal lymph node dissection has been closed primarily. The flap on the opposite side has now been drawn on the skin, and the same procedure is performed from Figures 2 through 18.

**20** A drain is placed in the space previously occupied by the gracilis muscle on this side, and this flap is rotated into position.

**21** Closure of the vulvar defect is completed. The leg opening on the opposite side is closed. The closed suction drains are removed between the eighth and twelfth postoperative days. Sutures are also removed during this time, depending on the condition of the edges of the flap.

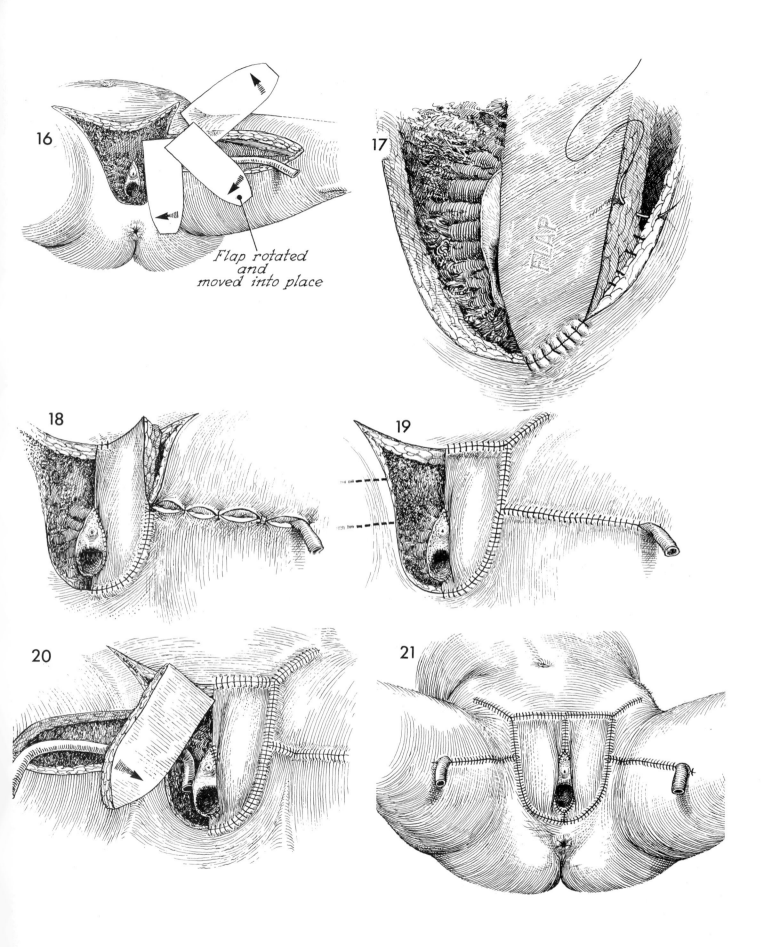

16

Flap rotated
and
moved into place

17

FLAP

18

19

20

21

# Transverse Rectus Abdominis Myocutaneous Flap and Vertical Rectus Abdominis Myocutaneous Flap

Muscle flaps play a large role in pelvic reconstruction of the female patient who has had radical resection for malignant disease, particularly when associated with total pelvic irradiation. They offer the advantage of bringing a nonirradiated tissue with a nonirradiated blood supply into the pelvis for coverage of defects. The rectus abdominis muscle with its unique blood supply coming from the inferior epigastric vessels, right or left, and the anatomy of the vessels in the rectus abdominis muscle allow a muscle flap to be based on a long muscle pedicle with excellent blood supply. The transverse rectus abdominis myocutaneous (TRAM) flap and the vertical rectus abdominis myocutaneous (VRAM) flap have the smallest incidence of necrosis of any of the myocutaneous flaps associated with pelvic reconstructive surgery.

**Physiologic Changes.** The physiologic change is that an open wound has been covered with a myocutaneous or muscle flap that offers an excellent covering for a wound and, at the same time, brings in a muscle with an excellent blood supply, i.e., the inferior epigastric artery, a branch of the external iliac artery.

**Points of Caution.** The paddle-shaped skin flap should not be separated from the anterior rectus fascia in order to preserve the perforator vessels from the muscle to the skin. Extreme care should be taken to ensure the integrity of the inferior epigastric vessels as they branch off the external iliac vessels. When the neurovascular bundle of the inferior epigastric artery has been interrupted, it would be extremely unusual for the VRAM flap to survive.

## Technique

**1** The abdominal wall shows the VRAM flap and the TRAM flap.

**2** The VRAM flap is outlined. The rectus abdominis muscles are seen ghosted beneath the skin. The incision is noted. The skin island is designed appropriate to the defect to be filled within the pelvis.

**3** After the incision has been made along the medial border of the rectus fascia and the skin island is noted toward the superior portion of the proposed flap, the external oblique fascia, the lateral and medial borders of the fascia, is noted. The linea alba is seen. The left rectus abdominis muscle is ghosted under the rectus fascia. The incision follows a second incision in the rectus fascia and is outlined as above, keeping intact a 5-cm width of rectus fascia to be taken with the flap. This ensures that the perforators coming off the anterior surface of the muscle through the rectus fascia are not interrupted or damaged. The inferior epigastric vessels are shown ghosted on the lateral portion of the rectus muscle.

**4** A cross section looking cephalad from beneath the flap is shown. The skin island is cut at an angle to preserve blood supply to the surface of the skin. The rectus muscles are shown. The posterior rectus fascia is left intact; the muscle is dissected off the posterior rectus fascia. By not sacrificing the posterior rectus fascia, reduction in hernias is noted.

**5** The VRAM flap has been completed, the posterior rectus fascia is noted, and the small perforators coming off the posterior rectus fascia are ligated. The rectus muscle is transected at the pubic symphysis area. The entire muscle with its sheath of rectus abdominal fascia on the anterior portion of the muscle is intact. The skin island is now ready for rotation through the defect made in the posterior rectus fascia above the symphysis pubis to bring this into the pelvic area. The medial border of the right rectus muscle has been shown. The lateral border of the right rectus fascia is also noted.

**6** The entire rectus muscle is lifted out of its fascia covering the rotated 180° and mobilized inferior through the posterior fascia into the pelvic cavity. The blood supply is coming exclusively through the inferior epigastric artery, and the perforators are coming through the muscle as shown in Figure 4.

**7** The VRAM flap is now pulled through the abdominal cavity into the pelvis and will be brought out to cover the vulvoanal defect noted in this particular patient. Modifications can be made to cover the exact limits of the defect noted in specific patients.

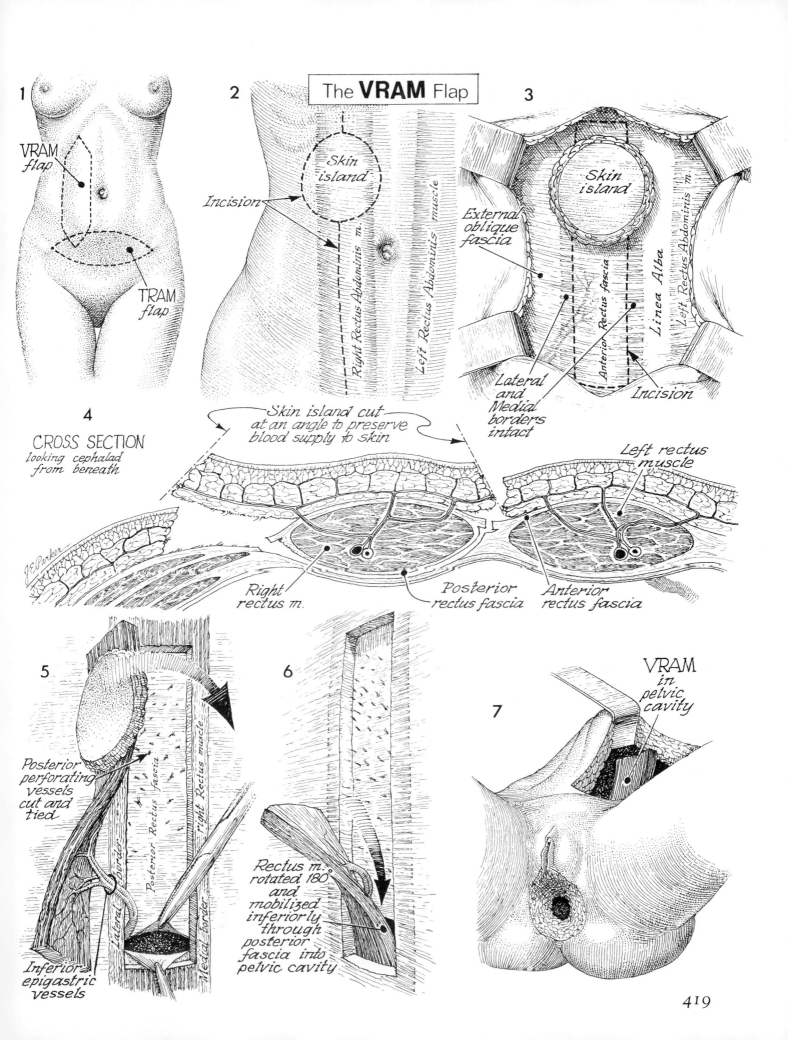

**1**

VRAM
flap

TRAM
flap

**2** The **VRAM** Flap

Skin
island

Incision

Right Rectus Abdominis m.

Left Rectus Abdominis muscle

**3**

Skin
island

External
oblique
fascia

Anterior Rectus fascia

Linea Alba

Left Rectus Abdominis m.

Lateral
and
Medial
borders
intact

Incision

**4**

CROSS SECTION
looking cephalad
from beneath

Skin island cut
at an angle to preserve
blood supply to skin

Left rectus
muscle

J.F.Parker

Right
rectus m.

Posterior
rectus fascia

Anterior
rectus fascia

**5**

Posterior
perforating
vessels
cut and
tied

Posterior Rectus fascia

Right Rectus muscle

Lateral border

Medial border

Inferior
epigastric
vessels

**6**

Rectus m.
rotated 180°
and
mobilized
inferiorly
through
posterior
fascia into
pelvic cavity

**7**

VRAM
in
pelvic
cavity

419

# Transverse Rectus Abdominis Myocutaneous Flap and Vertical Rectus Abdominis Myocutaneous Flap

## (Continued)

**8** The TRAM flap is made in a paddle-shaped manner from one anterior superior iliac spine to the opposite anterior superior iliac spine. The rectus abdominis muscles can be seen beneath the rectus fascia. Note that the right rectus abdominis muscle has been preserved in this particular case. The dissection is made underneath the anterior rectus fascia, which is preserved in a transverse fashion.

**9** The TRAM flap is supported by the left inferior epigastric muscles. Note that the left rectus muscle has been brought out of its fascia enclosure, preserving the anterior rectus fascia for 5 cm on each side of the muscle. The *dotted line* across the tip of the paddle is usually ischemic and can be proven so by the fluorescein and Wood's lamp test. Most of this usually has to be sacrificed.

**10** In this cross section of the TRAM flap looking caudad from above, the posterior rectus fascia is left intact. The inferior epigastric vessels are shown entering the rectus muscle. The right rectus muscle remains intact. The perforators coming off the anterior rectus fascia have been ligated. The skin is cut at an angle. The right side of this skin flap may have to be sacrificed if it is shown to be ischemic under the Wood's lamp with fluorescein dye injection.

**11** The TRAM flap is entering the abdominal cavity through an incision in the posterior rectus fascia. It can be brought down through the space of Retzius when the bladder has been removed, or if the bladder is in place, it can be brought down through the space of Retzius through the urogenital diaphragm and into the vagina for a variety of purposes.

**12** The anterior rectus fascia is closed up to the point of no tension. At this point, a synthetic mesh can be introduced into a defect and sutured into place.

**13** The skin is closed with stainless steel staples.

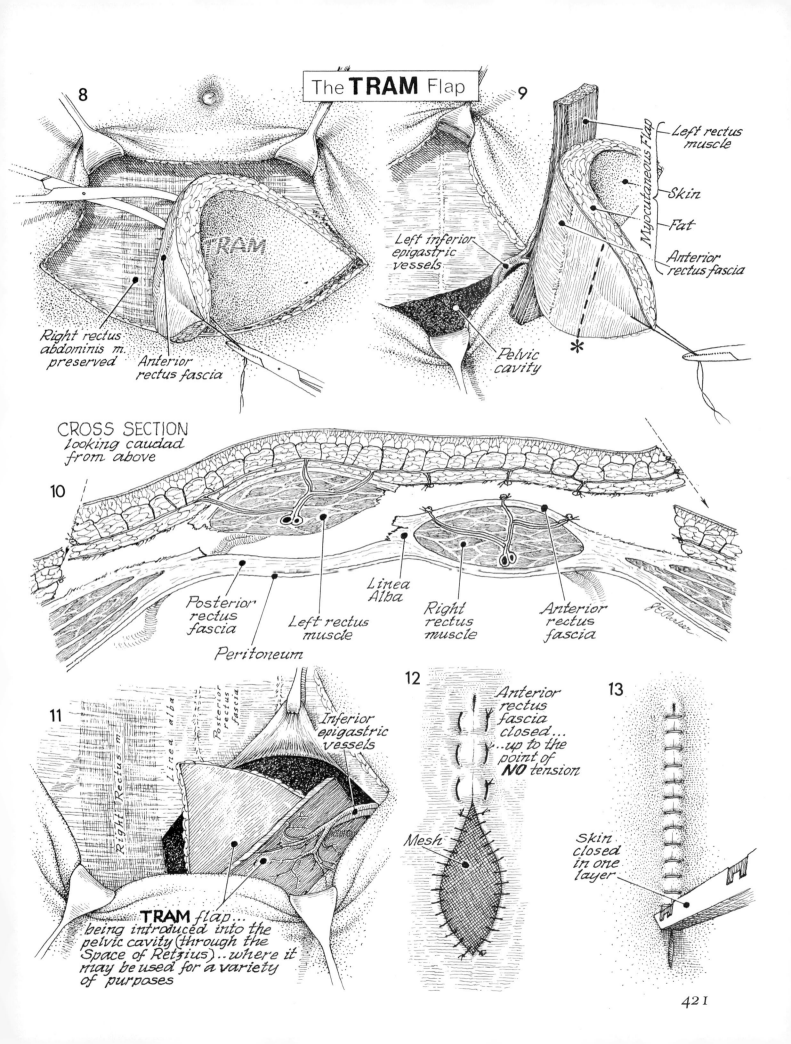

The **TRAM** Flap

**8**

*Right rectus
abdominis m.
preserved*

*Anterior
rectus fascia*

TRAM

**9**

*Left inferior
epigastric
vessels*

*Pelvic
cavity*

\*

*Left rectus
muscle*

*Skin*

*Fat*

*Anterior
rectus fascia*

*Myocutaneous Flap*

CROSS SECTION
*looking caudad
from above*

**10**

*Posterior
rectus
fascia*

*Peritoneum*

*Left rectus
muscle*

*Linea
Alba*

*Right
rectus
muscle*

*Anterior
rectus
fascia*

*P.C.Parker*

**11**

*Right Rectus m.*

*Linea alba*

*Posterior
rectus
fascia*

*Posterior
rectus fascia*

*Inferior
epigastric
vessels*

**TRAM** *flap...
being introduced into the
pelvic cavity (through the
Space of Retzius)...where it
may be used for a variety
of purposes*

**12**

*Anterior
rectus
fascia
closed...
...up to the
point of
NO tension*

*Mesh*

**13**

*Skin
closed
in one
layer*

# Radical Wertheim Hysterectomy With Bilateral Pelvic Lymph Node Dissection and With Extension of the Vagina

Radical Wertheim hysterectomy is performed predominantly for stage IB and early stage IIA carcinoma of the cervix and for stage I carcinoma of the vagina. It is also appropriate for stage II adenocarcinoma of the endometrium (corpus excervicus). The operation essentially includes removal of the uterus, upper vagina, and all the parametrial tissues to the pelvic side wall. The ureter and bladder are dissected free and left intact. Reconstruction of the vagina, if necessary, can be achieved by the techniques of extension of the vagina, making a pocket out of the vesical peritoneum and the rectal serosa.

**Physiologic Changes.** Carcinoma of the vagina, cervix, and uterus is removed.

**Points of Caution.** The major complications of the radical Wertheim hysterectomy are vesicovaginal and ureterovaginal fistulae in approximately 1.5% of patients.

Hemorrhage can be a problem. The danger areas from hemorrhage are the hypogastric vein and its tributaries (internal iliac vein), the vessels in the obturator fossa, and nuisance bleeding from the small vessels located in the tunnel of the ureter.

Postoperative urinary retention with bladder atony is a permanent problem in less than 10% of patients. It comes from transection of (1) the sympathetic nerves to the bladder in the upper portion of the web and (2) the ureterosacral ligaments.

# Radical Wertheim Hysterectomy With Bilateral Pelvic Lymph Node Dissection and With Extension of the Vagina

## (Continued)

## Technique

### RADICAL WERTHEIM HYSTERECTOMY

**1** The patient is placed in the modified dorsal supine lithotomy position (15° Trendelenburg) . The bladder is emptied with a Foley catheter. A thorough bimanual examination is always performed. The abdomen, perineum, and vagina are surgically prepared.

An abdominal incision is made in the midline and extended around the umbilicus. A Foley catheter is left in the bladder and connected to straight drainage.

**2** The abdomen is thoroughly explored. The peritoneum between the cecum and terminal ileum is opened, the common iliac and aortic area are exposed, and any suspicious lymph nodes are removed for biopsy.

The intestine is packed off in the upper abdomen.

A large thyroid clamp is placed on the uterine fundus and used as an elevator. The round ligaments are clamped at both pelvic walls, incised, and tied. The anterior leaf of the broad ligament is opened along with the vesicouterine peritoneal fold.

**3** This view, which is a cut through the pelvis in the posterior-anterior plane, demonstrates the pelvic spaces essential for all radical pelvic surgery.

In this view, the presacral space (PSS) is at the top. Advancing anteriorly, the surgeon finds the rectum (R) and the pararectal spaces (PRS). The surgeon can enter this space by displacing the ureter and moving between the ureter and internal iliac artery.

The rectovaginal space (RVS) is the next space anterior to the rectum. This area is entered by incising the peritoneum in the cul-de-sac of Douglas and dissecting the posterior vaginal wall from the perirectal fascia covering the rectum. The next space is the vagina (V).

After the vagina comes the vesicovaginal space (VVS). This is entered by retracting the bladder (B) anteriorly and dissecting this space with sharp dissection along the pubovesical cervical fascia. Note the position of the ureter and its relationship to this space.

The next significant space is the paravesical space (PVS). Between the pararectal space and the paravesical space is the lateral extent of the cardinal ligament, originally described as the "web" by Wertheim. The web contains the venous network of the internal iliac

vein. The superior portion of the web contains the sympathetic nerve fibers to the bladder along with the venous plexus. The inferior portion of the web contains the parasympathetic nerve fibers to the bladder.

In between the paravesical space is the bladder. Anterior to the bladder is the space of Retzius (SR), the retropubic space.

Prior to performing a radical Wertheim hysterectomy, the surgeon must completely dissect the paravesical and pararectal spaces.

**4** The round ligaments have been cut and divided. The anterior leaves of the broad ligament have been opened, and the vesicouterine peritoneum has been transected. The vesical peritoneum is grasped with two forceps and elevated. Scissors are used to dissect the vesicovaginal space between the bladder and the anterior vaginal wall. Elevation of the bladder can be facilitated by the placement of two sutures through the vesicoperitoneum to the skin incision above the symphysis pubis.

**5** The posterior leaf of the broad ligament is opened, exposing the infundibulopelvic ligament in the area of the pelvic brim. A finger is inserted under the infundibulopelvic ligament. The ureter is identified and dissected free of the infundibulopelvic ligament. Three clamps are applied to the infundibulopelvic ligament, and it is transected and doubly tied. The same procedure is carried out on the opposite side.

**6** The infundibulopelvic ligament, tubes, ovaries, and round ligaments are all tied to the thyroid clamp placed on the middle of the fundus. The surgical field is kept free of excessive instruments.

**7** The uterus is retracted caudad and medially. The base of the aorta is exposed, and the lymphatic tissue surrounding the common iliac artery and vein is removed with sharp dissection. The ureter is identified, dissected free of the artery, and retracted laterally. All lymphatic tissue surrounding the external iliac and common iliac blood vessels is removed from the bifurcation of the aorta to the inguinal ligament at the femoral canal.

The lymph nodes are carefully isolated in individual specimen containers for precise pathologic analysis.

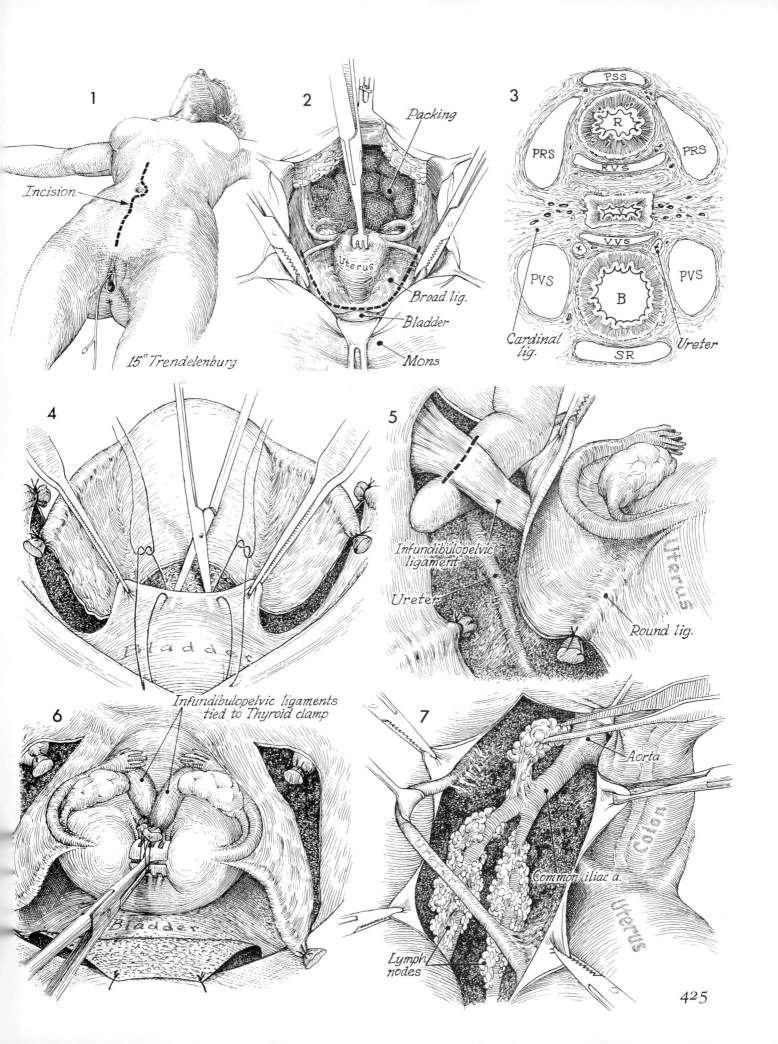

**1**

*Incision*

*15° Trendelenburg*

**2**

*Packing*

*Broad lig.*

*Bladder*

*Uterus*

*Mons*

**3**

*PSS*

*R*

*PRS*

*PRS*

*RVS*

*V*

*VVS*

*PVS*

*B*

*PVS*

*Cardinal lig.*

*Ureter*

*SR*

**4**

*Bladder*

**5**

*Infundibulopelvic ligament*

*Ureter*

*Round lig.*

*Uterus*

*Infundibulopelvic ligaments tied to Thyroid clamp*

**6**

*Bladder*

**7**

*Aorta*

*Ureter*

*Common iliac a.*

*Lymph nodes*

*Uterus*

*Colon*

425

# Radical Wertheim Hysterectomy With Bilateral Pelvic Lymph Node Dissection and With Extension of the Vagina

## (Continued)

**8** The common iliac, external iliac, and upper hypogastric vessels have been stripped of all lymphatic-bearing tissue. The obturator fossa and the lower branches of the hypogastric artery remain to be dissected.

**9** A vein retractor is used to retract the external iliac artery and vein laterally, and all lymphatic tissue is removed from behind these vessels and from the obturator fossa. The obturator nerve is preserved. Vessels deep in the obturator fossa may be ligated with hemoclips. The uterine artery is identified as it comes off the anterior division of the hypogastric artery before it enters the tunnel. It is transected and tied with 2-0 suture.

The same procedure is carried out on the left side.

**10** The pararectal space (PRS) and the paravesical space (PVS) are shown with the intervening web, which is the lateral extent of the cardinal ligament. The uterine artery on both sides has been transected and deviated medially. The distal stump of the uterine artery is seen as it enters the tunnel. Its relationship to the ureter within the tunnel is ghosted in this view. The ureter is seen as it enters the tunnel.

**11** The relationship of the ureter to the uterine artery is shown in the tunnel. The uterine artery has been transected as it branches from the anterior division of the hypogastric artery. It enters the tunnel laterally and crosses the ureter. Two horizontal curved clamps are inserted on top of the ureter

beneath the roof of the tunnel to include the uterine artery and vein. The tissue in the roof of the tunnel, consisting of the uterine artery and vein, is clamped, incised, and tied. In some patients, this may be performed in one step; in others, two to three successive bites with horizontal curved clamps on the roof of the tunnel are needed.

**12** The ureter is elevated with a small retractor. The filmy adhesions between the ureter and the floor of the tunnel connecting the ureter to the superior portion of the web are gently lysed and dissected laterally. The pararectal and the paravesical spaces, with the web in between, are visualized. The hypogastric artery and vein, along with the external iliac artery and vein, are retracted laterally. Note that in this particular patient the roof of the tunnel has been taken down in three successive bites between the horizontal curved clamps and been incised and tied.

**13** The external iliac artery and vein and the hypogastric artery and vein are retracted medially. The pararectal and the paravesical spaces are exposed. After the ureter has been dissected laterally (Fig. 12), the floor of the tunnel can be visualized. Two horizontal curved clamps are placed across the floor of the tunnel and excised. This completely frees the ureter from any attachment to the web.

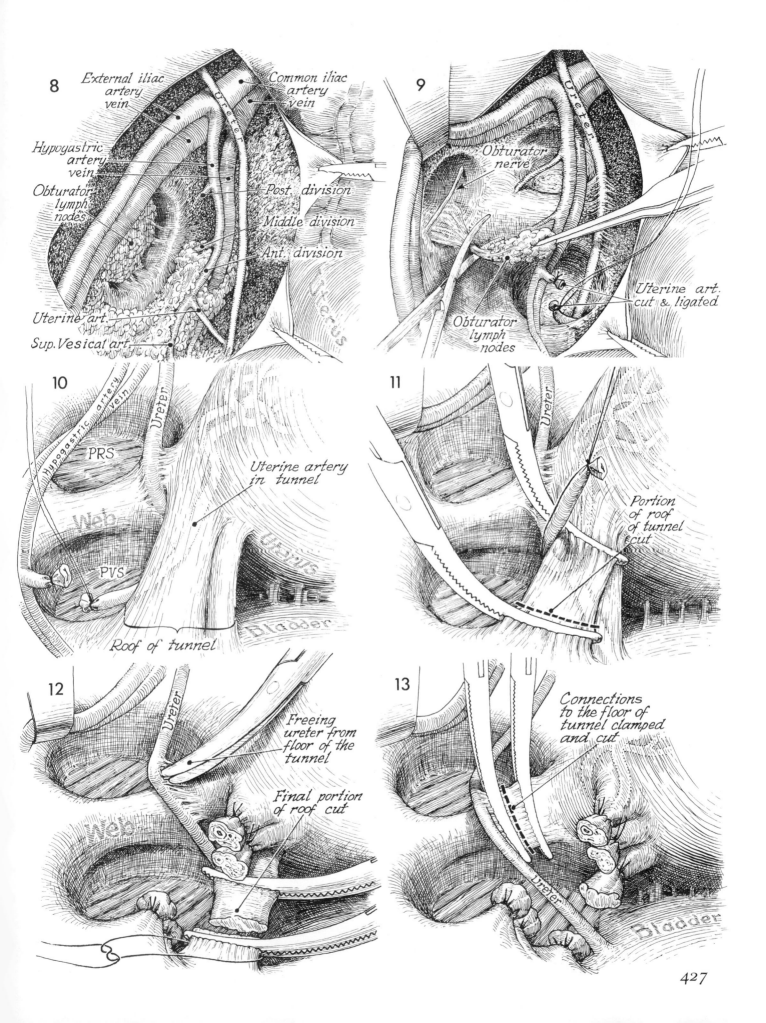

**8**
External iliac artery vein
Common iliac artery vein
Hypogastric artery vein
Obturator lymph nodes
Post. division
Middle division
Ant. division
Uterine art.
Sup. Vesical art.
Ureter
Corpus

**9**
Ureter
Obturator nerve
Uterine art. cut & ligated
Obturator lymph nodes

**10**
Hypogastric artery vein
Ureter
PRS
Web
PVS
Uterine artery in tunnel
Corpus
Bladder
Roof of tunnel

**11**
Ureter
Portion of roof of tunnel cut

**12**
Ureter
Freeing ureter from floor of the tunnel
Final portion of roof cut
Web

**13**
Connections to the floor of tunnel clamped and cut
Ureter
Bladder

# Radical Wertheim Hysterectomy With Bilateral Pelvic Lymph Node Dissection and With Extension of the Vagina

## (Continued)

**14** The uterus and the stumps of the tunnel, roof, and floor are seen on the right. The ureter is retracted laterally with a vein retractor. Both portions of the web are noted. The superior portion of the web, containing the hypogastric venous plexus and sympathetic nerves to the bladder, is separated from the lower portion containing the parasympathetic nerves to the bladder. In most cases, transection of only the upper portion is required to achieve the goal of the radical Wertheim hysterectomy.

We prefer to place a straight vascular clamp medial to the ureter on the medial portion of the web. A curved clamp can be placed on the lateral portion of the web at the pelvic wall. The superior portion of the web is transected and tied. The lower portion is left intact.

**15** The uterus is retracted upward and caudad. The incision in the posterior leaf of the broad ligament is extended across the cul-de-sac and the peritoneum overlying the cul-de-sac between the cervix and rectum.

**16** The uterus is retracted cephalad, a finger is inserted between the uterosacral ligaments, and the posterior wall of the vagina is dissected off the anterior rectal wall. Retraction on the uterus is changed to the anterior caudad position, plac-ing the uterosacral ligaments on tension. The upper portion of the uterosacral ligaments is clamped, incised, and tied. The lower portion of the uterosacral ligaments, containing the parasympathetic nerves to the bladder, is left.

**17** The lateral, posterior, and anterior attachments of the uterus and its parametria have all been transected and tied. Two right-angle Heaney clamps are placed on the paravaginal tissue on each side, and a scalpel is used to transect the remaining paravaginal tissue and vagina between these clamps. The paravaginal tissue pedicle is tied with a 0 synthetic absorbable suture. Approximately 5 cm of vagina should be removed.

**18** The Sakamoto sling suspends the ureters medially, out of the dissected pararectal and paravesical spaces. Several 0 synthetic absorbable sutures are used for this maneuver, which prevents the ureter from forming adhesions deep in the lateral pelvic wall spaces.

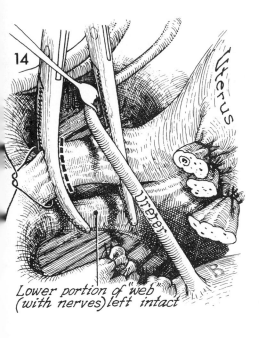

**14**

Lower portion of "web"
(with nerves) left intact

Uterus

Ureter

B

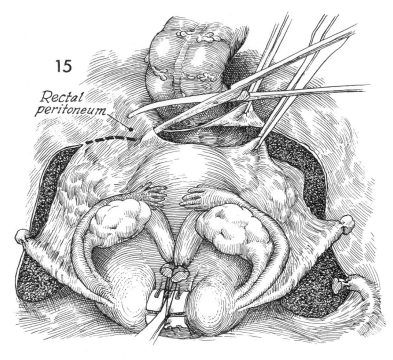

**15**

Rectal
peritoneum

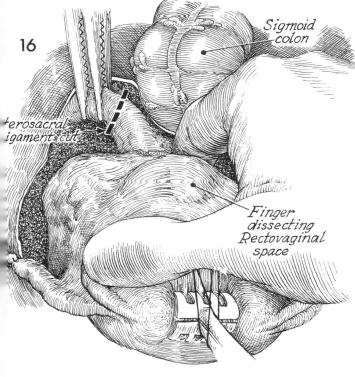

**16**

Uterosacral
ligament cut

Sigmoid
colon

Finger
dissecting
Rectovaginal
space

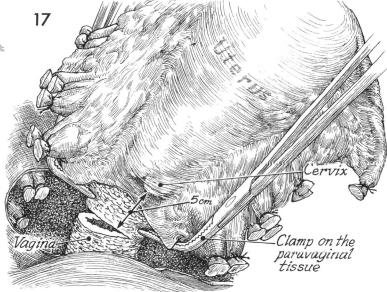

**17**

Uterus

Cervix

5 cm

Vagina

Clamp on the
paravaginal
tissue

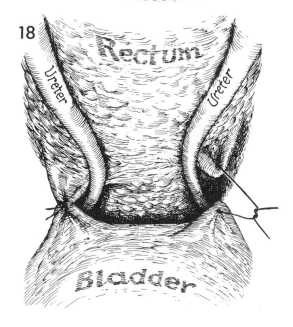

**18**

Rectum

Ureter

Ureter

Bladder

429

# Radical Wertheim Hysterectomy With Bilateral Pelvic Lymph Node Dissection and With Extension of the Vagina

## (Continued)

EXTENSION OF THE VAGINA

**19** This view shows, on the patient's left, the Sakamoto sling shown in Figure 18, page 429. If in younger patients following radical Wertheim hysterectomy in which 4–5 cm of upper vagina were excised a longer vagina is desired, the following steps can be performed. The vesical peritoneum coming off the bladder can be sutured to the anterior vaginal cuff. The serosa from the rectosigmoid colon can be sutured to the posterior vaginal cuff.

**20** On the patient's right, the Sakamoto sling is completed from the serosa of the rectum to the vesical peritoneum. Synthetic absorbable sutures are being placed in a row in the serosa of the rectum 5 cm from the posterior vaginal cuff to a site chosen on the vesical peritoneum 5 cm from the anterior vaginal cuff. When this row of sutures is completed, there will be an extension of the vagina from the vaginal cuff up to the new apex of the vagina that initially will be lined by mesothelium. After several months, this mesothelium will undergo squamous metaplasia, and the upper vaginal extension will be similar to the traditional vagina.

**21** This sagittal view shows the 5-cm extension to the vagina lined initially by mesothelium from the vesical peritoneum and the serosa of the colon. We insert a soft foam rubber form covered with condoms to keep this extension open for 6 weeks following Wertheim hysterectomy. Sexual intercourse is allowed after the form has been removed in 6 weeks.

**22** In young women, one or both ovaries can be preserved by dissecting out the infundibulopelvic ligament with its ovarian artery and vein and suspending the ovary to the psoas muscle high in the abdomen under the inferior pole of the kidney. This removes the ovary from any potential field of radiation that may be utilized postoperatively.

**23** The third portion of the duodenum is seen at the top. The ovary is suspended under the inferior pole of the right kidney to the psoas muscle by several interrupted absorbable sutures. The pelvic peritoneum has been closed with interrupted absorbable sutures. Note that Silastic Jackson-Pratt closed suction drains are inserted into the paravesical and pararectal spaces on each side. These are brought retroperitoneally to the anterior abdominal wall.

**24** The Silastic closed suction drains are brought out, respectively, through the right and left lower quadrants of the abdominal wall. The midline incision, extended around the umbilicus, is closed in layers.

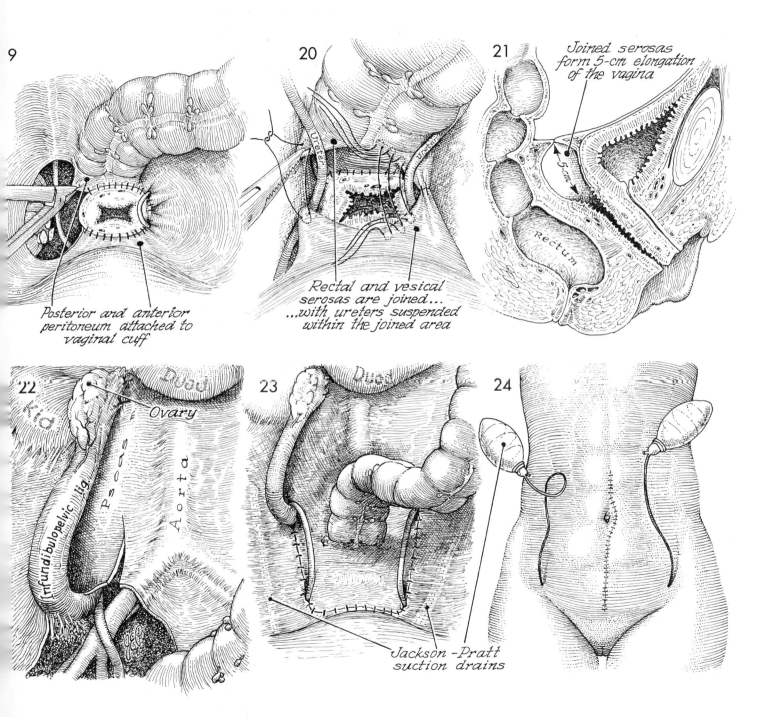

**9**
Posterior and anterior peritoneum attached to vaginal cuff

**20**
Ureter
Rectal and vesical serosas are joined...
...with ureters suspended within the joined area

**21**
Joined serosas form 5-cm elongation of the vagina
5-cm
Rectum

**22**
Kid
Duod
Ovary
Infundibulopelvic lig.
Psoas
Aorta

**23**
Duod
Jackson-Pratt suction drains

**24**

431

# Anterior Exenteration

When irradiation has failed in the treatment of pelvic cancers in the anterior plane of the pelvis, anterior exenteration may be performed. The operation is also efficacious for some cases of carcinoma of the urethra and bladder in which the vagina or cervix was invaded.

The purpose of the operation is to remove the bladder, urethra, vagina, uterus, and all tissue lateral to the pelvic side wall, including the tissue in the obturator fossa. The rectum and colon are left intact.

**Physiologic Changes.** The predominant physiologic alteration is elimination of the bladder and lower ureters and the formation of an urinary diversion.

**Points of Caution.** As soon as possible, the hypogastric artery on both sides should be identified and ligated to reduce blood loss. The ureter should not be transected until the surgeon is absolutely confident that the tumor is resectable. When the ureter is cut, it should be cut as low in the pelvis as possible, leaving ample ureter for construction of the urinary diversion.

The pelvis should be closed with a lid from an omental flap to prevent small bowel contents from falling into the denuded pelvis and adhering to the radiated tissue therein.

If the pelvis has been adequately irradiated, a complete lymphadenectomy is not performed.

## Technique

1 The patient is placed on the operating table in the modified dorsal lithotomy position with the hips abducted approximately 30°, exposing the perineum. The entire abdominal wall, vulva, perineal area, and vagina are surgically prepared. A Foley catheter is inserted in the bladder.

The abdomen is opened through a large lower midline incision that is extended around the umbilicus. The abdomen is thoroughly explored for tumor.

The bowel is packed off, exposing the pelvic brim. The peritoneum below the cecum and terminal ileum is opened, and the common iliac artery and aorta are exposed. The aorta is explored all the way to the renal vessels, and any suspicious lymph nodes are removed.

2 The peritoneum has been opened from the bifurcation of the aorta to the femoral canal, and suspicious lymph nodes have been dissected off the common iliac artery. The ureter crosses the common iliac artery on the right side, medial and inferior to the ovarian vessels.

3 The round ligaments on each side are cut at the pelvic wall, and the posterior and anterior leaves of the broad ligament are completely opened.

4 The external iliac vein is deviated laterally, exposing the obturator fossa from which all lymph nodes suspected of bearing tumor are removed. The ovarian vessels are clamped and doubly tied at the pelvic brim.

5 The ureter, with a generous portion of its peritoneal attachment left intact, is transected below the common iliac artery.

6 The ureter has been transected, and the distal ureter has been ligated. The obturator fossa has been cleaned of all contents. The hypogastric artery is cross-clamped, transected, and tied with 2-0 suture. The distal portion of the artery is elevated, and its branches are identified, clamped, and tied.

7 Attention is directed to the space of Retzius where the bladder is separated from the rectopubic space. Fine adhesions to the pelvic wall can be lysed with Metzenbaum scissors; and any small vessels in the plexus of Santorini can be clamped and tied with suture, or hemoclips may be applied.

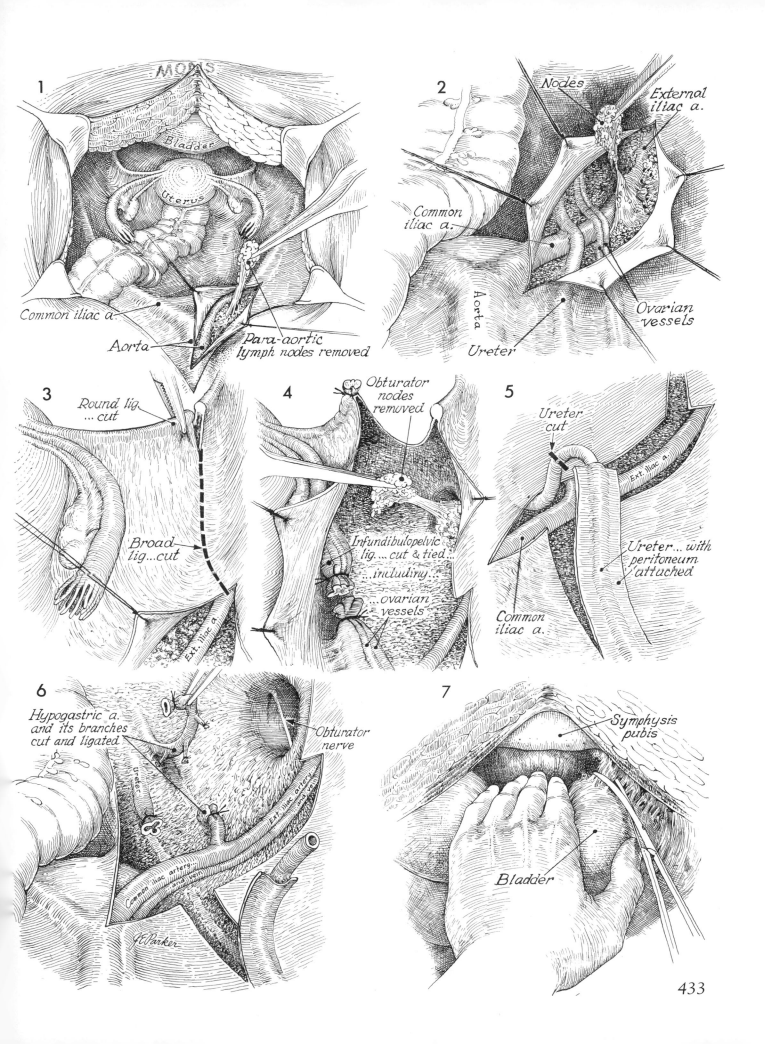

**1**

MONS

Bladder

Uterus

Common iliac a.

Aorta

Para-aortic
lymph nodes removed

**2**

Nodes

External
iliac a.

Common
iliac a.

Aorta

Ureter

Ovarian
vessels

**3**

Round lig.
...cut

Broad
lig...cut

Ext. iliac a.

**4**

Obturator
nodes
removed

Infundibulopelvic
lig. ... cut & tied ...
...including...

...ovarian
vessels

**5**

Ureter
cut

Ext. iliac a.

Ureter...with
peritoneum
attached

Common
iliac a.

**6**

Hypogastric a.
and its branches
cut and ligated

Obturator
nerve

Ureter

Ext. iliac artery
and vein

Common iliac artery
...and vein

J.E.Parker.

**7**

Symphysis
pubis

Bladder

# Anterior Exenteration

## (Continued)

**8** This view illustrates the pelvic spaces. In an anterior exenteration, both the paravesical spaces *(PVS)* and the pararectal spaces *(PRS)* are seen. The lateral extent of the cardinal ligament (the web) is demonstrated with countertraction from the first two fingers of the surgeon's hand. The web is clamped, incised, and tied at the pelvic wall. *B*, bladder; *PSS*, presacral space; *R*, rectum; *RVS*, rectovaginal space; *SR*, space of Retzius; and *VVS*, vesicovaginal space.

**9** The stumps of the ureterosacral ligament are seen transected adjacent to the pelvic wall, which includes the hypogastric venous plexus. Successive bites on the web at the pelvic wall are made with clamps and incised down to the levator ani muscles. The rectum remains intact.

**10** The hypogastric vein and artery have been cut and tied. The stumps of the web are seen on the pelvic wall. The specimen has been completely freed down to the levator sling and is retracted medially. The ureterosacral ligaments have been cut and tied at the pelvic wall. The peritoneum of the cul-de-sac of Douglas has been transected, and the posterior vaginal wall has been dissected off the rectum.

**11** The same procedure is carried out on the opposite side. The ligated ureter is seen. The specimen (bladder, uterus, tubes, ovaries, and vagina) has been freed from the anterior lateral pelvic wall.

**12** The specimen is now retracted cephalad. A scalpel is used to transect the urethra at the meatus.

**13** The vagina is transected across the introitus below the level of the levator sling. Any remaining rectal stalks attaching the posterior vaginal wall to the rectum are lysed, and the specimen is removed.

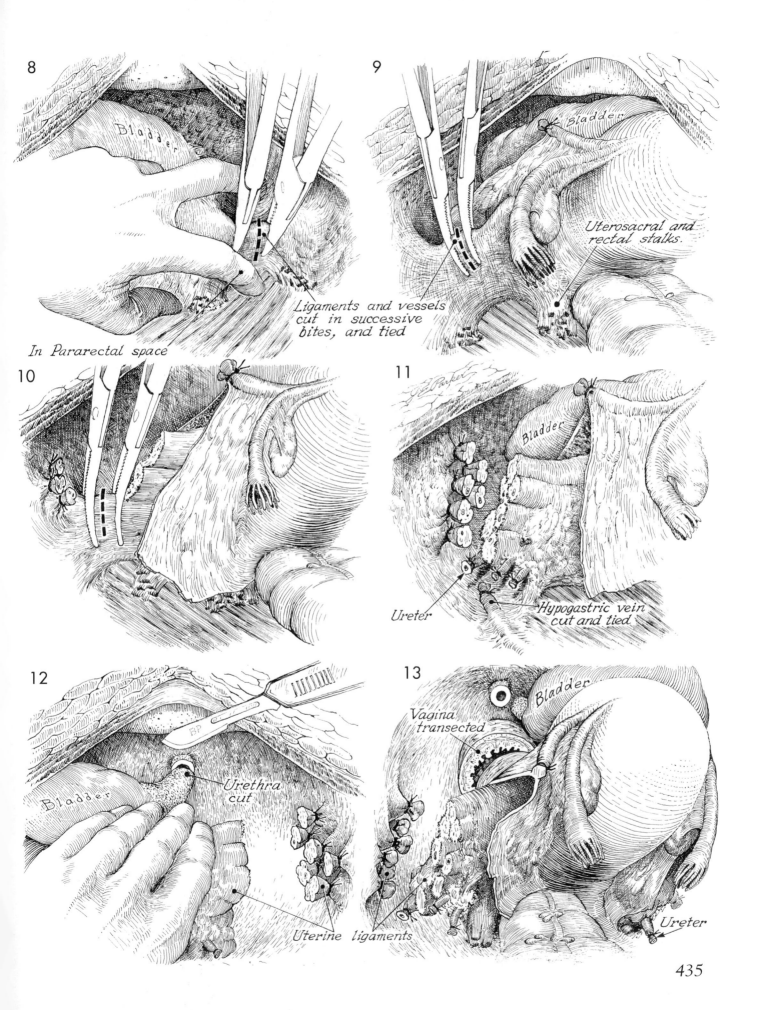

8

Bladder

In Pararectal space

Ligaments and vessels
cut in successive
bites, and tied

9

Bladder

Uterosacral and
rectal stalks.

10

11

Bladder

Ureter

Hypogastric vein
cut and tied

12

Bladder

Urethra
cut

Uterine ligaments

13

Bladder

Vagina
transected

Ureter

435

**14** The vaginal cuff has been closed with an interrupted 0 absorbable suture. The ureters are seen below the pelvic brim. The urethra has been transected at the meatus. Maximum attention at this stage is turned toward hemostasis within the pelvis.

**15** A continent urinary diversion (Kock pouch) will be made from small bowel. The terminal ileum with the respective links in centimeters for construction of the pouch is shown (see the Kock Pouch Continent Urostomy on page 463).

**16** The Kock pouch continent urostomy with afferent and efferent nipples has been completed. The letters A to A', B to B', C to C' delineate the order of suture that produces a spherical pouch.

**17** The continent pouch has been completed. The stoma is sutured to the subcuticular layer of the skin of the umbilicus with 3-0 polyglycolic acid (PGA) sutures. A No. 30 French Medena catheter has been placed through the stoma down the efferent limb and exits the efferent nipple into the pouch. This Medena catheter has been securely sutured in place with a No. 1 nylon suture that includes the margins of the skin, the entire intestinal wall of the stoma, the opposite intestinal wall, and the opposite margin of skin; it is securely tied around the Medena catheter with multiple half-hitch knots to hold the catheter in the pouch without slippage for 3 weeks. A second suture of No. 1 nylon is placed on the opposite side.

A Jackson-Pratt closed suction drain has been placed adjacent to the Kock pouch and is brought out through the abdominal wall. It is sutured with a 3-0 PGA suture to prevent removal for 3 weeks. Note that the afferent limb of the bowel and the afferent nipple have the ureters sutured in a mucosa-to-mucosa fashion with No. 8 French Finney "J" Silastic stents in place. The abdomen is closed. The Medena catheter is irrigated every 2–4 hours for the next 3 weeks to prevent mucus obstruction.

**18** An omental vascular pedicle "J" flap is created.

**19** The omental J flap is brought into the pelvis and sutured around the ileopectineal line and across the rectosigmoid colon as a pelvic lid. The abdomen is closed in layers. A sump nasogastric tube or a feeding gastrostomy tube is inserted in the stomach.

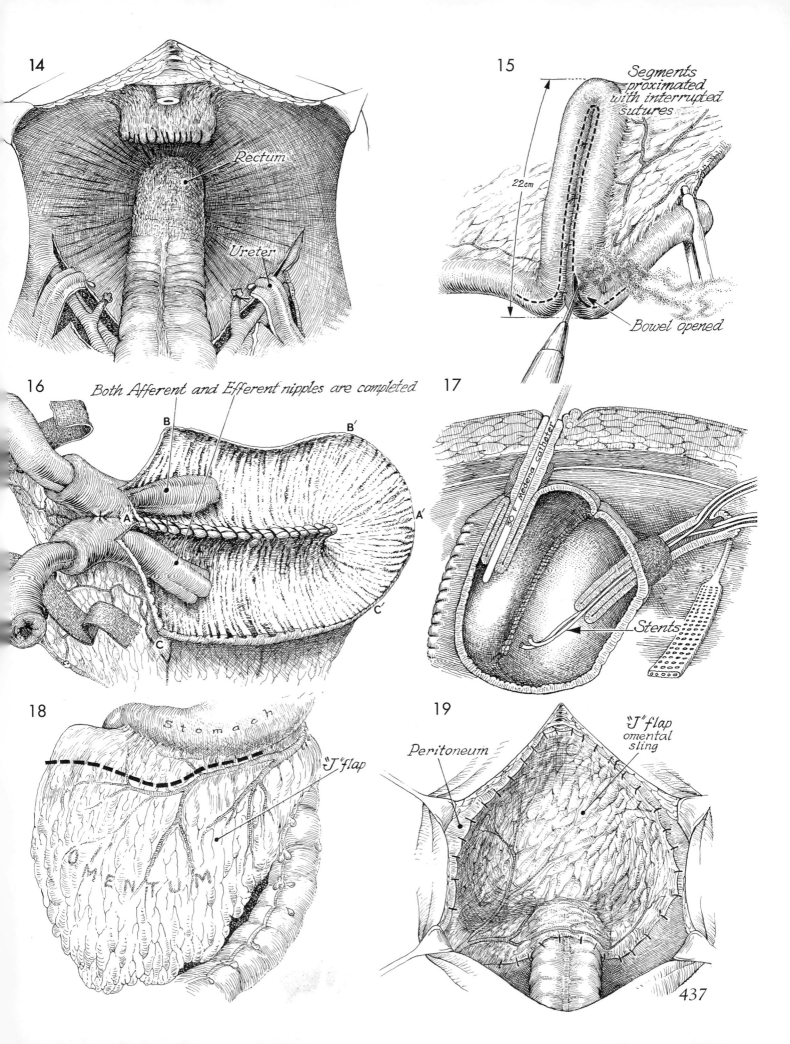

**14**

Rectum

Ureter

**15**

Segments
proximated
with interrupted
sutures

22cm

Bowel opened

**16** Both Afferent and Efferent nipples are completed

B

B'

K A

A'

C

C

**17**

30 F Medena catheter

Stents

**18**

Stomach

"J" flap

OMENTUM

**19**

Peritoneum

"J" flap
omental
sling

# Posterior Exenteration

Posterior exenteration is rarely indicated today in the treatment of carcinoma of the cervix and upper vagina. The patterns of presentation of malignancy frequently make this operation inadequate and leave the bladder denervated; and the frequency of fistulae is significant. In most cases, we would perform a total exenteration.

Where indicated, the opportunity for reconstruction with a permanent diverting colostomy was dramatically improved by the advent of the EEA (end-to-end anastomosis) automatic surgical stapler for very low colonic anastomoses. It is now possible to achieve the anastomosis of the descending colon to the rectum at levels at or below the levator sling, thus allowing the en bloc removal of some pelvic cancers without a permanent colostomy. Basically, a posterior exenteration is a combination of a radical Wertheim hysterectomy and an anterior resection of the colon or abdominal peritoneal resection of the rectosigmoid colon and anus.

The purpose of the operation is to remove the uterus, tubes, ovaries, rectosigmoid colon, and all parametrial tissue from the uterus to the pelvic wall.

**Physiologic Changes.** The predominant physiologic change is removal of the tumor from the pelvic cavity. Denervation of the urinary bladder in most cases occurs, but the actual loss of a small segment of rectosigmoid colon produces little clinical or physiologic change.

**Points of Caution.** The procedure should not be performed on patients with epidermoid cancer when there is metastasis to the common iliac and aortic lymph nodes.

The proximal colon should be transected as low in the pelvis as possible to permit the maximum amount of colon to be available for reanastomosis and construction of a rectal "J" pouch.

The surgeon should take care to identify the left ureter when opening the mesentery of the rectosigmoid colon.

The dissection of the ureter in the tunnel must be performed with meticulous surgical technique to avoid vesicovaginal fistula.

Throughout this operation, hemorrhage must be carefully controlled.

## Technique

**1** The patient is placed on the operating table in the modified dorsal lithotomy position with the hips abducted 30°. A Foley catheter is inserted into the bladder. The skin from the breast to the perianal area is surgically prepared.

The abdomen is opened through a lower midline incision extended around the umbilicus. Pfannenstiel incisions are not appropriate for this operation.

The abdominal cavity should be explored, and all suspicious areas of tumor should be identified and removed for frozen section analysis.

**2** Once the decision has been made to proceed with the operation, the peritoneum is opened along the right common iliac artery down to the external iliac artery. All lymphatic tissue is removed, with care taken to preserve the ureter. The ovarian vessels seen crossing the common iliac artery will be ligated.

**3** The round ligament is clamped, transected, and tied at the pelvic wall. The posterior leaf of the broad ligament is opened, and the entire external iliac artery is exposed.

**4** The lymph nodes are removed from the external iliac artery, vein, and obturator fossa. The ovarian vessels are clamped, transected, and tied. The same procedure is performed on the other side.

**5** The hypogastric artery is cleaned of lymph node tissue. The ureter can be seen medial to the hypogastric artery crossing the common iliac artery. The obturator nerve is seen in the obturator fossa.

**6** The obturator fossa has been cleaned of lymph nodes, and the obturator nerve has been preserved. The hypogastric artery is clamped, ligated, and incised with its branches. The same procedure is carried out on the opposite side.

**7** The mesentery of the rectosigmoid colon is opened in an avascular area, and a rubber drain is passed through this opening as a source of traction on the colon. The peritoneum covering the mesentery is opened. Care is taken at this point to identify the left ureter because the mesentery of the rectosigmoid colon generally points to the left ureter at its base.

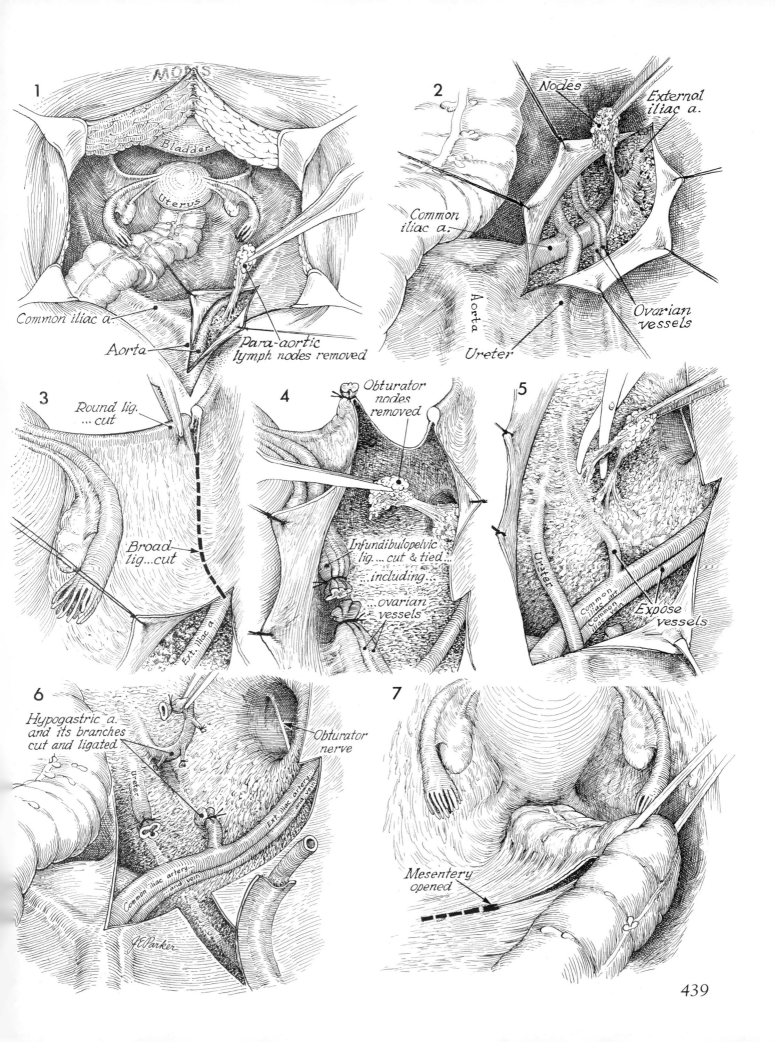

**1**

MONS

Bladder

Uterus

Common iliac a.

Aorta

Para-aortic
lymph nodes removed

**2**

Nodes

External
iliac a.

Common
iliac a.

Aorta

Ureter

Ovarian
vessels

**3**

Round lig.
...cut

Broad
lig....cut

Ext. iliac a.

**4**

Obturator
nodes
removed

Infundibulopelvic
lig....cut & tied...
...including...
...ovarian
vessels

**5**

Ureter

Common
iliac artery
Common
iliac vein

Expose
vessels

**6**

Hypogastric a.
and its branches
cut and ligated

Obturator
nerve

Ureter

Ext. iliac artery
and vein

Common iliac artery...
...and vein

J. E. Parker

**7**

Mesentery
opened

439

# Posterior Exenteration

## (Continued)

**8** The colon is retracted caudad. A finger has been inserted in the opening of the mesentery under the rectosigmoid colon. The peritoneum covering the medial side of the mesentery is opened.

**9** The vessels in the mesentery of the rectosigmoid colon have been clamped and tied with 2-0 suture.

**10** The linear stapler has been applied to the rectosigmoid colon slightly below the sacral promontory. It is activated, transecting the rectosigmoid colon between double rows of staples.

**11** The remaining portion of the mesentery attached to the rectum is clamped, incised, and tied with 2-0 suture.

**12** Cephalad retraction is made on the combined specimen of the uterus and rectosigmoid colon. A hand is inserted into the presacral space to dissect the rectum from the sacrum down to the coccyx.

It is important to keep the dissecting hand in the midline to prevent evulsion of the presacral veins on the lateral margin of the sacrum. These can be a source of troublesome bleeding if lacerated.

**13** The stalks of each side of the rectum are progressively clamped, incised, and tied with 2-0 suture. This frees the rectum from its lateral attachments.

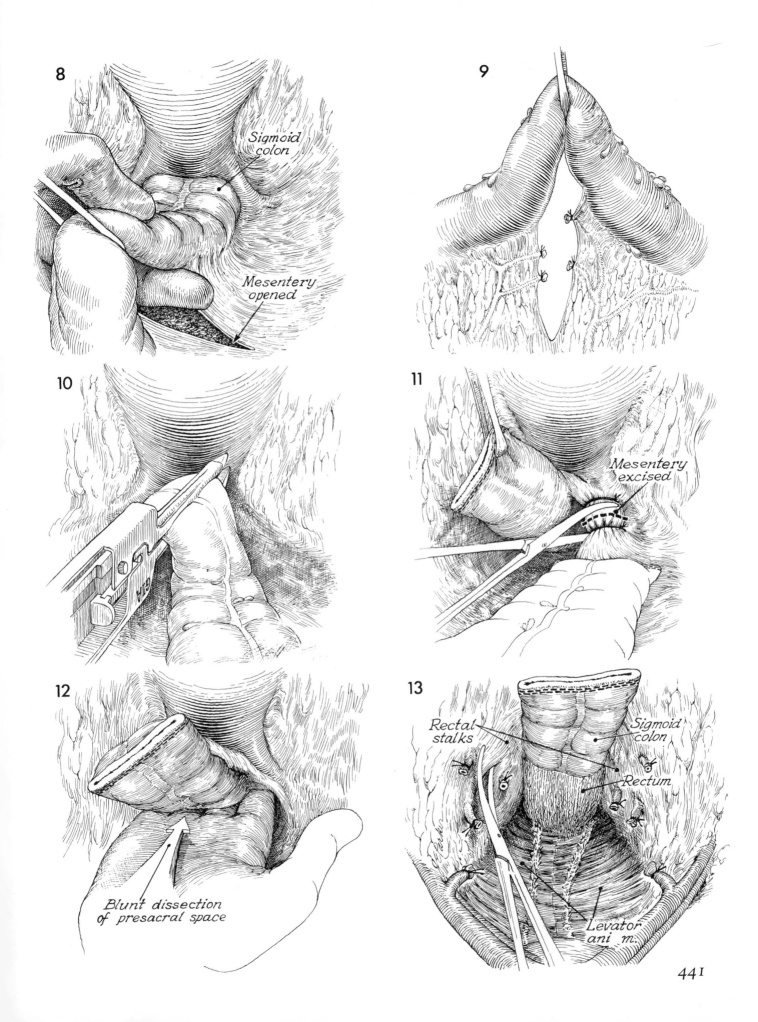

8

Sigmoid colon

Mesentery opened

9

10

11

Mesentery excised

12

Blunt dissection of presacral space

13

Rectal stalks

Sigmoid colon

Rectum

Levator ani m.

441

# Posterior Exenteration

## (Continued)

**14** The anterior leaf of the broad ligament is incised down and across the bladder peritoneum. The vesicoperitoneum is elevated and sutured to the skin for retraction, and the bladder is dissected off the lower uterine cervix and anterior vagina for a distance of at least 6–8 cm below the tumor level.

**15** The uterus is retracted medially. The paravesical and pararectal spaces are dissected. Notice that in taking down the rectal stalks the posterior wall of the pararectal space has been removed. The ureter crosses the superior medial portion of the web as it enters the tunnel. The hypogastric artery and vein have been retracted medially. The external iliac artery and vein have been retracted laterally, revealing the obturator fossa and nerve.

**16** The dissection of the ureter is carried down to the web by delicately elevating the ureter with a vein retractor. The attachments of the ureter to the web are lysed with Metzenbaum scissors. A Kelly clamp is inserted on top of the ureter underneath the tunnel toward the bladder. The *dotted line* indicates the incision to be made in the web adjacent to the pelvic wall.

**17** The tunnel is taken down in successive bites and tied with 3-0 synthetic absorbable suture. When the tunnel has been completely transected, the course of the ureter can be seen all the way to the ureterovesical junction. The web is taken down in successive bites and tied with 0 suture all the way to the levator muscle.

**18** The specimen is free of lateral attachments to the pelvic wall and, posteriorly, from the sacrum. The specimen, consisting of the uterus, its lateral attachments, rectum, and the ureterosacral and rectal stalk ligaments along with the hypogastric artery, vein, and its branches, can be elevated. The ureter is freed all the way to the bladder.

**19** By firm cephalad traction on the specimen, the vagina has been transected with a scalpel at the level of the levator muscle. The rectum is transected below the tumor but preferably above the levator sling.

**20** The completed operative field, the stumps of the various lateral attachments of the uterus and rectum, the dissected ureters, and the intact bladder are shown. The vaginal cuff is reefed with a 0 suture and left open. The rectum is available for reanastomosis of the descending colon.

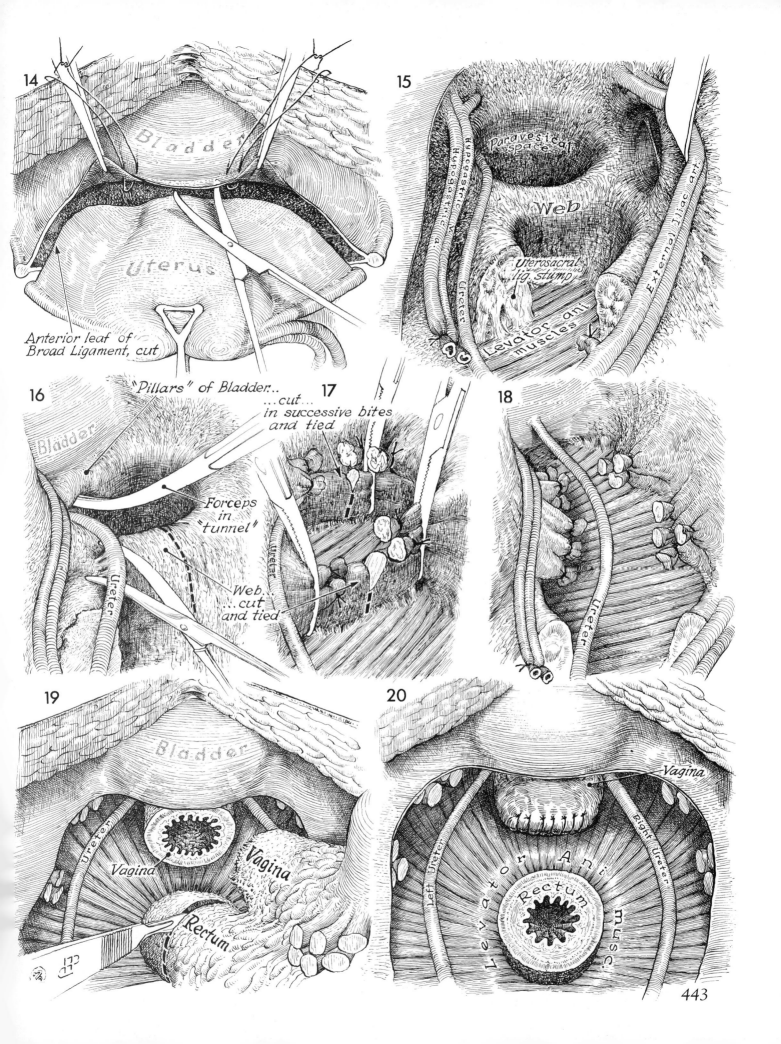

**14**

*Bladder*

*Uterus*

*Anterior leaf of Broad Ligament, cut*

**15**

*Paravesical space*

*Web*

*Uterosacral lig. stump*

*Hypogastric v.*

*Hypogastric a.*

*Ureter*

*External Iliac art.*

*Levator ani muscles*

**16**

"Pillars" of Bladder...

*Bladder*

*Ureter*

*Forceps in "tunnel"*

*Web... ...cut and tied*

**17**

...cut... in successive bites and tied

*Ureter*

**18**

*Ureter*

**19**

*Bladder*

*Ureter*

*Vagina*

*Vagina*

*Rectum*

**20**

*Vagina*

*Left Ureter*

*Right Ureter*

*Levator Ani muscle*

*Rectum*

443

# Posterior Exenteration

## (Continued)

**21** The descending colon is mobilized. The splenocolic ligament is clamped and tied. The peritoneum lateral to the descending colon is opened along the line of Toldt to the pelvic brim.

**22** The surgeon mobilizes the rectosigmoid and descending colon further by transecting the left colic branch of the inferior mesenteric artery. An attempt should be made to preserve as many of the branches of the inferior mesenteric artery as possible to give maximum blood supply to the descending colon at its anastomosis with the rectum. If the marginal artery of the colon is intact, however, the inferior mesenteric artery itself may be clamped and tied at the aorta to produce complete mobility of the colon. There must be no tension on the J pouch colorectal anastomosis. The marginal artery of the colon allows sacrifice of the superior hemorrhoidal and left colic branches of the inferior mesenteric artery if needed to achieve a tension-free anastomosis.

**23** A rectal reservoir colonic J pouch has been constructed. The opening in the inferior portion of the J pouch is stapled to the rectal stump with the automatic surgical stapler (EEA stapler) inserted through the anus and activated.

**24** The descending colon has been formed into a rectal J pouch colonic reservoir and stapled to the rectum. The vaginal cuff has been closed. The ureters have been suspended with the Sakamoto stitch.

**25** Maximum peritonealization has been achieved.

**26** In all radiated cases, and in any case in which there is some doubt about the healing properties of the anastomosis, a protective temporary diverting loop colostomy should be performed. This may be closed in 2–3 months, after the rectal J pouch colonic reservoir has healed.

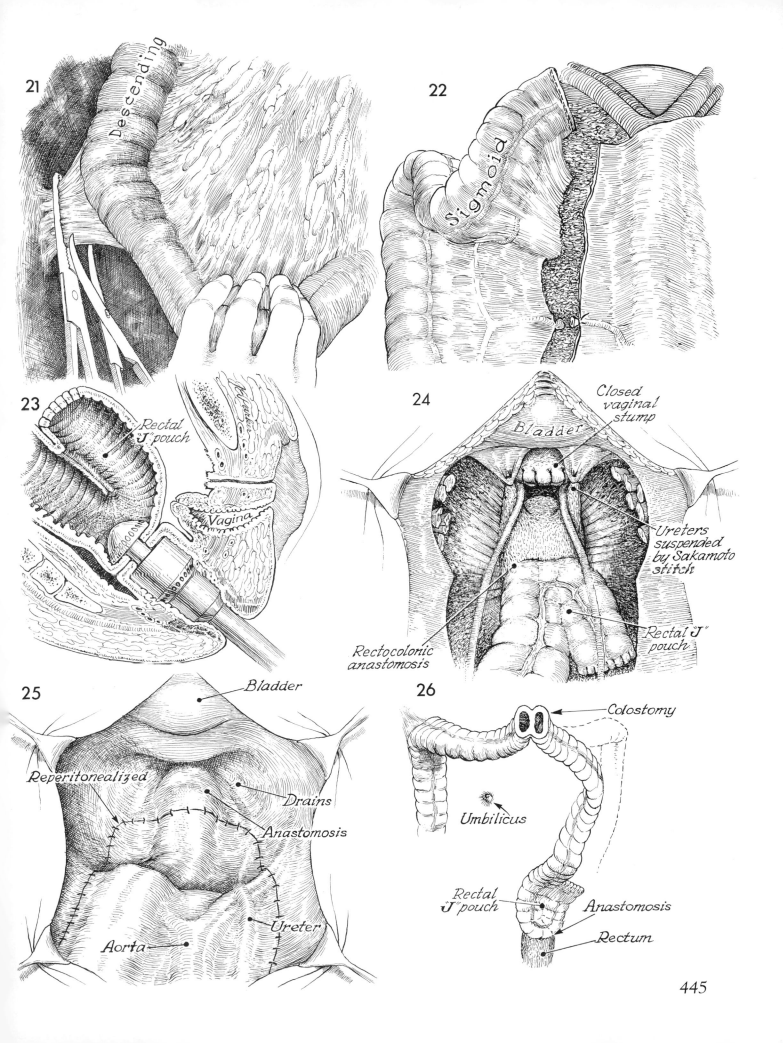

**21**

Descending

**22**

Sigmoid

**23**

Rectal "J" pouch

Bladder

Vagina

**24**

Closed vaginal stump

Bladder

Ureters suspended by Sakamoto stitch

Rectocolonic anastomosis

Rectal "J" pouch

**25**

Bladder

Reperitonealized

Drains

Anastomosis

Ureter

Aorta

**26**

Colostomy

Umbilicus

Rectal "J" pouch

Anastomosis

Rectum

445

# Total Pelvic Exenteration

Total pelvic exenteration is indicated in those patients with carcinoma of the cervix with recurrence after irradiation and in patients with primary stage IV disease in which tumor has advanced into the bladder and rectum but remains confined to the pelvis.

Total pelvic exenteration is indicated and performed more often than anterior or posterior exenteration. Thorough preoperative evaluation, correction of anemia and nutrition, and a thorough mechanical and antibiotic preparation of the intestines are prerequisites to surgery.

Recently, the EEA (end-to-end anastomosis) automatic surgical stapler has made it possible to leave many of these patients without permanent colostomies. For carcinoma of the cervix or vagina to invade the lower 5 cm of the rectum and anus is rare; therefore, it is possible to leave the anus and lower rectum in many patients without reducing their chance for cure. The descending colon can be mobilized, brought deep into the pelvis, formed into a "J" pouch colonic reservoir, and stapled to the rectum. This has had a significant psychologic benefit for the cancer patient who would otherwise require two permanent abdominal stomas.

The urine can be diverted into a continent urostomy. Therefore, external appliances (bags) in most patients can be eliminated. Neovagina construction can be made for those who desire it.

The purpose of the operation is to remove all cancer tissue from the pelvis and to construct an appropriate diversion for the urine and stool if the colon cannot be reanastomosed to the rectum.

**Physiologic Changes.** The most significant physiologic change associated with this operation is the removal of all cancer tissue.

Diversion of the urine may result in significant physiologic change. It may be associated with a higher incidence of renal disease from urinary tract infection and obstruction. These complications are less, however, than when the ureters are implanted into an intact sigmoid colon or when the ureters are implanted into an ileal or colonic loop.

**Points of Caution.** Hemorrhage can be a major complication of total pelvic exenteration. Bleeding will be decreased significantly by early ligation of the internal iliac artery at the bifurcation of the common iliac artery.

The ureters should be transected as low in the pelvis as possible to give the surgeon maximum flexibility in performing the continent urostomy. Reconstruction should start in the posterior pelvis with the rectal J pouch coloproctostomy, proceed anteriorly with the neovagina, and conclude with the Kock pouch continent urostomy. This order of surgery is needed to prevent getting boxed in "from anatomic exposure."

Postoperative care is of paramount importance and should be performed in a surgical intensive care unit. Intravenous hyperalimentation given preoperatively and postoperatively can improve the patient's metabolic balance. The nutritional status of these patients can influence wound healing.

# Total Pelvic Exenteration

## (Continued)

### Technique

The patient is placed on the operating table in the modified dorsal lithotomy position with the legs abducted 30°. The surgical preparation is carried from the breast over the mons pubis to the tip of the coccyx. A Foley catheter is left in the bladder, and urine output is monitored until the ureters are transected.

**1** The abdomen is entered through a low midline incision that is extended around the umbilicus. A thorough exploration of the upper abdomen is made, particularly along the aorta and common iliac arteries. The peritoneum below the terminal ileum and cecum is opened. The right common iliac artery and vein are identified. The incision into the peritoneum is extended along the aorta until the renal vessels are located. Occasionally, the third portion of the duodenum requires mobilization for exposure. The aortic lymph nodes are palpated, and any suspicious lymph node is removed for pathologic analysis.

**2** The peritoneal incision is extended caudad along the external iliac vessels to the femoral canal. All lymphatic tissue is dissected from the common and external iliac arteries and veins.

**3** The round ligaments are cut and tied at the pelvic wall, and the broad ligaments are opened.

**4** All lymphatic tissue is removed from the obturator fossa. The infundibulopelvic ligaments with the ovarian vessels are clamped, cut, and tied at the pelvic brim.

**5** The right ureter is transected below the pelvic brim. Steps 1–5 are then repeated on the left side.

**6** The obturator fossa external iliac and common iliac artery and veins have been cleaned of all lymphatic tissue. The hypogastric artery and vein are clamped and tied at the bifurcation of the common iliac vessels. The ureter has been cut, the distal segment has been tied, and the proximal segment is left open and free.

**7** The peritoneum of the mesentery of the rectosigmoid colon is opened. A soft Silastic drain is placed through an avascular opening in the mesentery and used for retraction of the colon.

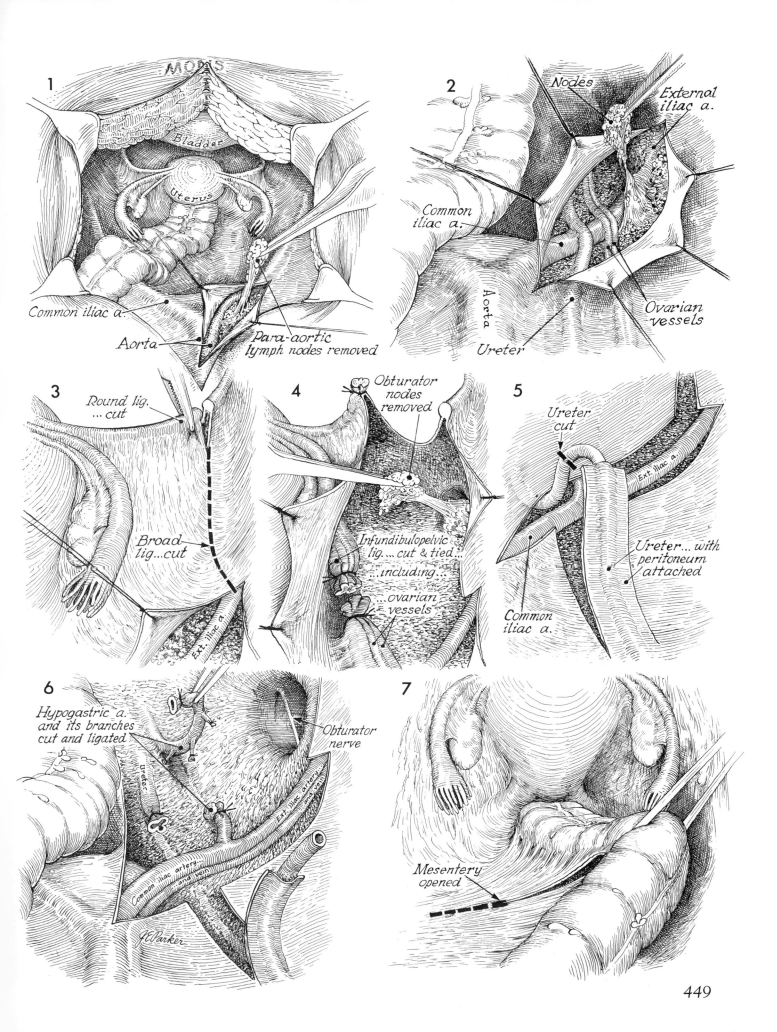

1

MODS

Bladder

Uterus

Common iliac a.

Aorta

Para-aortic
lymph nodes removed

2

Nodes

External
iliac a.

Common
iliac a.

Aorta

Ureter

Ovarian
vessels

3

Round lig.
...cut

Broad
lig...cut

Ext. iliac a.

4

Obturator
nodes
removed

Infundibulopelvic
lig. ... cut & tied ...

...including...

...ovarian
vessels

5

Ureter
cut

Ext. iliac a.

Ureter... with
peritoneum
attached

Common
iliac a.

6

Hypogastric a.
and its branches
cut and ligated

Obturator
nerve

Ureter

Ext. iliac artery
and vein

Common iliac artery
...and vein

J.E.Parker

7

Mesentery
opened

449

# Total Pelvic Exenteration

## (Continued)

**8** The peritoneum of the mesentery on the medial side of the rectosigmoid colon is opened.

**9** The vascular tissue in the mesentery is cross-clamped in successive pedicles, incised, and tied with 2-0 suture.

**10** The rectosigmoid colon is clamped and transected with the gastrointestinal anastomosis (GIA) automatic surgical stapler. This transects the colon and seals the distal and proximal segments.

**11** The remaining mesentery of the rectosigmoid colon is clamped and incised down to the sacrum.

**12** The rectum is dissected off the sacrum and coccyx by blunt dissection. This is performed by retracting the uterus and distal segment of the rectum anterior and cephalad, inserting a hand behind the rectum in the presacral space, and freeing the rectum down to the coccyx.

It is important not to allow the blunt dissection to proceed laterally, since the presacral veins may then be lacerated and may retract into the presacral foramen, causing copious bleeding.

**13** The rectal stalks on each side are clamped, incised, and tied with 2-0 sutures down to the levator muscles.

The specimen should now be free posteriorly.

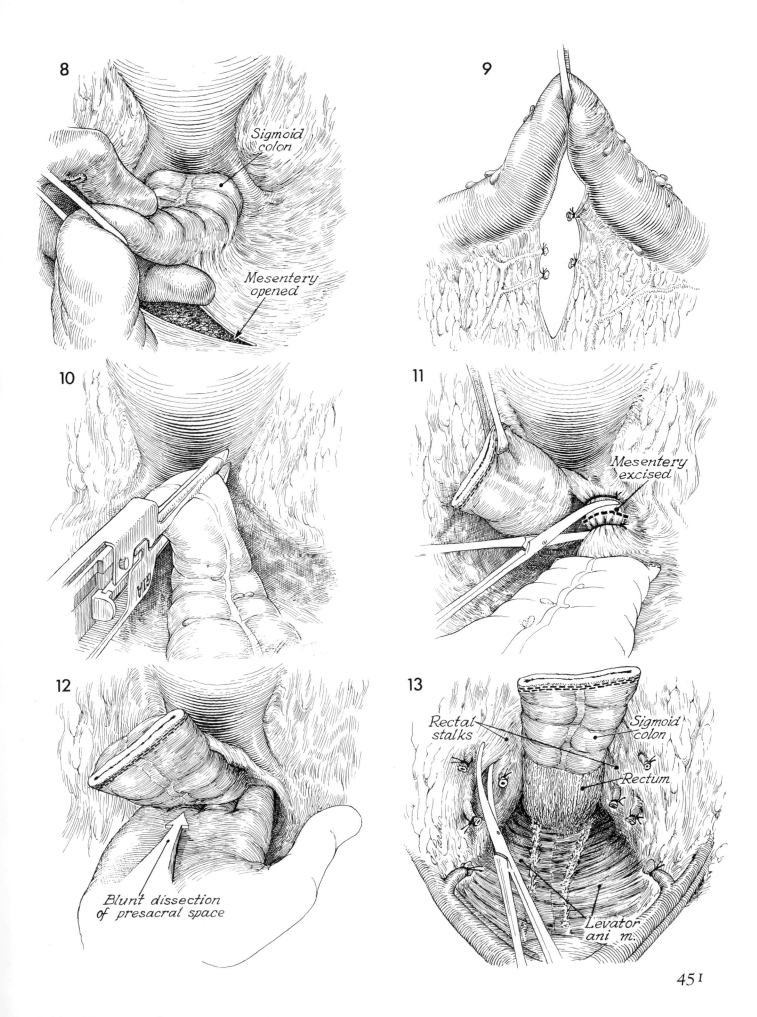

**8**

Sigmoid colon

Mesentery opened

**9**

**10**

**11**

Mesentery excised

**12**

Blunt dissection of presacral space

**13**

Rectal stalks

Sigmoid colon

Rectum

Levator ani m.

# Total Pelvic Exenteration

## (Continued)

**14** The bladder is separated from the pubic symphysis where the *dotted line* appears.

**15** The space of Retzius is entered, and the bladder and proximal two-thirds of the urethra are freed. The lateral attachments of the bladder are clamped and incised on both sides. The entire specimen can now be freed laterally, forming one large lateral attachment of bladder, rectum, and uterine parametria to the pelvic wall.

**16** The first and second fingers have been inserted into the paravesical and pararectal spaces, identifying both sides of the large lateral attachment to the pelvic wall. The anterior wall of the paravesical space and the posterior wall of the pararectal space have been removed with dissection of the rectal stalks and bladder attachments. The large pedicle contains the plexus of hypogastric veins. No attempt is made to isolate each vein individually. The pedicle is clamped, incised, and tied on the pelvic wall. Several successive bites are required to transect the pedicle to the levator ani muscles.

**17** This is a posterior view of the same step performed on the opposite side.

**18** The lateral attachment of the specimen is transected in successive bites. It is helpful for the assistant to retract the specimen medially during this maneuver.

**19** All lateral wall attachments have been clamped, incised, and ligated on each side. The specimen has been freed posteriorly, laterally, and anteriorly. The remaining attachments are the urethra, vagina, and rectum.

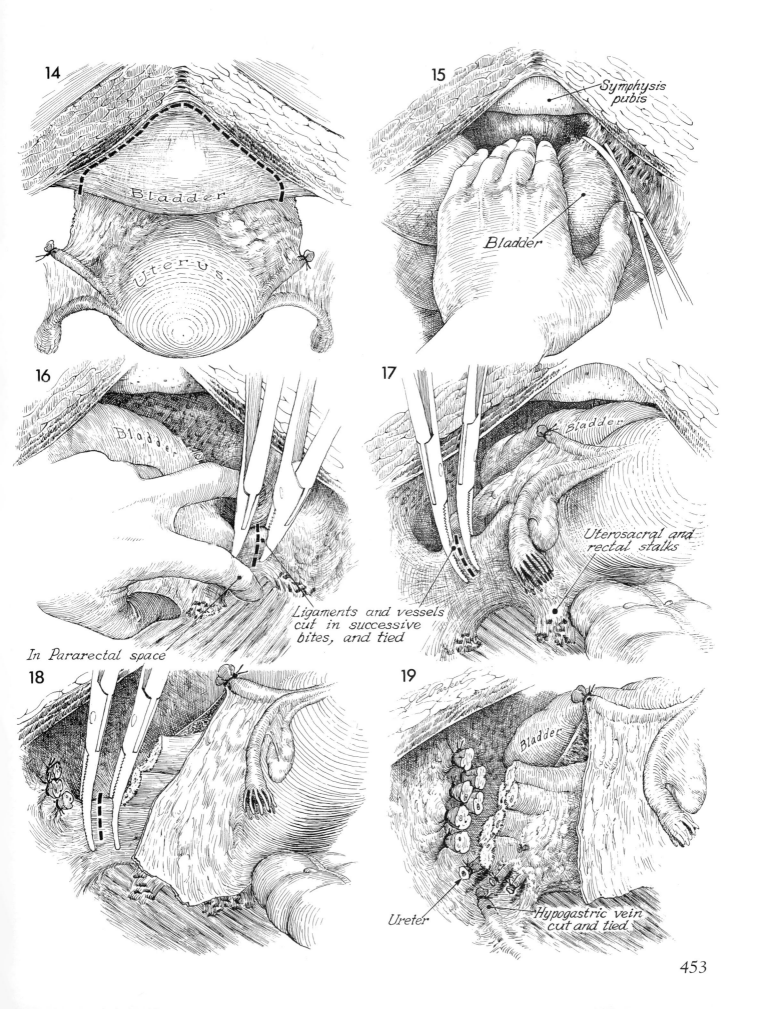

14

15
Symphysis
pubis

Bladder

Bladder
Uterus

16

17

Bladder

Bladder

Uterosacral and
rectal stalks

Ligaments and vessels
cut in successive
bites, and tied

In Pararectal space

18

19

Bladder

Ureter

Hypogastric vein
cut and tied

# Total Pelvic Exenteration

## (Continued)

**20** By cephalad retraction on the specimen, the urethra can be exposed and transected at the level of the levator sling.

**21** The vagina is transected.

**22** The rectum is transected at the level of the levator muscles or higher if an adequate margin from the tumor can be achieved.

**23** The exenterated pelvis is shown with the urethra transected near its meatus. The vagina has been transected and closed with 0 absorbable suture. The rectum is available for anastomosis for the descending colonic J pouch. A continent urostomy Kock pouch (see Section 10, page 464) will be constructed.

**24** Both afferent and efferent nipples have been completed. Note that the two strips of the polyglycolic acid (PGA) mesh pass through the windows of Deaver in the mesentery of both the efferent and afferent bowel limbs adjacent to the nipples. The letters A to A', B to B', C to C' delineate the order of suture placement that will produce a spherical rather than a tubular pouch shape.

**25** The continent pouch has been completed. The stoma is sutured to the subcuticular layer of the skin with 3-0 PGA sutures. The stoma is sutured to the subcuticular skin of the umbilicus with 3-0 PGA sutures. A No. 30 French Medena catheter has been placed through the stoma down the efferent limb and exits the efferent nipple into the pouch. This catheter has been securely sutured in place with a No. 1 nylon suture that includes the margin of the skin, the entire intestinal wall of the stoma, the opposite intestinal wall, and the opposite margin of skin; it is securely tied around the Medena catheter with multiple half-hitch knots to hold the catheter in the pouch without spillage for 3 weeks. A second No. 1 nylon suture is placed on the other side.

A Jackson-Pratt closed suction drain has been placed adjacent to the Kock pouch and brought out through the abdominal wall. It is sutured with a 3-0 PGA suture to prevent removal for 3 weeks. Note that the afferent limb of bowel and the afferent nipple have the ureters sutured in a mucosa-to-mucosa fashion with No. 8 French Finney "J" Silastic stents in place. The abdomen is closed. The Medena catheter is irrigated every 2–4 hours for the next 3 weeks to prevent mucus obstruction.

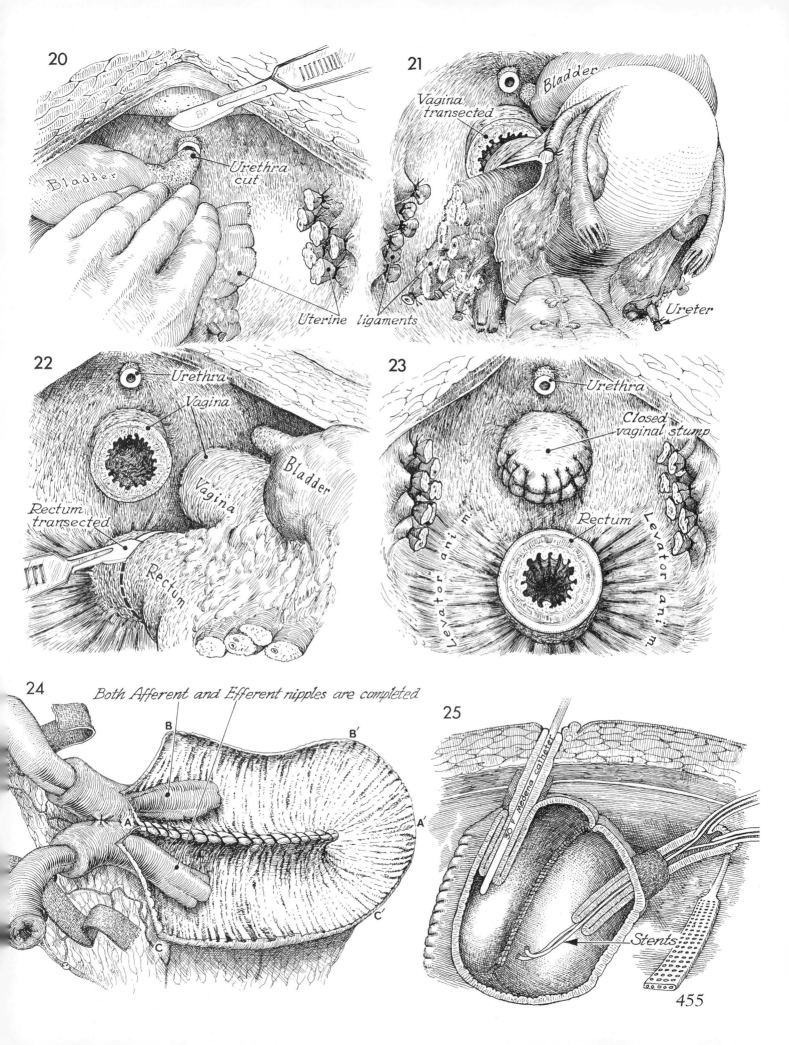

**20**

Bladder

Urethra cut

Uterine ligaments

**21**

Bladder

Vagina transected

Ureter

**22**

Urethra

Vagina

Vagina

Bladder

Rectum transected

Rectum

**23**

Urethra

Closed vaginal stump

Rectum

Levator ani m.

Levator ani m.

**24**

Both Afferent and Efferent nipples are completed

B

B'

A

A'

C

C'

**25**

30 F Medena catheter

Stents

455

# Total Pelvic Exenteration

## (Continued)

**26** A sagittal view is shown. The rectal J pouch has been stapled to the rectum with the EEA stapler. A diversionary loop colostomy has been performed.

**27** A pelvic view shows the rectal J pouch anastomosed to the rectum. The vagina is shown closed with suture.

**28** An omental J flap is initiated by transecting the omentum off the greater curvature of the stomach. The gastroepiploic artery is preserved.

**29** The omental J flap is sown into the pelvis as a lid.

**30** This sagittal view shows the omental J flap as a lid for the pelvis. It contains the small intestine and displaces it out of the pelvis in a sling made from omentum.

The colonic J pouch reservoir is anastomosed to the rectum. *V*, vagina.

**31** This shows the loop diversion colostomy placed in the transverse colon. The urine has been diverted into a continent Kock pouch. The colonic J pouch has been anastomosed to the rectum. *K*, kidney.

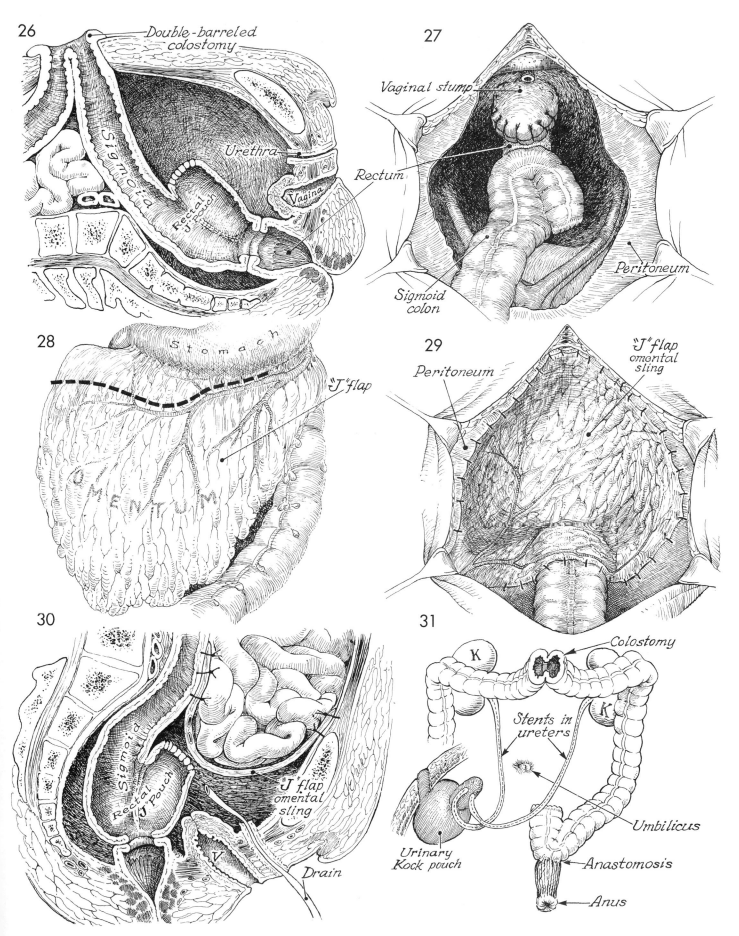

**26**
Double-barreled colostomy
Sigmoid
Urethra
Rectal "J" Pouch
Vagina
Rectum

**27**
Vaginal stump
Peritoneum
Sigmoid colon

**28**
Stomach
"J" flap
OMENTUM

**29**
Peritoneum
"J" flap omental sling

**30**
Sigmoid
Rectal "J" Pouch
"J" flap omental sling
V
Drain

**31**
K
Colostomy
K
Stents in ureters
Umbilicus
Urinary Kock pouch
Anastomosis
Anus

# Colonic "J" Pouch Rectal Reservoir

When the rectosigmoid colon must be removed in the treatment of genital cancer, an end sigmoid colostomy or a very low coloproctostomy may be performed. Very low anastomosis of the colon to the rectum may be associated with an unacceptable frequency of daily bowel movements. Although it is a social and esthetic relief to the patient to eliminate the colostomy stoma, having 6–8 bowel movements per day is an inconvenience and hardship. Treatment of the problem with opiates may produce addiction.

The purpose of the "J" colonic pouch is to provide a rectal reservoir, thereby reducing the number of bowel movements and eliminating the need for drugs.

**Physiologic Changes.** The J pouch rectal reservoir provides an increased storage area for feces. This may precipitate fluid absorption from the fecal stream and result in a firm but soft stool. The patient experiences a reduction in tenesmus.

**Points of Caution.** Adequate mobilization of the transverse and descending colon must be performed to allow the end-to-side Strasbourg-Baker anastomosis to be performed without tension. Since many of the patients undergoing this procedure have had pelvic irradiation, it is important to keep the inferior mesenteric artery and its superior hemorrhoidal branch intact if possible. These arteries will supply blood to the anastomosis, thereby aiding the wound healing process and reducing suture line leaks and fistulae.

Although it is possible to perform this procedure with a suture technique, the use of surgical staplers reduces tissue trauma, allows precise placement of sutures, and significantly reduces operative time.

If the patient has had pelvic irradiation or inflammatory bowel disease, a temporary diverting colostomy should be performed and kept in place until complete wound healing has been demonstrated. This is usually accomplished within 8 weeks.

## Technique

**1** The descending colon is adequately mobilized, and an appropriate site is selected for the side-to-end Strasbourg-Baker coloproctostomy. This site should be at the midpoint of at least 20 cm of distal colon. It should allow 10 cm of colon for the down side of the "J" pouch and 10 cm for the up side.

A stab wound is created at the midpoint lateral to the antimesenteric border. The gastrointestinal anastomosis (GIA) surgical stapler is inserted. The mesentery is cleared from the stapler, and the GIA instrument is fired. This establishes the distal 5 cm of the pouch.

**2** Frequently, it is difficult to reapply the GIA stapler from below for the second 5-cm portion of the pouch. Therefore, it is more convenient to open two small stab wounds on each segment of the J pouch from above and insert each blade of the GIA, connecting them so that they will match the procedure from below.

The surgeon can easily close the opening from the stab wound by picking up the margins of the wound with Allis clamps, placing a TA-55 (4.8 mm) stapler across the wound, and activating the stapler.

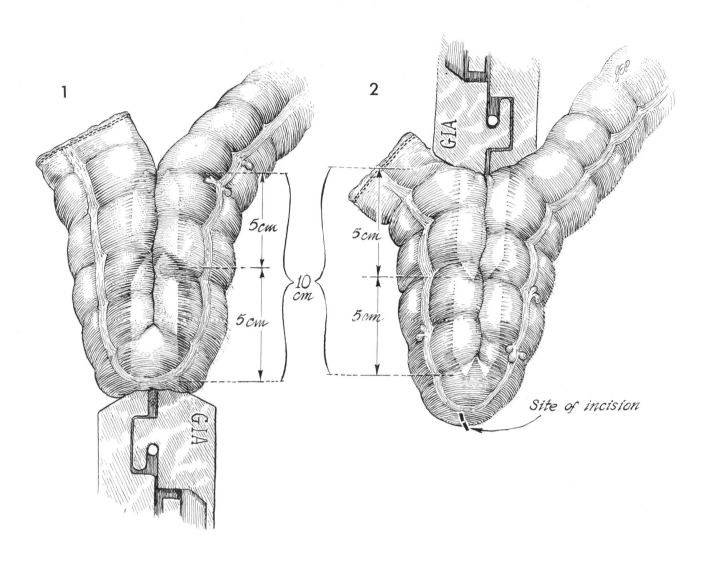

1

5cm

5cm

10 cm

2

5cm

5cm

GIA

GIA

Site of incision

# Colonic "J" Pouch Rectal Reservoir

## (Continued)

**3** A pursestring suture of 2-0 nylon is placed around the enterotomy at the midpoint at the bottom of the J pouch.

A pursestring suture of 2-0 nylon is placed around the margins of the rectal stump.

The EEA (end-to-end anastomosis) stapler is inserted through the anus. After opening the stapler, the surgeon ties both pursestring sutures around the central rod of the stapler. The EEA stapler is closed, then activated, and the coloproctostomy anastomosis is completed.

**4** This cutaway view shows the completed J pouch rectal reservoir.

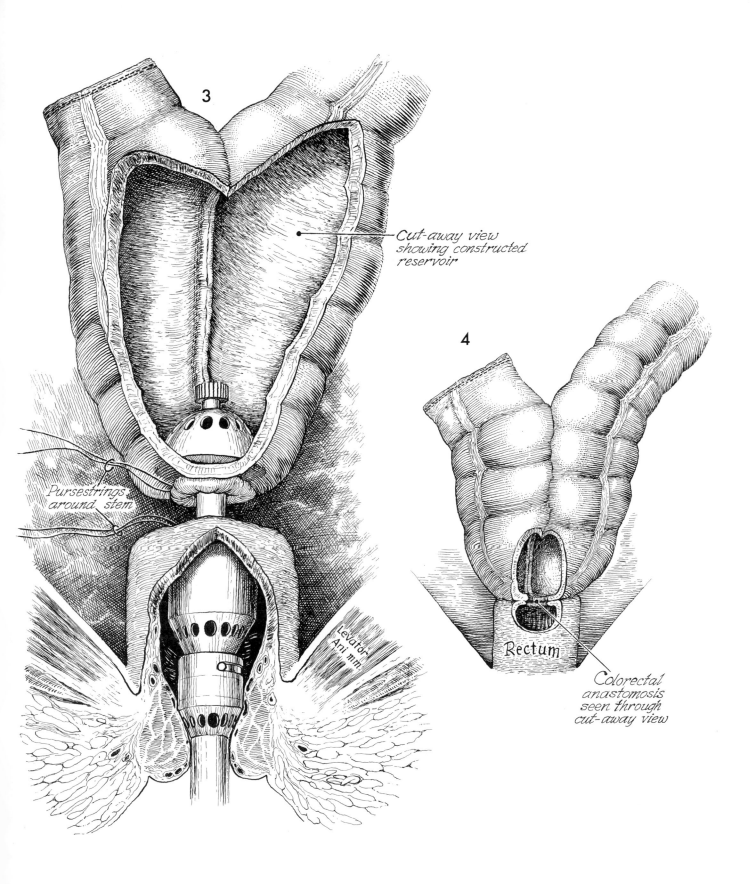

3

Cut-away view
showing constructed
reservoir

Pursestrings
around stem

Levator
Ani mm.

4

Rectum

Colorectal
anastomosis
seen through
cut-away view

# Kock Pouch Continent Urostomy

Patients who have lost the use of the bladder as a result of irradiation or surgical excision may be candidates for a procedure involving the construction of a continent ileal reservoir for cutaneous urinary diversion.

The Kock pouch, designed by Nils Kock in 1982, was devised as a continent urostomy. Modification by Donald Skinner provided a urinary diversion as a continent nonrefluxing urostomy. This alternative to urinary diversion deserves the consideration of gynecologic oncologists.

**Physiologic Changes.** Skinner et al. have shown that construction of an internal reservoir suitable for urinary bladder replacement must provide for (1) retention of 500–1000 mL of fluid, (2) maintenance of low pressure after filling, (3) elimination of intermittent pressure spikes, (4) true continence, (5) ease of catheterization and emptying, and (6) prevention of reflux.

The ileal mucosa of the pouch appears to adapt well to urine; villus height decreases, and in time, the mucosa becomes nearly flat, thereby reducing the absorption of electrolytes from the urine.

**Points of Caution.** Prerequisites to construction of the Kock pouch include reasonable renal function (creatinine less than 3.0 mg/dL); adequate length of small bowel, so that utilization of 80 cm of ileum will not result in a significant short bowel syndrome; and a patient who is motivated for the procedure and who understands the inherent risk (a 10–15% incidence of malfunction of the continent valve mechanism, requiring additional surgery).

The low pressure within the pouch and the high pressure within the nipples prevent reflux and allow the patient to remain continent. In accordance with Laplace's law, the low pressure within the pouch is maintained at high fluid volumes.

A midline incision is preferred for construction of a continent urostomy. The site of the stoma can be determined preoperatively. For young, slim women we prefer to place the opening below the underwear line immediately above the pubic hair. For older or obese patients, the stoma is often placed higher to facilitate catheterization. The surgeon should not feel bound by the preoperative stomal site marking, however, if the mesentery does not allow the pouch to reach that location. Since no appliance is worn for the collection of urine, the surgeon need not worry about skin folds. When the pouch procedure is done in conjunction with total pelvic exenteration or cystectomy, pelvic resection is performed first. For conversion of an existing ileal conduit, all the intra-abdominal wall adhesions must be taken down.

In summary, our motivation for using the Skinner modifications of the Kock pouch continent urostomy in gynecologic oncology has been 85% for medical reasons (i.e., to prevent contaminated reflux and thus deterioration of upper renal units commonly associated with ileal or colonic loops) and 15% for improvement in the quality of life. The elimination of the urinary bag with its attendant problems of awkwardness and odor has a positive effect on the quality of the patient's self-image and sexuality.

# Kock Pouch Continent Urostomy

## (Continued)

*Technique*

**1** In this view of the descending colon, cecum, and terminal ileum, note that the avascular plane of Treves has been entered after the terminal ileum was divided. The incision in the avascular plane of Treves was carried lateral to the ileocolic artery and medial to the superior mesenteric artery. The blood supply of the entire Kock pouch depends on the superior mesenteric artery and its branches. A 5-cm plug of ileum with its mesentery is removed at the upper limit of the Kock pouch to allow placement of the efferent limb of bowel at the preferred stoma site. The first 17-cm segment of the pouch is marked off and labeled for the efferent limb of bowel and the efferent nipple. The next 22-cm segment comprises one loop of the U-shaped pouch, and the last 22-cm segment forms the other limb of the U-shaped loop of the pouch. The last 17-cm segment is available for the afferent nipple and bowel limb of the pouch. This segment is not necessary if the surgeon is converting an ileal loop to the pouch.

**2** The two 22-cm U-shaped limbs are placed adjacent to each other, and interrupted 3-0 polyglycolic acid (PGA) sutures are placed in the bowel 1 cm above the junction of the two segments. A cautery is used to open the intestine approximately 2 cm from the junction of the mesentery, as indicated by the *dotted line*. This opening is extended on the efferent and afferent limbs for a distance of approximately 5 cm; the cautery electrocoagulates the small blood vessels on the edge of the bowel.

**3** A 3-0 PGA suture on a straight fine intestinal needle runs through the back wall of the pouch. A second layer of 3-0 PGA sutures is placed between these sutures.

**4** Construction of the nipples in the afferent and efferent limbs has begun. An 8-cm opening is created in the mesentery by opening the windows of Deaver, applying Hendren's rule that 4 cm of mesentery adjacent to the small bowel can be undercut because there is enough lateral vasculature in the small bowel wall to prevent necrosis. An opening of 8 cm is essential for nontraumatic intussusception and to prevent "extussusception," i.e., undoing of the intussusception. A Babcock clamp is inserted into the lumen of the bowel, and a small Kelly clamp is used to indent the bowel wall into the Babcock clamp.

Papaverine, 300 mg in 500 mL of normal saline, must be administered intravenously 10–15 minutes before intussusception for smooth muscle relaxation to allow intussusception without trauma to the small bowel. A slight drop in the patient's blood pressure should be expected; this rarely exceeds 20 mm Hg in systolic pressure and 10 mm Hg in diastolic pressure.

A 2-cm strip of PGA mesh is passed through the window of Deaver. This will be sutured in place after the nipple has been created.

**5** The intussusception is being performed under the influence of a smooth muscle relaxant. A segment of bowel is pulled out for a distance of 6–7 cm.

**6** The TA-55 4.8-mm stapler with 5 staples missing from the heel of the stapler is inserted on the nipple and stapled at the 2 and 10 o'clock positions.

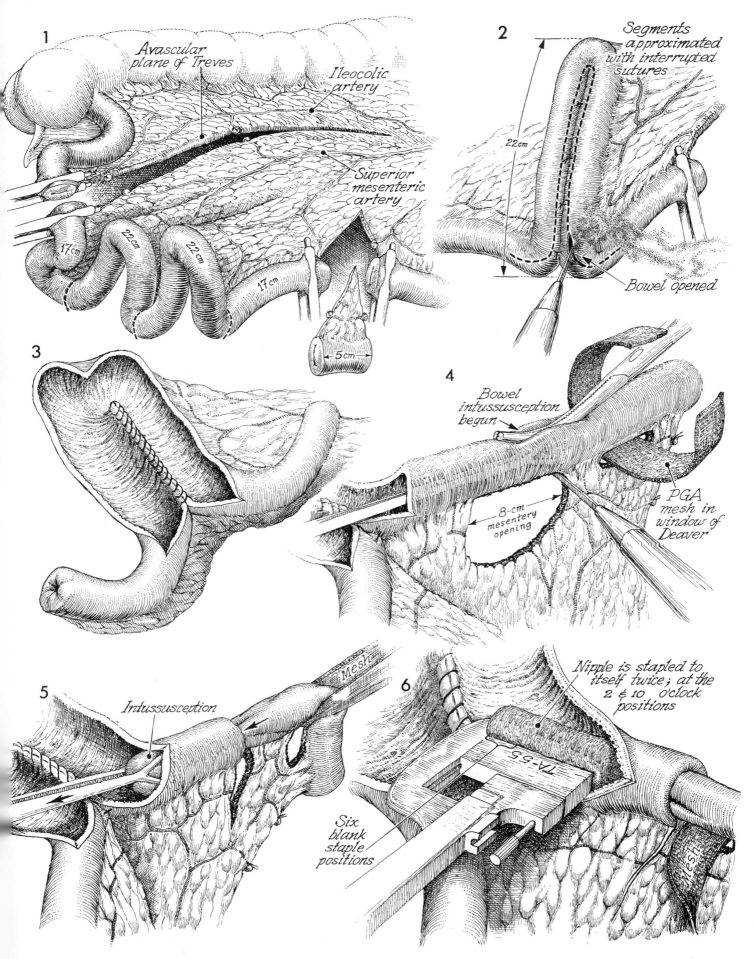

**1** Avascular plane of Treves · Ileocolic artery · Superior mesenteric artery · 17 cm · 22 cm · 22 cm · 17 cm · 5 cm

**2** Segments approximated with interrupted sutures · 22 cm · Bowel opened

**3**

**4** Bowel intussusception begun · 8-cm mesentery opening · PGA mesh in window of Deaver

**5** Mesh · Intussusception

**6** Nipple is stapled to itself twice; at the 2 & 10 o'clock positions · TA-55 · Six blank staple positions · Mesh

465

# Kock Pouch Continent Urostomy

## (Continued)

**7** The nipple is stapled to itself twice, at the 10 and 2 o'clock positions, with the S-GIA URO stapler (United States Surgical Corp.). The stapler contains no blade, and the inner rows of staples have been removed. It has the advantage of having no pinhole.

**8** An alternative method would be to perform a small enterotomy in the posterior wall of the pouch; place the stapler through the enterotomy and then through the nipple, and staple it. All pinholes from the TA-55 stapler must be sutured with interrupted 3-0 PGA sutures before proceeding. Note that the PGA mesh in the window of Deaver is still not sutured in place.

**9** Both afferent and efferent nipples have been completed. Note that the two strips of PGA mesh pass through the windows of Deaver in the mesentery of both the efferent and afferent bowel limbs adjacent to the nipples. The letters A to A', B to B', C to C' delineate the order of suture placement that will produce a spherical rather than a tubular pouch.

**10** With the pouch still open, the No. 30 French Medena catheter is inserted up the nipple in a retrograde fashion to allow accurate sizing for the PGA mesh. The mesh is sutured with interrupted 3-0 PGA sutures in a fashion that securely locks it at the junction of the intussusception to prevent extussusception.

**11** The pouch is closed with 3-0 PGA sutures by approximating points A to A', B to B', and C to C'.

**12** The remaining walls of the pouch are sutured with a running 3-0 PGA suture, and a second layer of running 3-0 PGA sutures is added.

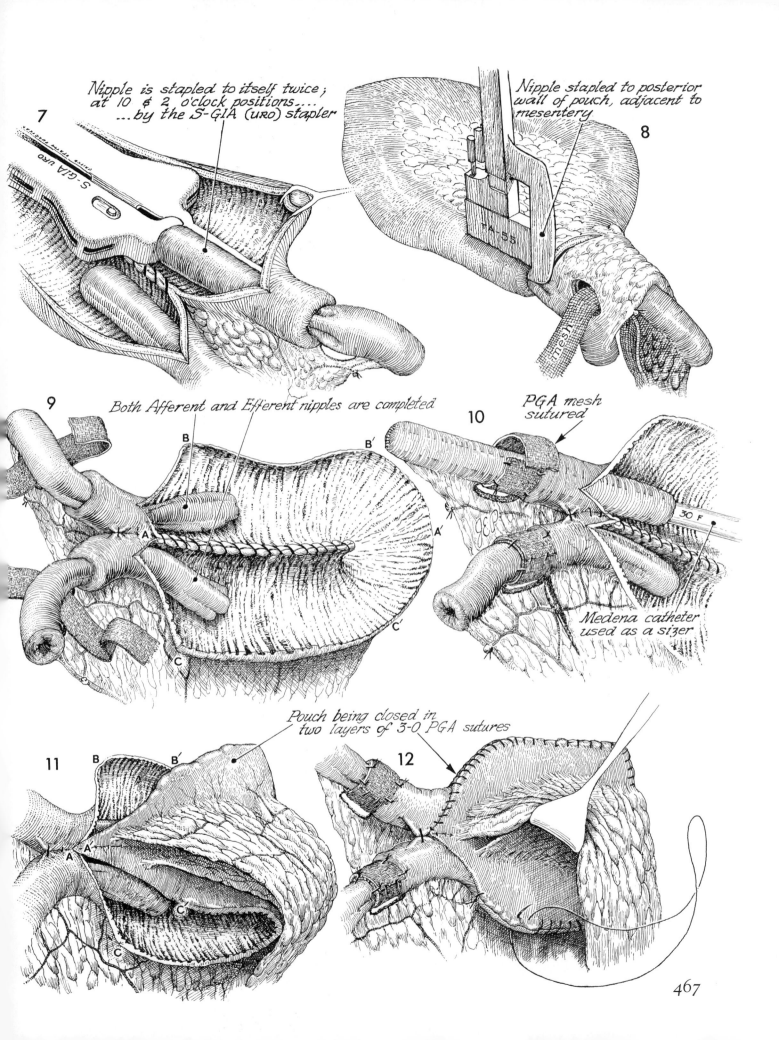

**7** Nipple is stapled to itself twice; at 10 & 2 o'clock positions.... ...by the S-GIA (URO) stapler

S-GIA URO

**8** Nipple stapled to posterior wall of pouch, adjacent to mesentery

TA-55

mesh

**9** Both Afferent and Efferent nipples are completed

B          B′

A          A′

C          C′

**10** PGA mesh sutured

30 F

Medena catheter used as a sizer

**11** B          B′

A          A′

C

C′

**12** Pouch being closed in two layers of 3-0 PGA sutures

467

**13** In the completed pouch, the PGA mesh is in place adjacent to the intussusception. Two enterotomies have been made in the afferent limb of the bowel. Two No. 8 French Finney J Silastic catheters are threaded through the enterotomies, down the afferent limb, through the afferent nipple, and into the pouch. The ureters previously mobilized have been spliced by incising the ureteral wall for a distance of approximately 3 cm.

**14** The Finney J Silastic catheter has been threaded up the ureters and into the renal pelvis. The ureter has been sutured to the enterotomy in the bowel with interrupted 4-0 PGA sutures in a mucosa-to-mucosa technique. Additional sutures are placed between the serosa of the bowel and the ureter. Indigo carmine dye, 3 mL, is administered intravenously. The suture line is thoroughly inspected to ensure that there is no leakage of blue dye-stained urine coming from the kidney and down the ureter. Note that the Finney J Silastic catheters are threaded into the loop. The J curled ends of the catheters indicate they are within the pouch and not in the nipple.

**15** The efferent bowel limb has been exteriorized through an umbilical ostomy defect. In addition, the efferent bowel limb has been tapered to fit a No. 20 French Medena catheter with the GIA instrument. Both of these procedures, exteriorization through the umbilicus and the tapering of the efferent bowel limb, are designed to reduce the diame-

ter of the efferent bowel limb and therefore raise the pressure of the overall efferent system to greatly exceed that in the pouch.

The efferent port is sutured on its medial and lateral borders to the anterior rectus fascia.

**16** The tapered efferent bowel limb is brought through the ostomy defect in the umbilicus. The sutures are tied to the umbilical ostomy defect.

**17** The efferent tapered nipple bowel limb is sutured to the edge of the umbilical defect.

**18** A No. 20 French Medena catheter is inserted through the efferent bowel limb through the efferent nipple into the pouch. The stoma has been matured in the umbilicus. The afferent bowel limb containing the ureters and the afferent nipple are shown on the right. Note the J Silastic stents coming from the renal pelvis down the ureters through the afferent bowel limb through the afferent nipple into the pouch. These are removed with a cystoscope 3 weeks following surgery.

The very important Jackson-Pratt suction drainage shown on the right remains in place until the pouch has completely healed and there is no leakage from the pouch or any of the anastomoses. This Jackson-Pratt drain is usually removed 3 weeks postoperatively.

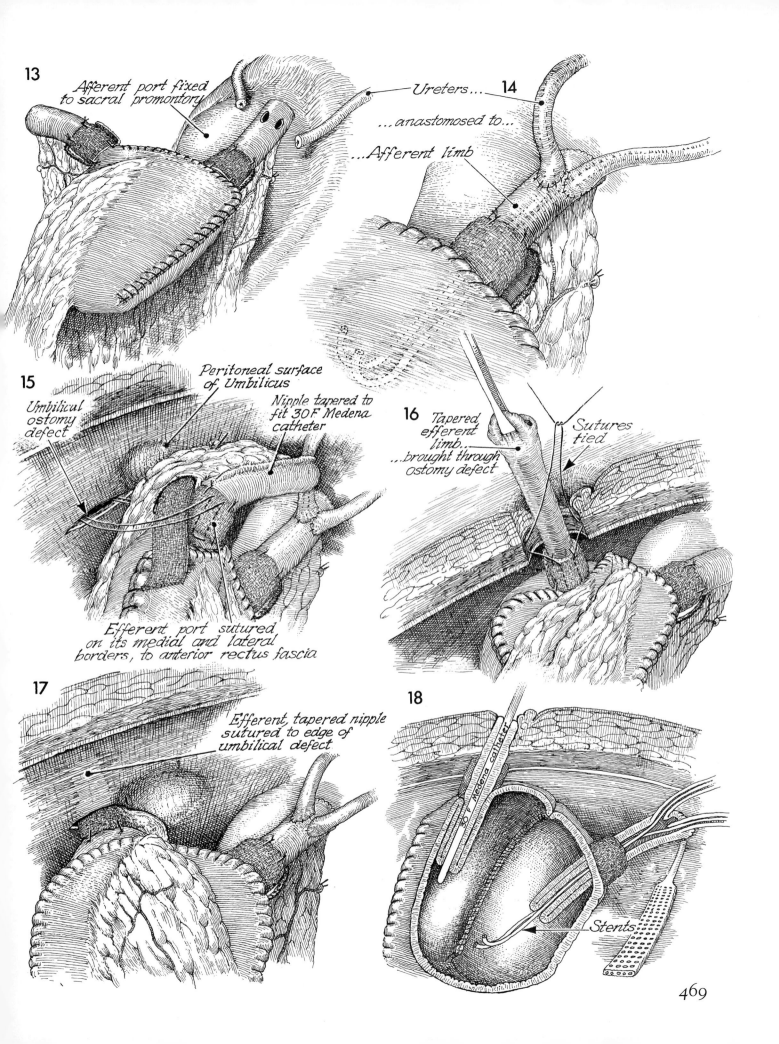

**13** *Afferent port fixed to sacral promontory*

**14** *Ureters...* *...anastomosed to...* *...Afferent limb*

**15** *Peritoneal surface of Umbilicus*
*Nipple tapered to fit 30F Medena catheter*
*Umbilical ostomy defect*
*Efferent port sutured on its medial and lateral borders, to anterior rectus fascia*

**16** *Tapered efferent limb... ...brought through ostomy defect*
*Sutures tied*

**17** *Efferent, tapered nipple sutured to edge of umbilical defect*

**18** *30 F Medena catheter*
*Stents*

469

# Omental "J" Flap Neovagina

Construction of a neovagina has been an accepted gynecologic procedure for many years. McIndoe (see Section 2, page 91) has described surgical techniques for construction of a neovagina when the bladder is in position anteriorly and the rectum and colon are in position posteriorly. These techniques are inapplicable, however, when patients have undergone total pelvic exenteration with or without low coloproctostomy. Under these circumstances, Berek and Hacker demonstrated that the anterior wall of the neovagina could be made from an omental flap.

By modifying the omental flap, which is normally used to close off the pelvic inlet after total pelvic exenteration with or without low coloproctostomy, the surgeon can create a cylinder providing anterior, posterior, and lateral walls for the neovagina. When the cylinder is sutured to the introitus and lined with a skin graft, it becomes a satisfactory functional vagina.

**Physiologic Changes.** The omentum that is enervated by the vagus nerve forms the wall of the neovagina. Normally, tugging or pulling on the omentum does not produce a sensation of pleasure that one would associate with sexual intercourse. Approximately 40% of the patients who have undergone this procedure, however, report that they experience sexual orgasm.

Another physiologic change is the development of estrogen hormone receptors on the split-thickness skin graft. Derived from skin on the buttocks or thigh that normally has no hormonal properties, the graft eventually becomes indistinguishable from normal vaginal mucosa on biopsy. At present, it is unknown whether the maturation index of the graft can be influenced by the administration of systemic estrogen, as can occur in normal vaginal mucosa.

**Points of Caution.** If the construction of the neovagina immediately follows total pelvic exenteration, it is important to ensure hemostasis in the pelvic wound before applying the skin graft. If hemostasis is uncertain, the omental neovagina should be packed with gauze or foam rubber covered by a contraceptive condom. Then, when hemostasis is maintained, in approximately 6–12 postoperative days a skin graft can be taken and applied to the vaginal form.

After the skin graft has been inserted, the neovagina must remain dilated with a vaginal form until healing is complete. Thereafter, a soft Silastic vaginal form should be worn for 6 months except during intercourse. After this time, the soft Silastic vaginal form is worn only at night if sexual intercourse is not a part of the patient's life.

## Technique

**1** This sagittal view shows a patient who has undergone a total pelvic exenteration. In this patient, the rectal stump was left, and the descending colon was brought down for a very low coloproctostomy. The urethra and vagina below the levator sling remain in place. The omentum has been brought down as a flap and has been sutured to the sacral promontory posteriorly and the pubic symphysis anteriorly.

**2** In the upper part of this figure can be seen the omental flap with the intestines lying in the pelvic lid sling. In the lower part of this figure can be seen the distal portion of the flap rolled into a cylinder. The lateral wall of the cylinder has been sutured with interrupted 3-0 polyglycolic acid (PGA) sutures.

**3** This perineal view shows the vulva and vaginal introitus. The wall of the omental cylinder has been sutured to the vaginal introitus with interrupted 3-0 PGA sutures.

**4** The omental cylinder has been completed and sutured to the vaginal introitus.

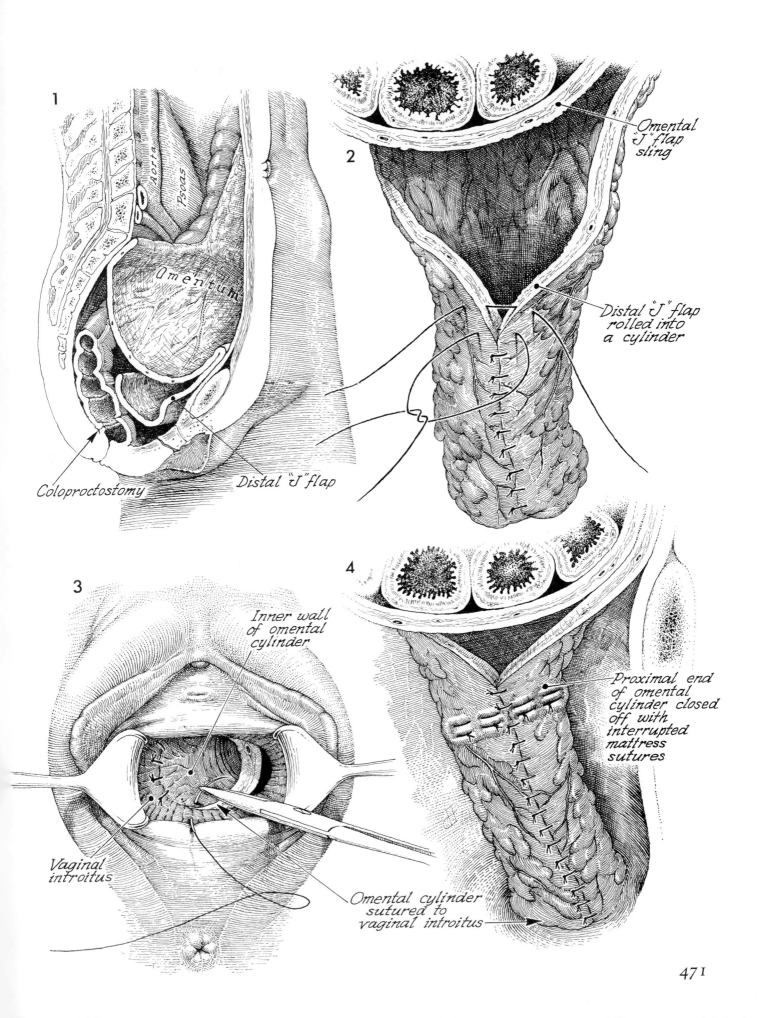

**1**

Aorta

Psoas

Omentum

Coloproctostomy

Distal "J" flap

**2**

Omental "J" flap sling

Distal "J" flap rolled into a cylinder

**3**

Inner wall of omental cylinder

Vaginal introitus

Omental cylinder sutured to vaginal introitus

**4**

Proximal end of omental cylinder closed off with interrupted mattress sutures

# Omental "J" Flap Neovagina

## (Continued)

**5** The dermatome can be seen in this view. *STSG*, split-thickness skin graft.

**6** The graft is laid out, and a vaginal form is fashioned from foam rubber stuffed into a contraceptive latex condom. The vaginal form has been shaped to an appropriate size, length, and diameter. This is laid on the graft; the graft is folded over the vaginal form, and the edges of the graft are sutured with interrupted 4-0 PGA sutures.

**7** The graft-covered form is inserted through the vaginal introitus into the omental cylinder.

**8** This sagittal section shows the omental "J" flap as the pelvic lid and the residue of the omental flap that forms the outer walls of the neovagina. The graft-covered vaginal form has been introduced into the neovagina.

**9** The labia majora have been approximated loosely by several 2-0 nylon sutures. These remain in place for 10 days. The stump of the condom covering the vaginal form protrudes through the suture line.

On the tenth postoperative day, the patient is returned to the operating room for an examination under anesthesia. The vulvar sutures and vaginal form are removed, and the graft covering the neovagina is inspected.

The patient is fitted with a soft Silastic vaginal form that must be worn for approximately 6 months.

The vaginal form is removed each day and washed, the neovagina is douched, and the form is replaced. Failure to be sexually active and/or to use the vaginal form as prescribed will result in contracture of the neovagina.

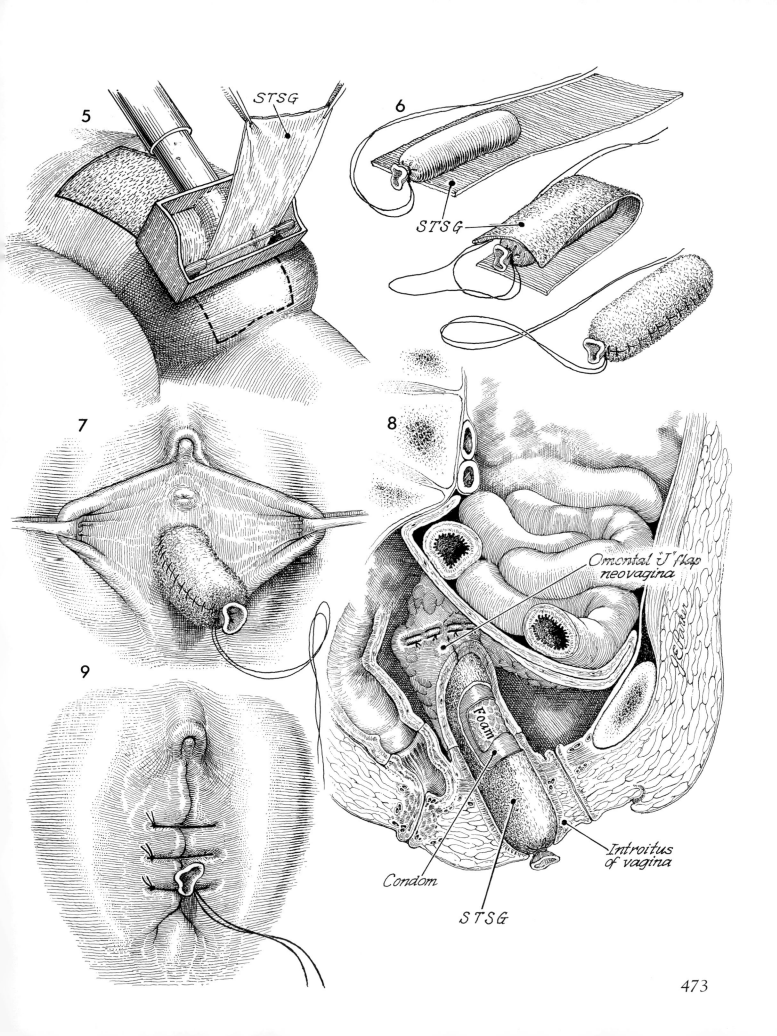

5

STSG

6

STSG

7

8

Omental 'J' flap
neovagina

Condom

Foam

STSG

Introitus
of vagina

9

# Ileocolic Continent Urostomy (Miami Pouch)

Continent urostomy of the ileal or ileocolic variety (Miami pouch) has become an essential part of urinary diversion in oncology patients. The mechanical engineering phenomenon of a pouch that has pressure lower than the ureteral pressure entering it and pressure lower than the efferent bowel limb leaving it has the advantage of having no urinary reflux. That, in turn, should reduce the incidence of chronic subclinical pyelonephritis among these patients and, consequently, reduce the loss of upper renal units. The continent efferent system allows a better quality of life for a patient and avoids the social disadvantages of a urinary ostomy bag.

**Physiologic Changes.** The continent urostomy should be a low pressure pouch with pressures in the range of 30 cm of water. At the same time, there should be a nonrefluxing ureteral anastomosis into the pouch. If the normal ureter has pressures of approximately 60 cm of water, there should be little reflux from the pouch to the kidney. The combination of these pressure differentials should allow the patient to be continent and have little or no urinary reflux to the kidney.

Removal of a large portion of the right colon, a significant portion of the transverse colon, and a portion of the terminal ileum can cause various physiologic phenomena in the gastrointestinal tract. Removal of the right colon and some of the transverse colon may produce a watery diarrheal stool. Removal of the terminal ileum results in problems with bowel salt metabolism, and absorption of fat-soluble vitamins and vitamin $B_{12}$. Loss of the ileocecal valve may involve reflux of contaminated stool back into the proximal ileum, which, in turn, can lead to problems with chronic small bowel infection and various metabolite changes.

**Points of Caution.** The blood supply to the Miami pouch is dependent on the ileocolic artery, particularly the right colic branch of the ileocolic artery, and the middle colic artery. These arteries connect with the marginal artery of the colon. Extreme care must be exercised so that the ileocolic or the middle colic artery is not compromised. When performing the anastomosis, the surgeon must be careful to place the ureter into the colonic pouch. The ureter must prolapse 3 cm into the pouch to reduce urinary reflux. We have changed the point of exteriorization of the efferent limb onto the abdominal wall from the right lower quadrant to the umbilicus. This gives a better cosmetic effect and also reduces incontinence of the efferent bowel limb.

# Ileocolic Continent Urostomy (Miami Pouch)

## (Continued)

## *Technique*

**1** An outline of the colon and the small bowel is shown with the key anatomical points: the ileocolic artery, the superior mesenteric artery, the avascular plane of Treves between the superior mesenteric artery and the ileocolic artery, the terminal ileum, and the right and transverse colon. The line of Toldt is outlined in the pericolic gutter *(dotted line)*. The *dotted line* shows the incisions to be made to create the pouch. In these cases, the larger portion of transverse colon is used to create a larger pouch. In radiated bowel, a large pouch will have a lower pouch pressure because irradiated bowel lacks compliance and, therefore, larger volumes of urine create excessive pouch pressure.

**2** The midileum is anastomosed to the transverse colon in a functional end-to-end anastomosis using the stapler.

**3** The transverse colon is brought along the side of the right colon and sutured with several interrupted 3-0 synthetic absorbable sutures. The colon is then opened in the midline with the cautery.

**4** After opening the colon down to the cecum, the surgeon sutures the posterior wall of the pouch with interrupted 3-0 synthetic absorbable sutures.

**5** The posterior wall of the colon can be either sutured or stapled. It is faster and easier to staple it with a TA-55 Polysorb staple using multiple bites and suturing in between each application of the stapler.

**6** The right and left ureters have been mobilized and are brought through the posterior wall of the pouch via a Leadbetter anastomotic technique. The ureter must prolapse 3 cm inside the colon after being anastomosed to allow protection from urinary reflux. Finney double-J Silastic catheters are inserted up the ureters into the kidney and brought out into the pouch.

**7** The Leadbetter anastomosis is demonstrated by a mucosa-to-mucosa anastomosis after spatulating the ureter to prevent iris contracture postoperatively.

**8** The pouch is folded over on to itself, *point A'* is brought alongside *point A'*, and *point B* is brought alongside *point B'*. The segment of terminal ileum that will eventually become the efferent bowel limb is shown.

**9** The ureters have been anastomosed to the pouch. The TA-55 polysorb stapler is used to close the margins of the pouch.

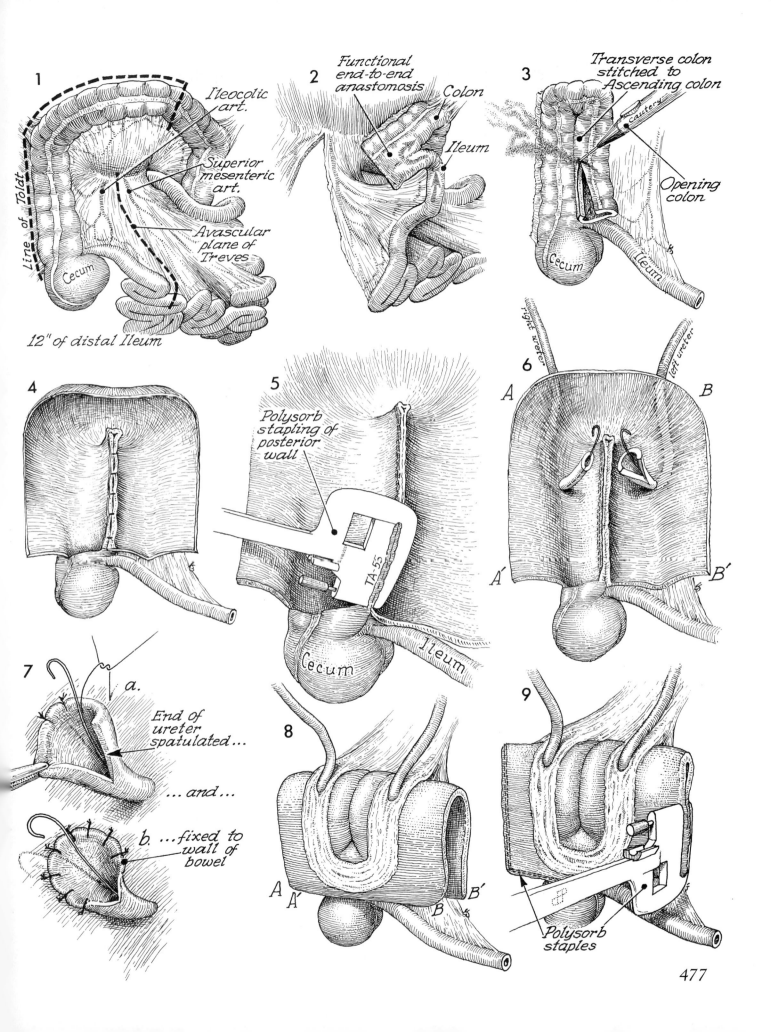

**1**
Line of Toldt
*Ileocolic art.*
*Superior mesenteric art.*
*Avascular plane of Treves*
Cecum
*12" of distal Ileum*

**2**
*Functional end-to-end anastomosis*
*Colon*
*Ileum*

**3**
*Transverse colon stitched to Ascending colon*
Cautery
*Opening colon*
Cecum
Ileum

**4**

**5**
*Polysorb stapling of posterior wall*
TA-55
Cecum
Ileum

**6**
right ureter
left ureter
A
B
A'
B'

**7**
*a.*
*End of ureter spatulated...*
*...and...*
*b. ...fixed to wall of bowel*

**8**
A
A'
B'
B

**9**
*Polysorb staples*

**10** The ureters have been implanted. The margins of the pouch have been stapled with a polysorb stapler. Small areas that are awkward for the stapler to anastomose can be sutured with 3-0 synthetic absorbable suture.

**11** Attention is turned to the efferent bowel limb. A No. 14 French catheter is inserted down the terminal ileum into the pouch. Two parallel pursestring sutures 1 cm apart are placed at the ileocecal junction with delayed synthetic absorbable suture.

**12** The pursestring sutures have been placed. The No. 14 French catheter is seen traversing the efferent bowel limb into the pouch.

**13** The GIA stapler with 4.8 staples is used to taper the terminal ileum on its antimesenteric border to narrow the lumen of the efferent bowel limb to the size of a No. 14 French catheter. This dramatically raises the pressure inside the lumen, such that the pressure in the lumen of the efferent bowel limb is more than twice the pressure in the pouch.

**14** The efferent bowel limb has been tapered with the stapler. Excessive ileum is discarded.

**15** The inferior rim of the umbilicus is excised enough to allow the efferent bowel limb to be pulled through the abdominal wall at that site.

**16** The efferent bowel limb has been brought through the inferior rim of the umbilicus, and the excessive ileal length has been excised. The remaining stump is sutured with 3-0 synthetic absorbable suture.

**17** In this transverse view of the completed Miami pouch, the ureters are implanted and prolapsed into the pouch. Finney J Silastic stents are placed in the pouch, and the efferent bowel limb has been sutured to the umbilicus. It is best to leave an indwelling Medena catheter inserted through the efferent bowel limb into the pouch for at least 2 weeks to allow complete healing of all suture lines. The pouch should be protected by a Jackson-Pratt closed suction cannula and irrigated every four hours with 30 mL of warm saline.

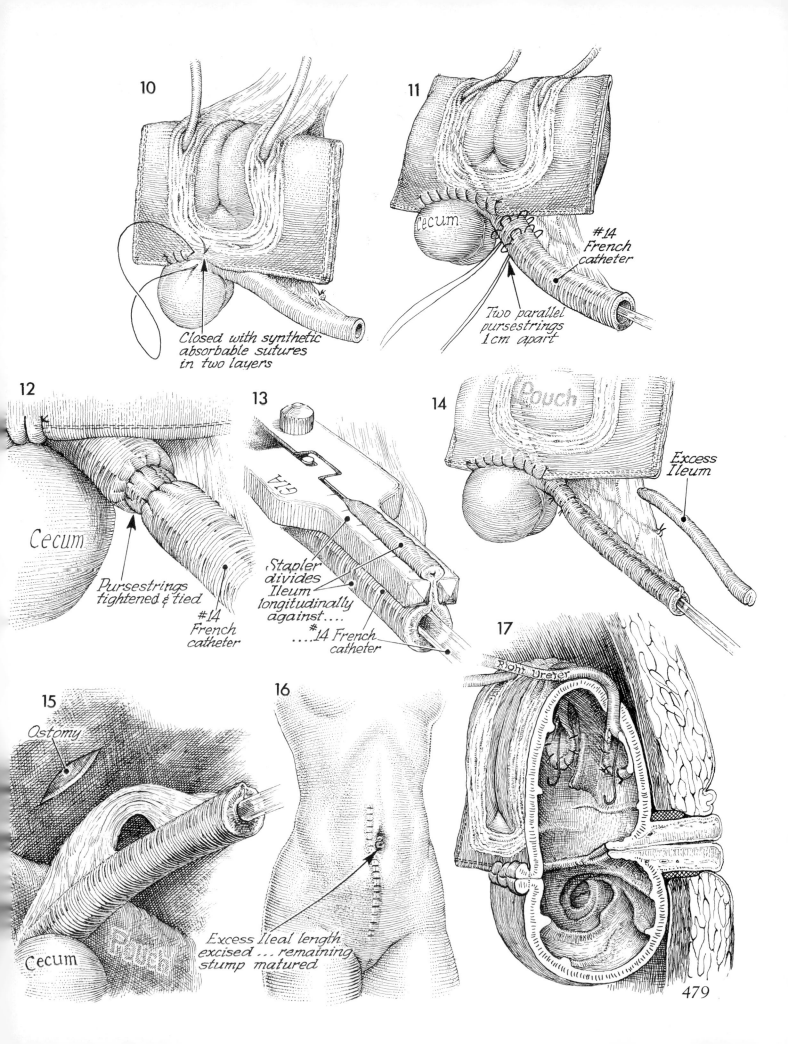

**10** Closed with synthetic absorbable sutures in two layers

**11** Cecum
#14 French catheter
Two parallel pursestrings 1 cm apart

**12** Cecum
Pursestrings tightened & tied
#14 French catheter

**13** GIA
Stapler divides Ileum longitudinally against....
....#14 French catheter

**14** Pouch
Excess Ileum

**15** Ostomy
Cecum
Pouch

**16** Excess Ileal length excised...remaining stump matured

**17** Right Ureter

# Construction of Neoanus Gracilis Dynamic Anal Myoplasty

In cases where the anal sphincter has become incompetent or when both the anus and anal sphincter have been removed (as in sublevator total pelvic exenteration or abdominoperineal resection), the surgeon may perform a neoanus dynamic anal myoplasty. The operation has been performed in Europe for 8 years and will come to the United States, pending Food and Drug Administration (FDA) approval.

**Physiologic Changes.** The dynamic anal myoplasty operation attempts to restore the anus so that normal defecation can occur by using the gracilis muscle and a modified cardiac pacemaker. The anus and anal sphincter are rebuilt with the gracilis muscle, and a pacemaker is attached to the muscle. When the muscle is electronically stimulated, it produces an anal pressure that is greater than the colonic pressure, allowing the patient to maintain continence. When the electrical current is withdrawn, however, the gracilis muscle relaxes, the anal pressure falls to a level below that of the colon, and the patient pushes down and defecates. The on-and-off switch for the modified cardiac pacemaker is a simple magnet.

**Points of Caution.** The integrity of the neurovascular bundle of the gracilis muscle must be carefully preserved, as it is dissected from the leg. Adjustment of the cardiac pacemaker for voltage and frequency can be made externally.

## Technique

**1** The patient is shown having had a laparotomy following abdominal perineal resection. With the patient in the dorsal supine modified lithotomy position with the leg extended and knee flexed, the gracilis muscle is palpated. An incision is made of approximately 30 cm, extending from the pubic ramus to the tubercle on the knee.

**2** The adductor longus, the gracilis, and the adductor magnus muscles are identified. The vital neurovascular bundle of the gracilis muscle is located and dissected. The gracilis muscle is transected at the so-called "goose foot" as it inserts on the knee and is transected proximally, adjacent to the ramus of the ischium. Care must be taken to identify the sartorius muscle and not confuse this with the gracilis muscle. The stump of the distal gracilis muscle tendon is seen adjacent to the knee.

**3** A tunnel is made under the posterior fourchette of the vagina, under the perineal body, and around the anus with sharp and blunt dissection. If it is a case of anal sphincter incompetence or a pull-through procedure from a previously existing abdominal perineal resection, the muscle is pulled through, with the gracilis neurovascular muscle kept intact.

**4** The entire gracilis muscle is pulled through the tunnel and wrapped around the colon or defective anal sphincter and is fixed in place with interrupted sutures. The margin of the anal skin incision is shown for those cases where the anus and the anal sphincter have been completely removed. The wire leads from the modified cardiac pacemaker are attached to the gracilis muscle at the junction of the neurovascular bundle to the muscle and confirmed in this position by electronically stimulating the device while the incision is open.

**5** The neoanus is shown with the sigmoid colon anastomosed to the border of the anus or perianal skin. The gracilis muscle is shown ghosted underneath.

**6** The wire leads are brought through the subcutaneous tunnel to a site that is selected for the modified cardiac pacemaker on the abdominal wall. The wound in the left leg has been repaired over Jackson-Pratt suction drains.

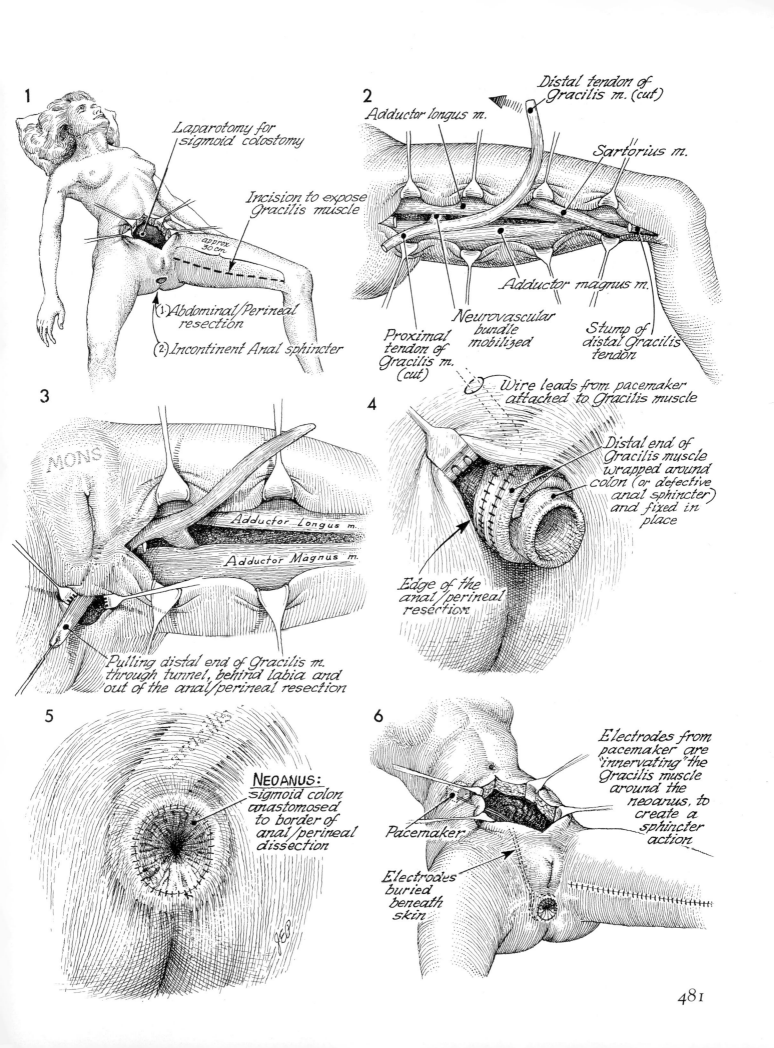

**1**

Laparotomy for sigmoid colostomy

Incision to expose Gracilis muscle

approx 30 cm.

(1) Abdominal/Perineal resection

(2) Incontinent Anal sphincter

**2**

Distal tendon of Gracilis m. (cut)

Adductor longus m.

Sartorius m.

Adductor magnus m.

Neurovascular bundle mobilized

Proximal tendon of Gracilis m. (cut)

Stump of distal Gracilis tendon

**3**

MONS

Adductor Longus m.

Adductor Magnus m.

Pulling distal end of Gracilis m. through tunnel, behind labia and out of the anal/perineal resection

**4**

Wire leads from pacemaker attached to Gracilis muscle

Distal end of Gracilis muscle wrapped around colon (or defective anal sphincter) and fixed in place

Edge of the anal/perineal resection

**5**

NEOANUS: sigmoid colon anastomosed to border of anal/perineal dissection

**6**

Electrodes from pacemaker are "innervating" the Gracilis muscle around the neoanus, to create a sphincter action

Pacemaker

Electrodes buried beneath skin

481

# Skin-Stretching System Versus Skin Grafting

Skin grafting has been an unusual but needed procedure in gynecologic oncology surgery. The physiology of wound healing is dramatically improved if wounds are covered as soon as possible and not left granulating over a period of months.

A new instrument has been added to the gynecologic surgeons armamentarium, the skin-stretching device known as Sure-Closure (MedChem, Woburn, Massachusetts).

The purpose of the operation is to cover an exposed defect on the abdominal wall, vulva, or sacrum.

**Physiologic Changes.** The predominate physiologic change is closure of the wound to prevent contraction and epithelialization. Loss of fluid and protein from open wounds allowed to granulate over a period of time is a major metabolic and nutritional problem.

**Points of Caution.** Care must be taken to adequately mobilize the edges of the wound. The wound should never be covered under tension.

The air dermatome should be held at an angle of 45–60°. Holding the air dermatome at an angle of less than 45° produces (1) a split-thickness skin graft that is chopped into pieces and (2) a donor site with an irregular surface.

The technique of skin-stretching via the device known as Sure-Closure takes advantage of the processes of the "mechanical creeping" produced by the Sure-Closure device, which applies a controlled amount of tension evenly along two open wound margins of skin. The mechanical stretcher uses the vesicoelastic properties of skin to stretch in a reasonable time while minimizing the skins tendency to recoil. Repeated cycles of stretching are performed over a 30–45-minute period of time until the skin margins can be brought in opposition for suturing without tension.

## Technique

1. In an open wound of the abdominal wall with the underlying rectus fascia closed with interrupted sutures, the skin on either side of the defect is undermined for 2–3 cm with the electrocoagulation device.

2. An air dermatome is demonstrated taking a split-thickness skin graft. Note that the dermatome occupies a 45° angle to the level of the donor site. The graft is grasped with Allis forceps or skin hooks. The air dermatome is set to produce a graft of 0.2 mm.

   The donor site is covered with a fine mesh gauze to prevent epithelial cells from growing through the pores on regular gauze, debriding the donor wound with each dressing change.

3. The graft is laid on the open wound, and the margins of the open wound are sutured to the margins of the split-thickness skin graft (STSG).

4. The elements of the Sure-Closure skin-stretching system can be seen here. They consist of two straight needles, the two parts of the stretching device with hooks that engage the two needles under the platform of the stretching device. On one stretching device there is a strain gauge that prevents the skin from stretching too rapidly. The upper platform of the stretching device shows the needles but also shows the locking system that prevents the device from unlocking after the skin has been stretched.

5. The needles have been inserted along the margins of the skin parallel to the wound. The stretching system has small retained needles on the bottom of their platforms stuck under the linear needles to provide a solid stretching system. The strain gauge portion of the stretching system is engaged into the receiving end and locked in place. The wheel screw of the stretching system is turned, and the margins of the skin are stretched. The strain gauge will show when the skin is being stretched beyond its capacity. There is a clutch in the stretching system that disengages the wheel crank when too much stretching pressure has been applied to the skin; this allows for the skin to recover before further stretching is allowed.

6. When the margins of the wound have been approximated to each other, the wound is closed with interrupted mattress sutures.

7. The devices have been set in place for a radical vulvectomy incision. After stretching, tension has been removed from the skin of the inguinal node dissection. The skin of the vulva resection can be stretched to close the skin to the margins of the vagina without tension through the skin-stretcher process.

8. The wound is closed following the stretching process.

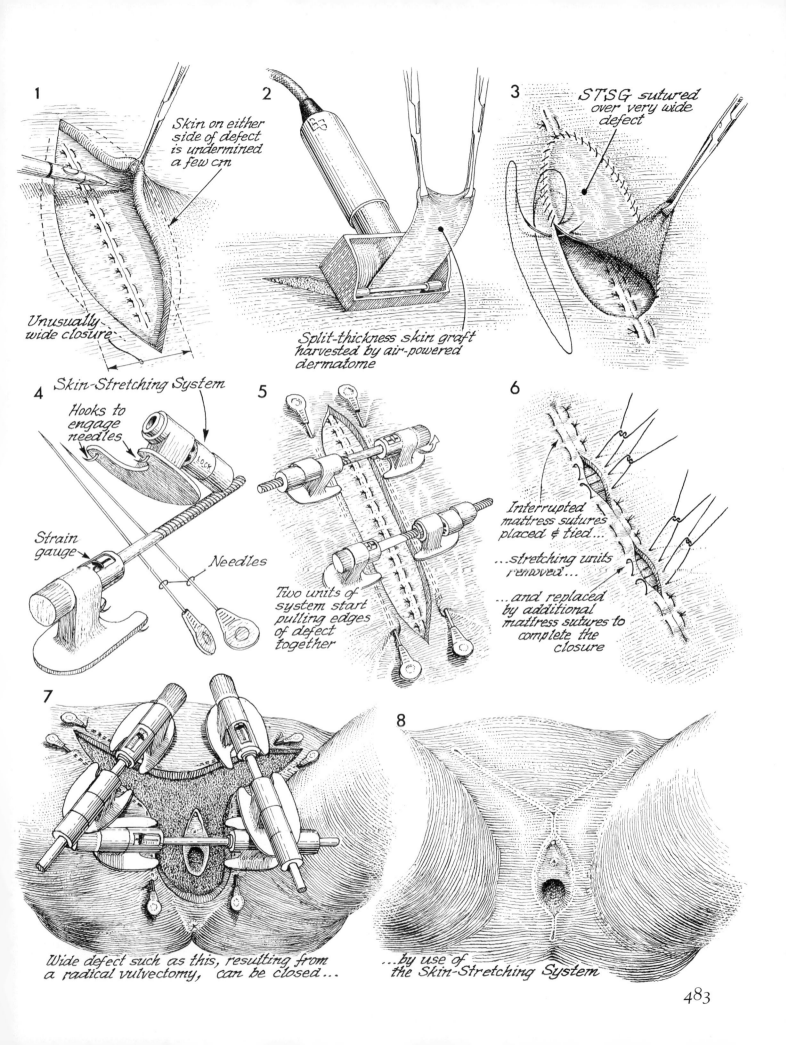

**1** Skin on either side of defect is undermined a few cm

Unusually wide closure

**2** Split-thickness skin graft harvested by air-powered dermatome

**3** STSG sutured over very wide defect

**4** Skin-Stretching System

Hooks to engage needles

Strain gauge

Needles

**5** Two units of system start pulling edges of defect together

**6** Interrupted mattress sutures placed & tied...

...stretching units removed...

...and replaced by additional mattress sutures to complete the closure

**7** Wide defect such as this, resulting from a radical vulvectomy, can be closed...

**8** ...by use of the Skin-Stretching System

# Gastric Pelvic Flap for Augmentation of Continent Urostomy or Neovagina

Radiation therapy is one of the keystone treatments in gynecologic cancer. A sequela of radiation therapy, however, can be endarteritis with fibrosis and ischemia to the pelvic tissues as well as the rectosigmoid colon and terminal ileum. When a continent urostomy is made out of irradiated bowel, the compliance of this radiated tissue is frequently low; therefore, because it cannot stretch under filling with urine, the pressure in a continent urostomy pouch will be elevated, which may lead to incontinence.

Neovaginas made out of radiated sigmoid colon have the same compliance features as continent urostomies. The compliance is low, secondary to radiation fibrosis, and the distensibility is minimal.

A source of highly compliant nonirradiated bowel is frequently needed to allow a reconstructed organ such as a continent urostomy and neovagina to have an excellent blood supply and function as desired.

The stomach is a resource available for both. It has not been irradiated. It has a copious blood supply. It secrets hydrochloric acid that reduces urinary tract infections in the continent urostomy and provides an acid secretion for the neovagina.

**Physiologic Changes.** Removal of a small flap of gastric tissue from the greater curvature of the stomach has few sequelae. The stomach is a highly vascular organ and reanastomosis of the stomach heals very well. Gastrointestinal physiology is not significantly reduced by the use of a small gastric flap. Using the gastric flap as part of a continent urostomy changes the physiology of the urine from alkaline to an acid, compromising the environment for growth of bacteria.

The acid secretion of a flap augmenting a sigmoid neovagina makes the secretions more acid and allows greater distensibility through compliance to the sigmoid neovagina.

**Points of Caution.** The main point of caution is the protection of the gastroepiploic artery and the short gastric arteries that provide the blood supply to the gastric flap.

A second point of caution is the careful removal of all staples in the gastric flap. If present in the suture line in contact with urine, they will be a source of stone formation.

Third, the stainless staples should never be left in a neovagina. If present, they can cause a penile laceration.

# Gastric Pelvic Flap for Augmentation of Continent Urostomy or Neovagina

## (Continued)

*Technique*

**1** The esophagus, spleen, and stomach with the omentum and the right and left epigastric arteries in place are shown. The right or left gastroepiploic arteries can be ligated. The short gastric arteries proximal or distal to the proposed flap are individually ligated and tied. The flap is marked off with a skin-marking pencil. The reader is referred to the "clam" gastrocystoplasty for the two steps involved in stapling and cutting the flap with the gastrointestinal anastomosis (GIA) linear stapler cutter. As seen in Figure 1 of the clam gastrocystoplasty (Section 3, page 172), the first GIA stapler is placed over the drawn triangular area across the anterior and posterior stomach wall. It is fired and cut. As seen in Figure 2 of the "clam" gastrocystoplasty (page 172), a second GIA stapler is placed on the pencil markings of stomach. The stapler is fired and cut. This leaves a triangular flap of the anterior and posterior gastric wall approximately 5–6 cm at the base and approximately 5 cm into the stomach.

Figure 3 of the clam gastrocystoplasty (page 172) shows the missing wedge-shaped flap from the greater curvature of the stomach. Two small gastrostomies are created adjacent to the staple line. These incisions in the stomach next to each staple line edge of resection allow the placement of another GIA stapler for reanastomosis.

**2** The GIA stapler is inserted into the small gastrotomy incisions. In this figure, the GIA stapler is ghosted as it approximates the edges of the previous staple line and, when it is closed and activated, transects the septum created by taking the wedge of gastric flap. In Figure 5 of the clam gastrocystoplasty (page 172), the two gastrotomy defects are picked up with Babcock clamps, and a TA-55 stapler is placed

across these defects in the stomach wall. Excess tissue is trimmed away. The stomach is now continuous. All incisions have been closed with staples.

A feeding tube gastrostomy is performed as demonstrated in Figures 6–8 of the clam gastrocystoplasty (page 172).

**3** The transverse colon is retracted caudad, and a retractor is placed under the reconstructed stomach, revealing the vena cava (VC). The celiac artery and its branches are also shown.

A defect is made in the mesentery of the transverse colon medial to the middle colic vessels. The omentum with the gastric flap attached is passed through the defect in the mesentery of the transverse colon.

The right gastroepiploic artery has been used in this case with the short gastric branches attached. If the left gastroepiploic vessels are used, the omentum and its flap are placed lateral to the left colon.

**4** Shown here is the passage of the omentum with its gastric flap through a defect in the transverse colon mesentery, proceeding to a second defect created in the avascular plane of Treves of the mesentery of the terminal ileum. Shown also are the middle colic vessels in the transverse colon mesentery and the superior mesenteric artery. The right gastroepiploic artery selected in this case and the stomach wedge-shaped flap are passed through the second opening created in the avascular plane of Treves. This step drops the gastric flap deep in the pelvis and makes it available for an augmentation patch for continent urostomies or neovaginas.

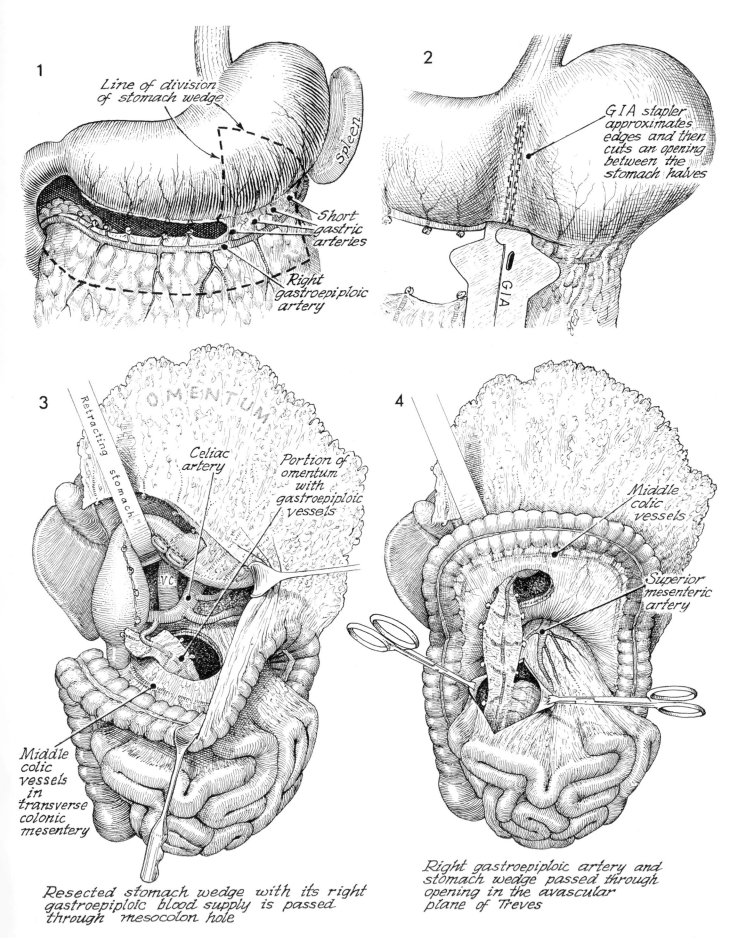

**1**

Line of division of stomach wedge

Spleen

Short gastric arteries

Right gastroepiploic artery

**2**

GIA stapler approximates edges and then cuts an opening between the stomach halves

GIA

**3**

Retracting stomach

OMENTUM

Celiac artery

Portion of omentum with gastroepiploic vessels

IVC

Middle colic vessels in transverse colonic mesentery

Resected stomach wedge with its right gastroepiploic blood supply is passed through mesocolon hole

**4**

Middle colic vessels

Superior mesenteric artery

Right gastroepiploic artery and stomach wedge passed through opening in the avascular plane of Treves

487

# Gastric Pelvic Flap for Augmentation of Continent Urostomy or Neovagina

## (Continued)

---

**5** Shown here are the right gastroepiploic vessel with its short gastric branches to the stomach and the wedge-shaped gastric flap. Each staple is removed with sharp dissection.

**6** The triangular gastric flap is now opened into a diamond-shaped flap. At the bottom, a Kock pouch continent urostomy has been constructed out of small intestine that may have been irradiated.

Instead of folding the intestine over on itself to make a classic Kock pouch (see Kock Pouch Continent Urostomy, page 463), the open diamond-shaped stomach flap can be placed over the intestine of the Kock pouch as shown, and the corresponding edges can be sutured with synthetic absorbable suture.

**7** The colonic ileal pouch (Miami pouch) has been made at the bottom. Also shown are the open right colon and the terminal ileum, below which

will become the afferent bowel limb of the Miami pouch. At the far right, the ureters have been implanted into a segment of ileum that has been sutured to the medial opening of the right colon. At the top, the omental flap with the right gastroepiploic vessels can be seen, with the gastric flap sutured to the open colon, giving the resultant pouch more capacity at lower pressure.

**8** A sigmoid neovagina has been created and sutured to the vaginal introitus. The gastric flap can be sutured to the sigmoid neovagina in a fashion that would augment the sigmoid neovagina that has been irradiated. This allows greater distensibility of the vagina with improved blood supply from a nonirradiated source.

**5**

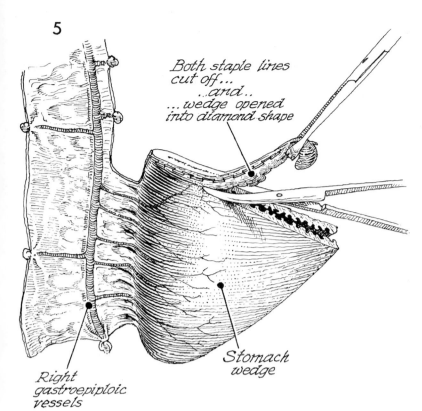

Both staple lines
cut off...
...and..
...wedge opened
into diamond shape

Stomach
wedge

Right
gastroepiploic
vessels

**6**

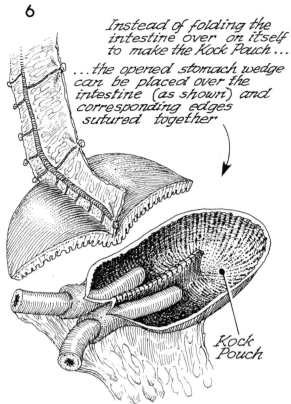

Instead of folding the
intestine over on itself
to make the Kock Pouch...
...the opened stomach wedge
can be placed over the
intestine (as shown) and
corresponding edges
sutured together

Kock
Pouch

**7**

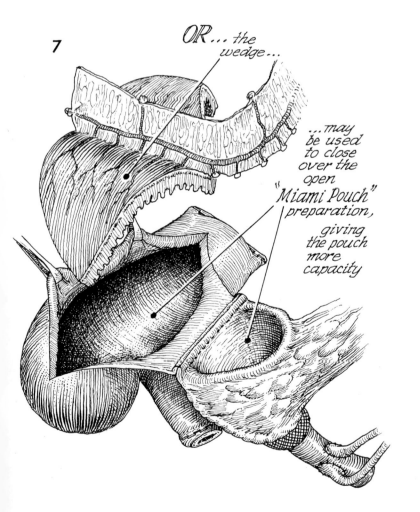

OR...the
wedge...

...may
be used
to close
over the
open
"Miami Pouch"
preparation,
giving
the pouch
more
capacity

**8**

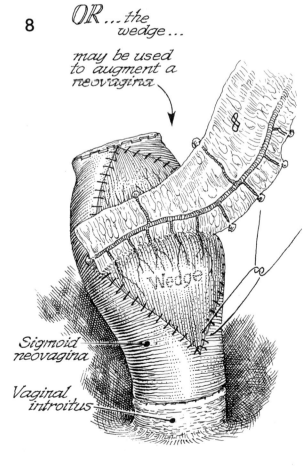

OR...the
wedge...

may be used
to augment a
neovagina

Wedge

Sigmoid
neovagina

Vaginal
introitus

# Control of Hemorrhage in Gynecologic Surgery

The gynecologic surgeon operating in the pelvis and abdomen is constantly performing surgery in the vicinity of large vital blood vessels. Occasionally, one of these large blood vessels will be accidentally entered, producing profuse hemorrhage.

Large abdominal and pelvic arteries should be repaired. Small defects in abdominal and pelvic veins should likewise be repaired with surgical suturing. Difficult laceration in large veins that cannot be repaired easily must be tied off. The only vein in the abdominal and pelvic cavity that cannot be tied off is the portal vein. Tying the vena cava may produce temporary bilateral leg edema until collateral circulation is established.

The basics of hemorrhage control should be mastered by all abdominal and pelvic surgeons. This topic has been divided into following parts:

- Repair of the Punctured Vena Cava
- Ligation of a Lacerated Internal Iliac Vein and Suturing of a Lacerated Common Iliac Artery
- Hemorrhage Control in Sacrospinous Ligament Suspension of the Vagina
- Presacral Space Hemorrhage Control
- What Not to Do in Cases of Pelvic Hemorrhage
- Packing for Hemorrhage Control
- Control of Hemorrhage Associated With Abdominal Pregnancy

**Physiologic Changes.** The typical 70-kg female will have approximately 5000 mL of blood before surgery. A blood loss of 1000–2000 mL, i.e., 40% of the patient's blood volume, may be tolerated without transfusion or potential hypovolemic shock. Patients with blood loss greater than this, however, must have immediate replacement of whole blood. Crystalloids are a poor substitute for whole blood.

An excellent rule to follow is that for every 6 units of packed red cells infused, 2 units of fresh frozen plasma should be infused to replace factor VIII, which is frequently diluted with large blood transfusions. This dilution can create a disseminated loss of blood from small punctures of blood vessels by needles as well as from sharp dissection. The total platelet count may be reduced; the prothrombin time (PT) and partial thromboplastin time (PTT) may be normal or elevated.

**Points of Caution.** If transfusion exceeds 10–12 units and bleeding is not under control by standard surgical techniques, a clear assessment must be made in consultation with the anesthesiologist. If the patient is cold, has metabolic acidosis, and continues to bleed, it may be wise to totally pack off that portion of the abdominal cavity that is bleeding; to close the skin of the abdomen, only not the rectus fascia; to send the patient to the surgical intensive care unit for correction of all vital signs, temperature, electrolytes, and clotting factors; and to return the patient in 48 hours under good surgical conditions to remove the packs and control any residual hemorrhage if found.

# Repair of the Punctured Vena Cava

## Technique

**1** The surgeon is frequently faced with small circular defects in the wall of the inferior vena cava above the bifurcation caused by evulsion of the perforator vein entering the para-vena cava lymph nodes. Hemorrhage is copious and immediate. The first step in control of this hemorrhage is to apply pressure with the finger, the second step is to gain exposure by suctioning blood from the abdominal cavity, extending the incision, etc., and the third step is to obtain proper vascular instruments.

**2** The small circular defect in the vena cava can be grasped with smooth vascular pickups.

**3** A stainless steel hemoclip can be applied to the tented portion of the vena cava (VC). Excess blood should be washed from the area with saline.

**4** The repaired puncture should be observed for several minutes. We have discontinued resuturing the incised peritoneum over the vena cava. The remaining aortic and vena cava lymphadenectomy should continue.

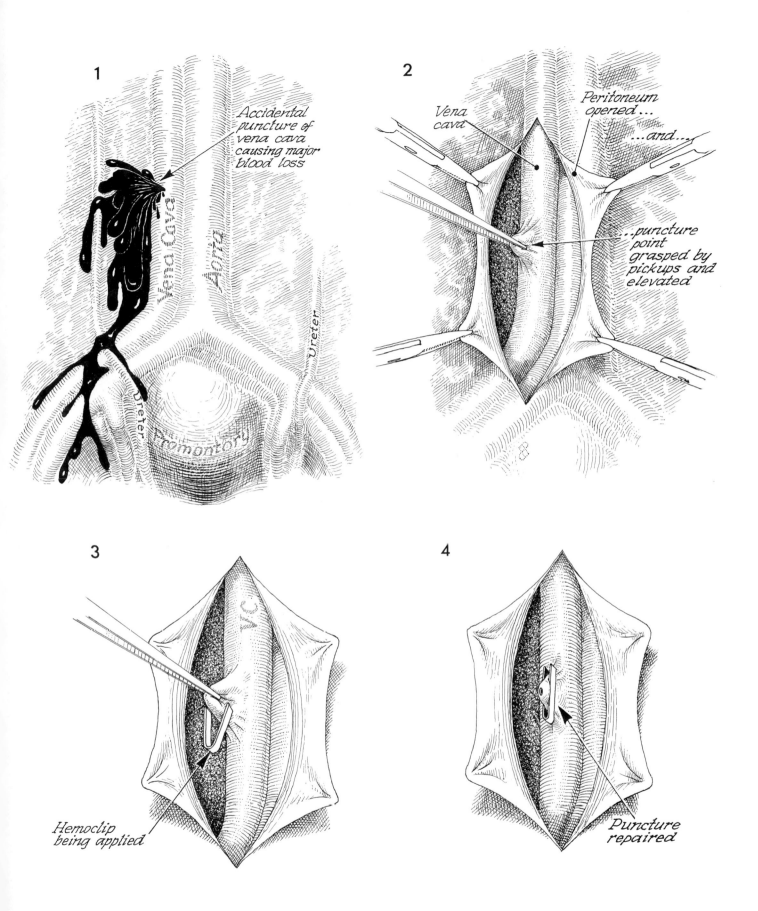

**1**

Accidental puncture of vena cava causing major blood loss

Ureter

Ureter

Promontory

**2**

Vena cava

Peritoneum opened...

...and...

...puncture point grasped by pickups and elevated

**3**

Hemoclip being applied

**4**

Puncture repaired

# Ligation of a Lacerated Internal Iliac Vein and Suturing of a Lacerated Common Iliac Artery

Laceration of a common iliac vein or artery can occur during insertion of the trocar and sleeve with laparoscopy or can occur with lymph node dissection for cancer.

## Technique

### METHODS COMMON TO BOTH LIGATION AND SUTURING

**1** The most common site for laceration of the common iliac artery is generally on the right side, as shown here, because most surgeons are right-handed and insert the laparoscopic trocar with the right hand. At the bottom, the internal iliac (hypogastric) vein is shown lacerated, with copious bleeding coming from both sites.

**2** The first step any surgeon should utilize is placing the finger over the laceration of the artery or vein. Note the proximity of the right ureter to both the right common iliac artery and the right common iliac vein.

### LIGATION OF A LACERATED INTERNAL ILIAC VEIN

**3** Every laparotomy kit contains sponge sticks. Sponge sticks can be used for proximal and distal pressure against the lacerated vessel, whether it be the internal iliac vein, as shown here, or the common iliac artery, as shown in Figure 2.

Blood flow through the open vessels must be controlled. Do not attempt to suture a large blood vessel while copious volumes of blood are flowing.

**4** Ligation of a lacerated vein can be more difficult than suturing of a lacerated artery. The internal iliac vein can be tied off without sequela. Here, DeBakey vascular clamps are placed proximal and distal on the vein laceration. The vein is tied off at the proximal and distal ends with synthetic absorbable suture. Collateral venous drainage will develop between the lower extremity and the ligated internal iliac vein.

### SUTURING OF A LACERATED COMMON ILIAC ARTERY

**5** Sponge sticks can also be used to control hemorrhage from a lacerated right common iliac artery. The artery must be repaired with suture. Blood flow must be controlled. Suturing an open artery is inaccurate and poor technique.

Sponge sticks are always available in laparotomy kits. Often, proper vascular instruments are not. It is a serious mistake to use Kelly, Ochsner, or Kocher clamps on large arteries or veins that need to be sutured.

**6** Figure 6 illustrates the proper way to repair a common iliac artery. DeBakey vascular clamps are placed proximal and distal to the site. When the bleeding ceases, a proper closure is made in the transverse plane of the vessel with 5-0 synthetic monofilament permanent suture on a cardiovascular needle. The 5-0 Prolene with a cardiovascular needle frequently comes in a double-tipped needle at both ends of the suture. This allows a running suture that everts rather than inverts the suture line in the artery. Inversion may produce eddy currents that may cause blood clots.

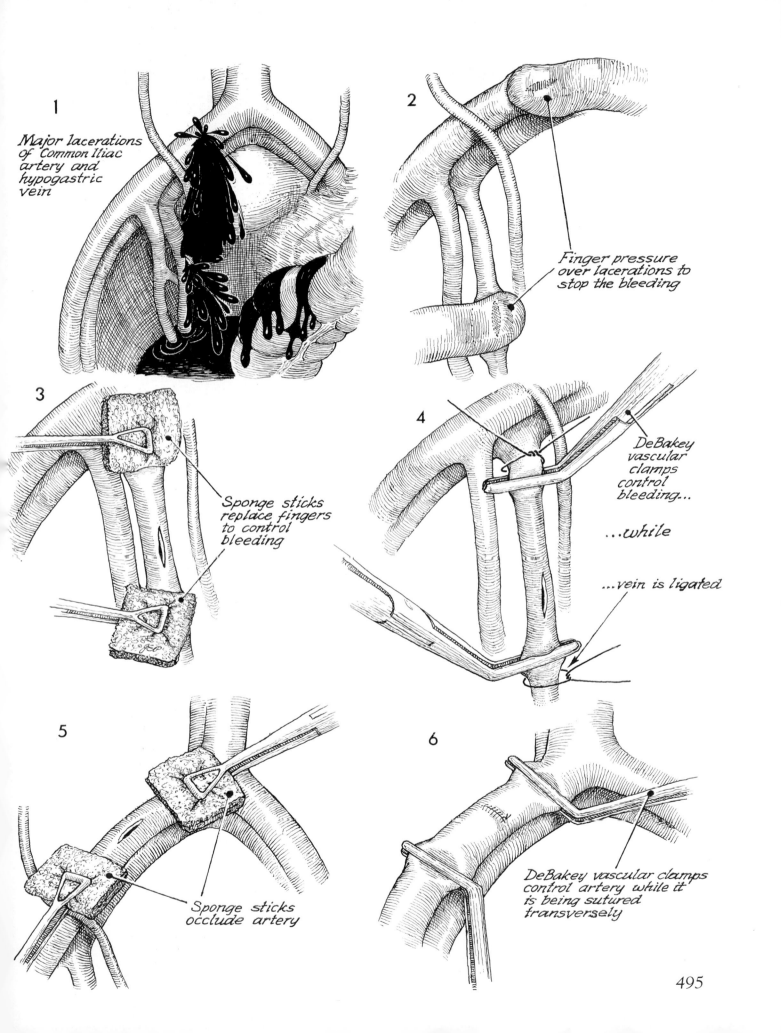

**1** Major lacerations of Common Iliac artery and hypogastric vein

**2** Finger pressure over lacerations to stop the bleeding

**3** Sponge sticks replace fingers to control bleeding

**4** DeBakey vascular clamps control bleeding...

...while

...vein is ligated

**5** Sponge sticks occlude artery

**6** DeBakey vascular clamps control artery while it is being sutured transversely

495

# Hemorrhage Control in Sacrospinous Ligament Suspension of the Vagina

Control of hemorrhage from branches of the internal iliac vein in sacrospinous ligament suspension of the vagina can be difficult. Dissection anterior to the iliac spine can enter the lateral extension of the cardinal ligament (the web). This structure is filled with branches of the internal iliac veins. Disruption of these veins produces copious hemorrhage.

## Technique

Figure 1 illustrates the anatomy in the posterior pelvis. At the top is the external iliac vein with the internal iliac vein (hypogastric vein) coming off cephalad to the sacrospinous ligament. The ischial spine is seen with the attached sacrospinous ligament traveling to the sacrum. The sigmoid colon is located on the left. The surgeon has placed sutures in the top of the prolapsed vagina and the pulley stitch as well as the secure stitch to the sacrospinous ligament approximately 4 cm (2 finger widths) from the ischial spine to avoid the pudendal artery nerve and vein. The vaginal vault has been closed after the hysterectomy has been performed; the pedicles from the hysterectomy are shown tied. The so-called web, the lateral extent of the cardinal ligament, is shown in the brackets between the pararectal space and the rectovaginal space. This web contains a dense complex of veins that are branches of the internal iliac (hypogastric) vein.

Hemorrhage can occur by blunt dissection through opening the posterior vaginal wall. The dissection enters the rectovaginal space. This can occur when the surgeon carries the dissection too far anteriorly rather than extending the finger dissector posteriorly toward the sacrum and palpating the ischial spine. When the dissection is carried into the web and the branches of the internal iliac (hypogastric) vein have been lacerated, copious hemorrhage will occur through the vagina. Individual identification with clamping and tying of individual venous branches of the hypogastric vein is rarely possible.

The solution to this problem is the placing of packs immediately into the pararectal space against the bleeding branches of the veins. When hemorrhage is under control the packs can be rolled slightly laterally and inferiorly. With a long Allis clamp the branches of these veins can be picked up individually. It is extremely difficult to tie off each branch separately. Therefore, a fine synthetic absorbable suture is used to suture-ligate the plexus. After each lacerated venous plexus has been sutured, the pack is further rolled inferiorly and laterally until all branches of the hypogastric vein have been grasped with the long thoracic Allis clamp and each one of the branches is sutured with fine synthetic absorbable suture. This procedure carries some risk to the ureter. At this point, the anesthesiologist should administer 1 ampule of indigo carmine dye intravenously. A water cystoscope should be inserted transurethrally into the bladder. The ureteral orifice on the affected side should be observed for the production of blue urine through the ureteral orifice. If after 10 minutes of observation no urine is seen, a ureteral catheter should be inserted up the ureter on the affected side. If the hemorrhage is controlled and the ureter has been sutured, the surgeon faces two possibilities: (1) to individually unligate the sutured veins until the ureter can be identified and a ureteral stent passed up to the kidney, or (2) to proceed above, open the abdomen, and dissect out the ureter, removing the offending sutures. The veins can be religated under direct observation after opening the paravesical and pararectal spaces.

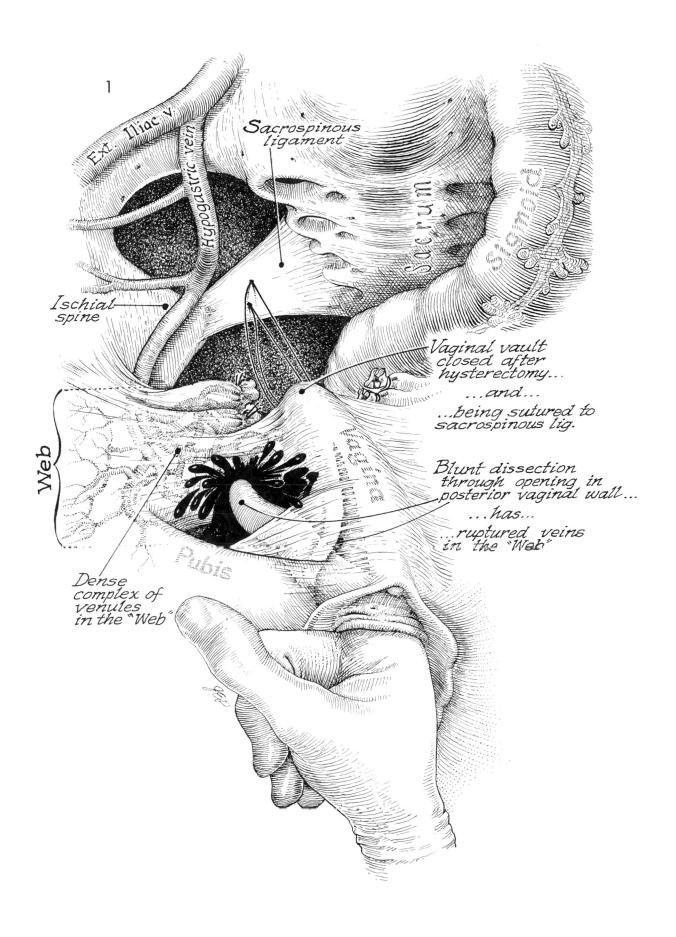

1

Ext. Iliac V.

Hypogastric vein

Sacrospinous ligament

Sacrum

Ischial spine

Web

Pubis

Dense complex of venules in the "Web"

Vaginal vault closed after hysterectomy...

...and...

...being sutured to sacrospinous lig.

Blunt dissection through opening in posterior vaginal wall...

...has...

...ruptured veins in the "Web"

497

# Presacral Space Hemorrhage Control

Bleeding from the presacral space arteries and veins, particularly branches of the middle sacral artery, can be copious and difficult to control. This is particularly true if the venous or arterial structures retract into the foramen of the sacrum. Surgeons can become frustrated by attempted electrocoagulation, suturing, clamping, and tying.

## Technique

**1** The sacrum is shown with arteries and veins in the periosteum.

**2** The finger is placed over the lacerated artery and vein. Conservative methods such as fulguration and suturing can be tried but are often unsuccessful.

**3** A thumbtack from the bulletin board grasped in a straight Kocher clamp can be placed in the laceration of the vessels in the presacral space. It is inserted through the vessel wall and embedded into the bone of the sacrum. It remains permanently in the bone.

**4** Thumb pressure is used to drive the thumbtack firmly into the sacral bone, occluding the lacerated artery.

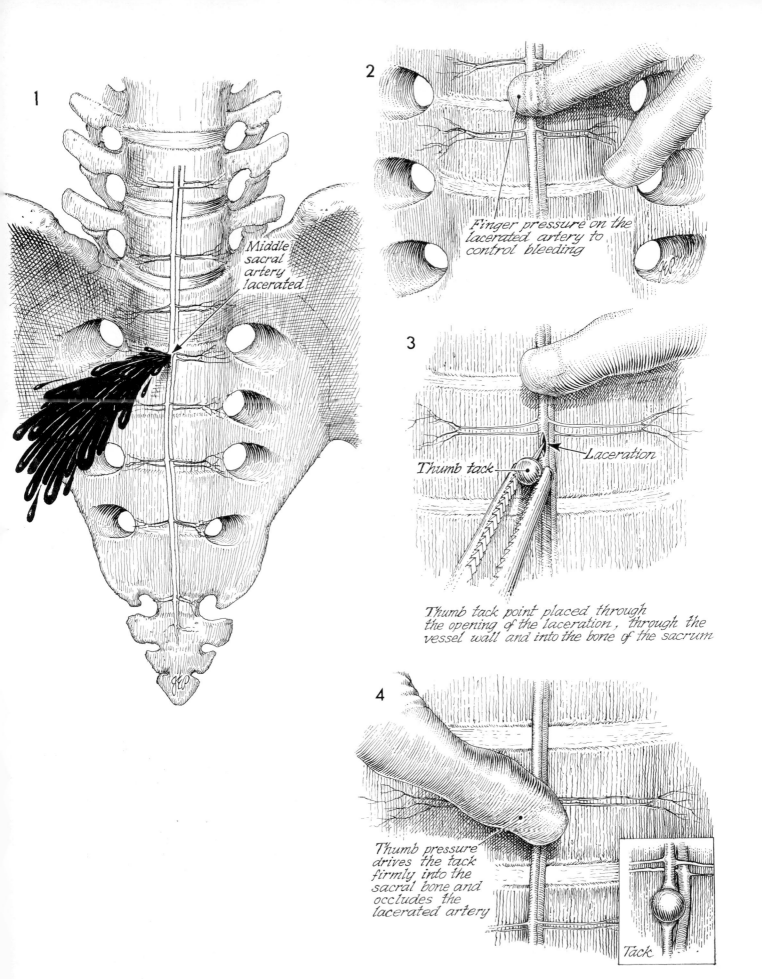

**1**

Middle sacral artery lacerated

**2**

Finger pressure on the lacerated artery to control bleeding

**3**

Lacération

Thumb tack

Thumb tack point placed through the opening of the laceration, through the vessel wall and into the bone of the sacrum

**4**

Thumb pressure drives the tack firmly into the sacral bone and occludes the lacerated artery

Tack

# What Not to Do in Cases of Pelvic Hemorrhage

What not to do in cases of pelvic hemorrhage is important to the gynecologic surgeon. Laceration of a large pelvic vein, external iliac artery, external iliac vein, internal iliac artery, or internal iliac vein can produce copious hemorrhage that will fill the pelvis immediately (Fig. 1). Suction with location of the lacerations is the first step. Finger pressure is important and will stop the hemorrhage in most cases.

**What Not to Do.** Nonvascular clamps such as the Kelly clamp crush arteries and veins and should not be used. Sutures on large needles placed blindly beneath the pool of blood not knowing precisely what tissue and what structure is being grasped, pinched, or sutured should not be used. Finger and pack pressure should be used until proper exposure of the vessel laceration can be made. This allows the operating room team to obtain proper vascular instruments, vascular suture, and cardiovascular needles. More damage can be created to the lacerated artery and vein by typical gynecologic clamps. Gynecologic suture and needles are frequently inappropriate in vascular surgery. Trying to place a suture in a hemorrhaging vein or artery is not a proper technique for repairing that artery or vein.

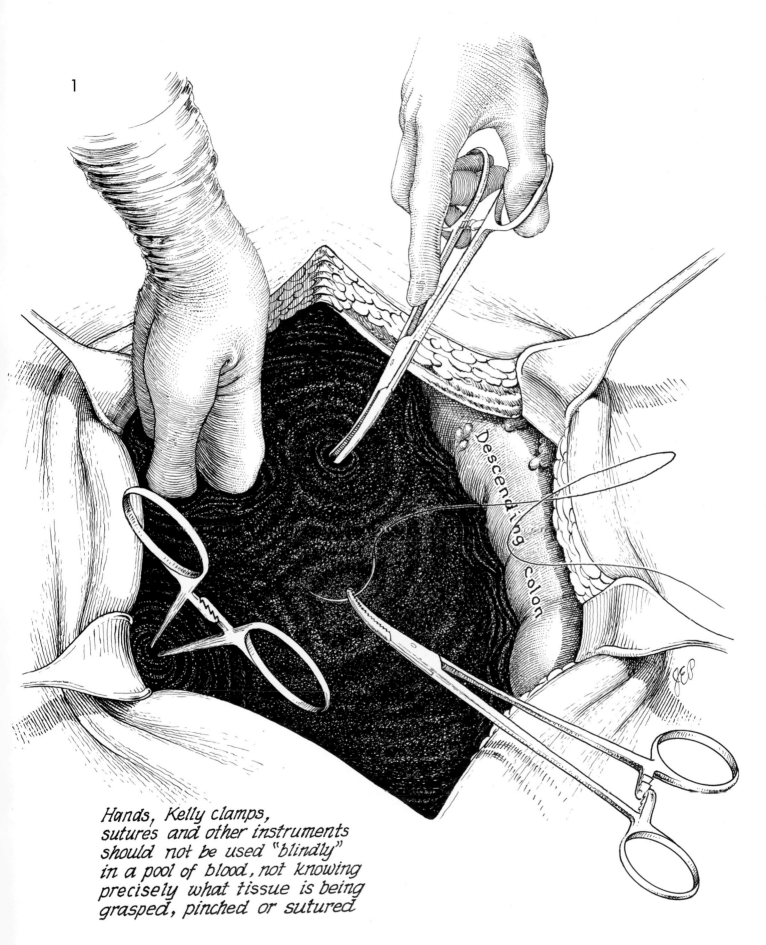

1

Descending colon

Hands, Kelly clamps,
sutures and other instruments
should not be used "blindly"
in a pool of blood, not knowing
precisely what tissue is being
grasped, pinched or sutured

# Packing for Hemorrhage Control

Packing has made a popular return to trauma and pelvic surgery, based on objective data. Every operative team should have its basic rules concerning packing. Basically, when a hemorrhage has occurred and cannot be controlled with the techniques mentioned in this section of the *Atlas* and more than 10 units of blood have been administered, the patient will start developing the signs and symptoms of hypovolemic shock. They will be hypothermia and/or acidosis. The patient will also develop dilutional coagulopathy with bleeding from other sites.

At this point, further attempts at vascular control are usually fruitless, and it is efficacious to pack this area of the body with any large sterile pack available. Extensive use of large packs is required; there is no role for 4 × 4 sponges. Laparotomy packs may include tools, sheets, and other aids to pack off this area in a proper manner.

In closing the patient's abdomen the rectus fascia should not be closed. The skin should be closed with towel clips. The patient should be taken to the surgical intensive care unit. She should remain intubated and on a mechanical respirator. Central venous access must be made, and corrections must be started for all the signs and symptoms of hypovolemic shock.

The fascia should not be closed to prevent compartmental syndrome. The large amount of packing necessary to control large vessels in the pelvis can make ventilation extremely difficult, resulting in compartmental syndrome.

Forty-eight hours later, when all vital signs, electrolytes, hemoglobin, prothrombin time (PT), and partial thromboplastin time (PTT) levels have been corrected, the patient can be brought back to the operating room, the skin clamps and the packing can be carefully removed, and the surgeon may frequently find little if any hemorrhage. If there is hemorrhage, it can be properly controlled at this time with adequate operative personnel and instruments.

## Technique

**1** Uncontrolled bleeding can occur from laceration of pelvic veins and the external and internal iliac arteries. *IVC*, inferior vena cava.

**2** The pelvis is packed tightly with any sterile material available. The open veins are seen ghosted under the packs.

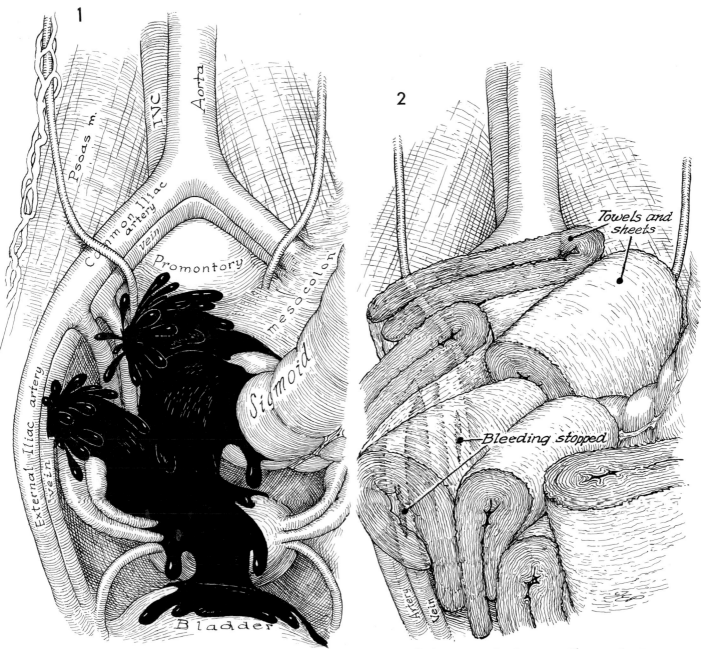

**1**

Psoas m.

IVC

Aorta

Common Iliac artery

vein

Promontory

mesocolon

Sigmoid

External Iliac artery

External Iliac vein

Bladder

Lacerations in the Hypogastric vein
and the External Iliac vein produce
massive bleeding

**2**

Towels and
sheets

Bleeding stopped

Artery

Vein

Pelvic cavity is rapidly packed
with large numbers of towels and
sheets, under high pressure, which
tightly compress the vessels and
control hemorrhage

# Control of Hemorrhage Associated With Abdominal Pregnancy

Control of hemorrhage associated with abdominal pregnancy is an important technique in obstetrical care. Every labor or delivery room should have a protocol as to the management of abdominal pregnancy. There are several available protocols, but none is perfect, and all have sequelae and long-term complications.

## Technique

**1** In this patient, the fetus shows multiple placental attachments to the mesentery of the descending colon. In this patient also, the placentae are attached in one particular area. Placentae can be attached all over the abdomen, however, from the liver to the pelvis. Each of these placentae has its own blood supply.

**2** Several of the placentae have been dislodged and torn away from the attachments. Profuse hemorrhage results. Individual clamping or ligating of these hemorrhaging sites is frequently impossible. The most efficacious management of this problem is to clamp the main umbilical cord immediately adjacent to the fetus, remove the fetus, and pack off the bleeding sites with large abdominal packs, sterile sheets, or whatever is available.

**3** If the hemorrhage cannot be controlled with the usual surgical techniques and the patient has lost more than 5000 mL of blood, hypovolemic shock will result. The most efficacious procedure in this situation consists of packing the pelvis, admission of the patient to the surgical intensive care unit, and return of the patient to the operating room in 48 hours. The rectus fascia should not be closed; the skin should be closed with towel clips.

In 48 hours, she can be returned to the operating room with the proper vascular surgery team and instruments. The towel clips can be removed from the skin, the abdomen can be opened, packing can be removed, and in most cases, the hemorrhage is contained. Occasionally, small bleeding points can be oversewn or overligated.

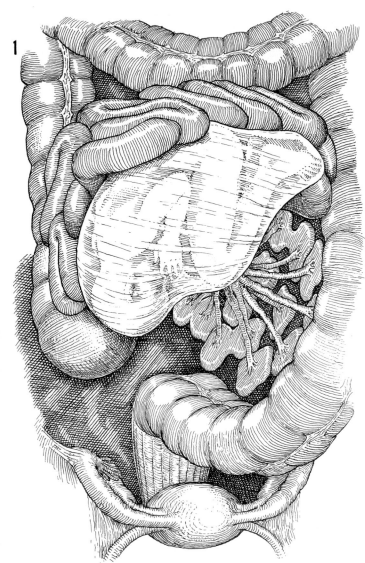

1

Multiple small placentae attached
to abdominal wall, mesenteries
and bowel

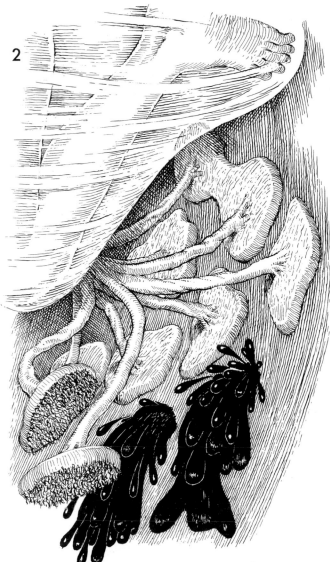

2

If the small placentae are torn
away from their attachments,
profuse hemorrhaging results

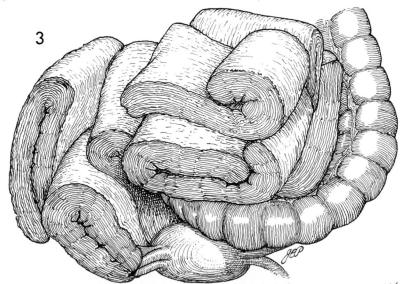

3

Pelvic cavity must be rapidly and tightly packed with
towels and sheets under great pressure in order to
control the hemorrhage

505

# Index

Page numbers in *italics* denote figures.